I like plastic surgery, it's fun.
— a 19-year-old Los Angeles woman who had
breast implants, a nose job, and liposuction, said
while waiting for her implant check-up

Some turn out great. Some turn out lousy. You win
some, you lose some. Every, every doctor makes mistakes.
If they tell you they have never had an operation that
turned out like they did not want it to, they are lying.
— A Beverly Hills plastic surgeon

I used to be a very happy, active and social person.
Now there is not a day that goes by that I do not think
about suicide.
— A Los Angeles woman who had botched facial
plastic surgery

Untold numbers of patients seeking the fountain of
youth through a face-lift, a tummy tuck or an acid peel
sometimes get more than they bargain for, suffering
infection, stroke, and occasionally death following
procedures that are advertised as safe, easy, and
painless.
— Congressman Ron Wyden, from Congressional
subcommittee hearings on plastic surgery industry,
1989

Also by John McCabe

Surgery Electives: What to Know before the Doctor Operates
Published by Carmania Books, 1994

Plastic Surgery

Surgery

Hopscotch

A Resource Guide for Those Considering Cosmetic Surgery

by John McCabe
edited by Miriam Ingersoll

Plastic Surgery Hopscotch: A Resource Guide for Those Considering
Cosmetic Surgery
By John McCabe, Edited by Miriam Ingersoll

Carmania Books
P.O. Box 1272
Santa Monica, CA 90406–1272

All company names and products should be considered registered
trademarks.

Printed in the United States of America

Published only in soft cover
by Carmania Books – 1995
10 9 8 7 6 5 4 3 2

Health   Medicine   Self-Help

Library of Congress Catalog Card Number 93-74927

ISBN   1-884702-32-5 (USA) $19.95 softcover

The elective surgery version of this book, *Surgery Electives: What To Know
Before The Doctor Operates* ($14.95), and additional copies of this book
($19.95) are available from Carmania Books. To order, send a check or
money order for the price of the book, plus $3 for the first book and $1 for
each additional book for shipping to Carmania Books at the address listed
above. Books being sent to a California address must also add sales tax.

This book is available to the bookstore and library market through the
major book wholesalers. For further information contact Carmania Books
at the address above.

Disclaimer

The information contained in this book has been compiled from thousands of sources and is subject to differences of opinion and interpretation. Every attempt was made to present accurate information as it could be gathered and cross-referenced before the publication date. This book is sold with the understanding that the publisher, author and any related parties are not rendering medical or legal services. The opinions, suggestions, and advice given in this book are meant to inform readers and to provoke thought only and should not be used as a substitute for needed healthcare. Neither the publisher, author nor any involved and interested parties assume any liability for omissions or errors in this book, and therefore are not responsible for the interpretation or implementation of information contained in this book and are not liable for any damages or loss caused or alleged to be caused directly or indirectly by information contained in this book including, but not limited to, legal disputes.

Because medical information is continuously being updated; many records are incomplete; new methods of treatment continue to be found; new laws are constantly being put into effect; and many scientists and others dedicated to the study of the human body have their own findings, beliefs and opinions, the information contained here should not be considered the final say on any subject.

Though doctors, lawyers, editors and others have adjusted some of the wording in this book, it was written by the author using his understanding of the issues covered. Therefore, some subjects may not be explained as fully as some readers may need for their specific health needs. As with any work this size, there is the possibility that typographical and content errors exist.

This book is focused on non-emergency health concerns. When experiencing a health emergency, a person should do what it takes to preserve their health and seek prompt medical attention. A person who is experiencing severe pain or a high fever, has suffered a broken bone, has been inflicted with an injury, such as a deep cut or burn, or any ailment that is interfering with the normal functions of their body, such as those that interfere with vision or breathing, should seek immediate medical care. Even in non-emergency situations it is important to seek the correct treatment early in the disease process or when any health concern arises rather than to wait for the problem to deteriorate before finding treatment.

Each reader is encouraged to do their own research of issues that interest or concern them. For information on particular health subjects, referring to the many books and organizations listed in the Research Resources section of this book may prove to be helpful.

For physical and psychological issues, contact a properly licensed and certified, responsible doctor or health professional who is well-trained in the area of your health concern.

The legal information here is not to be used as a substitute for private legal advice. For legal matters, contact a legitimate lawyer who is familiar with the laws in your area. (Some information on seeking legal counsel is given in the Research Resources section of this book under the heading of Legal Assistance. Persons interested in the legal concerns of healthcare consumers may want to read the book *The Consumer's Legal Guide to Today's Healthcare: Your Medical Rights and How to Assert Them*, by Stephen L. Isaacs, JD, & Ava C. Swartz, MPH; Houghton Mifflin Co., 1992)

It is not the intent of the author to express any sexual bias. Because most plastic surgeons are men (about 95%), this book uses the masculine pronoun when referring to them.

My thanks to the people and groups who supplied me with medical and legal advice, assisted in editing, read and re-read the manuscript, sent me information, connected me with the right people, and helped me in their own various ways.

Some of them include Nancy S., Jonathon K., Terry M., Debbie T., Christina A., Trudie C., Marion C., Ray S., Marilyn M., Cheryl D., Steven H., Hugh B., Amy C., Jane C., Trent D., Daniel and Amy B.W., Marjorie B., Julie B., Lynda R., Dan P., Courtney H., Megan F., Lorin L., Bernard K., Brant L., Janet V., Bill S., Bill E., Curt F., Bill P., Peter K., Judy S., Joyce P., Tom and Cheryl R., Patrick D., Lee S., Renae R., and Miriam I.

Thank you to Callahan and to David Letterman's WORLDWIDE PANTS for adding some of the humor to this book.

I especially want to thank the many victims of medical negligence who I interviewed for this book and who wish to remain anonymous. Without their input this book would not be what it is.

— John McCabe

CONTENTS

Introduction

While growing up in the 70s I thought that surgery was something you did only when you absolutely had to. Back then, it seemed that just the thought of undergoing surgery was supposed to make you shudder. Yet, I was hearing more and more of people who were going under the knife voluntarily for no reason other than to change their appearance. My first run-in with cosmetic surgery was in 1980 when a friend of my girlfriend gave me a hug that I will not forget because it felt like she had a baseball in each breast. I was later told that her parents had let her get breast implants and the implants had caused her breasts to become hard.

In the 80s cosmetic surgery became increasingly popular and the faces of some famous people became billboards for good and bad results of the this type of surgery. Now, in the 90s it seems you cannot open a newspaper or magazine without seeing a cosmetic surgery advertisement or some mention of cosmetic surgery. If you don't hear about it on a TV talk show, it is being discussed on the radio, is the subject of gossip columns or is being pushed by models in commercials. It is now being talked about as if it is so simple that it is like getting a new pair of pants.

Where I live, in Los Angeles, cosmetic surgery has made a big impact. You can overhear people talking about it and notice people who have obviously been surgically altered. Women who have faces younger than their hands and have telltale scars behind their ears stand in front of you at the store and bank. There are people who you know were born with dark hair, brown eyes and classic noses who now sport blond hair, wear contact lenses to make their eyes blue or green and have undergone surgery to make their noses smaller and their chests larger. On the beaches there are women who feature breasts that look more like balloons. Seeing all of this makes me wonder how popular cosmetic surgery will become. Will people who look a certain way be expected to undergo surgical changes? Will a new standard of appearance be established? Will there be a class division between those who have and those who have not undergone cosmetic surgery?

It reminds me of an episode of the old TV show *The Twilight Zone* called *The Private World of Darkness*. In the opening scene, doctors and nurses are gathered in a dimly-lit room where they are unwrapping the face of a patient and talking about how they hope the operation cured her of her hideous appearance. When the bandages come off it is revealed that the patient is a beautiful woman and as the camera backs away from her it is revealed that the medical team all have faces of hellish beasts. They live in a world where the beautiful woman and everyone around her think she is hideous because she does not look like anyone else. She is eventually banned to live in a colony of people who are considered visually repulsive but who most people today would consider to be physically beautiful.

Cosmetic surgery may have become popular, but what seems to be transpiring all around seems weirder than that *Twilight Zone* episode. The whole scenario of thousands of people who have undergone cosmetic surgery leaves me to wonder what the great renaissance painters would think of these modern people running in for operations that remove their character.

A person who is foreign to the issue of cosmetic surgery would have to wonder what kind of satisfaction can result from undergoing this unnecessary surgery. Does it make a person happy? Does it stop them from getting old? Does it mean they are going to live longer? Is it some kind of cure for death? Is it some form of eugenics?

As cosmetic surgery involves placing a person under anesthesia and cutting into their body tissues, one would have to wonder what kind of risks are involved. And, mostly, because the procedures do involve risks, one would have to wonder what the motives are of the people who undergo cosmetic surgery and especially of the people who perform the operations.

This book was written to provide information about the cosmetic surgery industry to people who are considering cosmetic surgery and to suggest to them what questions to ask, to educate them about the risks and to direct them toward the information they need to make well-balanced, informed decisions regarding whether to undergo cosmetic surgery.

When I started this book project I though it would take several months to accomplish. It eventually took over three years as I found so much material relating to cosmetic surgery. During this time I have spoken with both satisfied and unsatisfied cosmetic surgery patients, medical doctors, psychologists, lawyers, consumer advocates, lawmakers, librarians, government workers, magazine editors and journalists. The books, pamphlets, articles and videos these people have provided me along with what they have told me helped this project slowly grow into the book that you now hold in your hands. Many of these people also read and reread the manuscript as I was writing it and many of their comments have been written into the text.

Some people might say that this book is alarmist and presents an image of the medical industry that will scare people away from needed medical care. But with the topic of this book being vanity surgery, I do not see where I would be endangering anybody's life by providing information about risks, dangers and so forth that are present when a person decides to undergo unnecessary surgery. It is very wise for a person to know what can happen to them during surgery and I think most people will be able to assess what does and does not apply to their situation.

The first step to success with any choice is becoming informed. A person undergoing medical care should not assume the doctor will tell them every important piece of information regarding their care. It is often hard to determine what aspects of certain procedures are most important for each patient, as what may seem unimportant at one moment may become life altering at another time.

Just as the subtitle of this book states, this is an information resource guide for those considering cosmetic surgery. I knew that some of the people who would be referencing this book would be depressed teenagers, desperate and lonely adults, people obsessed with their appearance and others who, for their own reasons, think they would be happier if they let some doctor surgically alter their face or body. To be safe I have included information for people who are considering plastic surgery for any reason.

The type and quality of medical care a patient receives, in large measure, depends on the patients' taking the initiative to become educated about their health and asking the right questions whenever they are in need of healthcare.

A study published in the November 23, 1994, issue of the *Journal of the American Medical Association* reported that patients are more likely to be satisfied with their medical care if they communicate well with the doctor from the very start. Many other studies have shown that patients who are informed about their options and know what to expect when undergoing medical care, and who become active participants in their own treatment recover faster than patients who are not informed about or involved with their medical care. Doctors are told by their associations and insurance companies that open communication with patients is helpful in reducing medical malpractice suits and that patients who understand their diagnosis and prescribed treatment are more realistic in their expectations of what a doctor can do.

There is a wide range of doctors who work in the area of plastic surgery, from those such as Dr. William Magee, a highly praised plastic surgeon who performs miraculous procedures on children with facial deformities, to those at the other end of the spectrum whose only concentration seems to be on the process of making money off of insecure people.

Probably everyone who has ever lived to adulthood has thought that some aspect of his or her physical appearance could be improved. There has also probably always been some type of crude surgery performed to change the appearance of anyone who was willing. Not until today has appearance-altering surgery been so prevalent and made to look so simple and pleasurable through clever marketing. Never have so many people taken such serious health risks to make medically unnecessary and permanent alterations to the appearance of the human body. And never has there been so much money to be made by providing a way for people to possibly look younger, prettier and skinnier. These risky procedures are being done by cosmetic surgeons who prey off of today's appearance-obsessed society. These cosmetic surgeons who are untrustworthy opportunists help to build up the unrealistic expectations of what cosmetic surgery can do for people. The result is that patients sometimes literally die in their efforts to become beautiful.

When I was writing this book I received phone calls from people who found out about the subject of this book and who were considering cosmetic surgery. They wanted to read chapters of the book that would help them in their decision. Several wanted to know which doctor they should go to. I am not interested in referring people to cosmetic surgeons. Though I have spoken with people who are very satisfied with the result of their cosmetic surgery, I have also spoken with too many people who have had horrible experiences with this surgery and also know of dozens of people who have died undergoing cosmetic surgery.

Those who decide to undergo cosmetic surgery should realize that it is always a gamble. The outlandish claims of some cosmetic surgeons and the nightmarish stories of some patients are proof enough that anyone planning on undergoing cosmetic surgery should know what the limitations and risks are.

In any situation where surgery is suggested, the final authority of whether surgery takes place should be none other than a well-informed alert patient who knows their options, who has had more than one professional opinion and who understands and has weighed the physical, emotional and financial risks.

— John McCabe

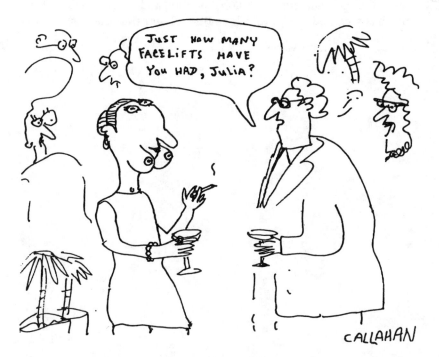

1 • PLASTIC SURGERY

What Plastic Surgery Is

The word "plastic" in plastic surgery does not refer to the use of plastic. It is used in the sense of the Greek word "plastikos," which means "to mold." But even the word "mold" would give a false impression of what plastic surgery does because there is no actual molding done. At least not in the way a person would mold Jello or plaster.

Plastic surgery is done by altering, removing or repositioning skin, fat, muscle, blood vessels, cartilage and bone or some combination of these. Tissues are sometimes taken from one area of the body or head and then used as an implant or graft to build up another area or to replace damaged or lost tissue. These grafts taken from one part of a person's body and used in another part are called "autogenous" grafts. They do not always do what they are meant to do, may be reabsorbed by the body, become infected or make more surgery necessary.

Man-made materials are sometimes used in plastic surgery. Some implants are made of silicone rubber, as in the silicone sacs used for breast implants and solid silicone implants used on the cheeks, chin, nose, forehead, male pectoral muscles, buttocks and calves. These can cause problems and may not last a lifetime. There are also some doctors who use natural materials such as bovine (cow) cartilage and sea coral, which have been processed for use inside the human body.

The term "plastic surgery" is commonly used to describe surgery performed to improve function, often with the goal of creating normal appearance on structures that are abnormal due to a birth defect or because of some type of trauma, disease or infection. The difference between "plastic" surgery and "cosmetic," or what I refer to as "vanity" surgery, is that "cosmetic" surgery is plastic surgery done to satisfy the vanity of an essentially healthy person with normal structures.

Cosmetic surgery cannot stop or reverse the aging process. It also cannot give a person an entirely new body. Alterations can be made to change the appearance of various parts of the face and body by rearranging the tissues. Sometimes the outcome is very pleasing to the patient. Some of the surgeries may be relatively simple compared with others, but all surgery involves risks, and surgeons have botched even the simplest operations. Even with the best medical attention, there is no guarantee that the desired appearance will be obtained. Health, skin type, age, bone structure, heredity, healing, the operational techniques of the doctor and his medical team and the care taken during the healing all play a part in the final result.

Cosmetic surgery inflicts trauma on the body and involves making a healthy person temporarily unwell, and this should never be taken lightly. Undergoing cosmetic surgery is not like getting a haircut. All of the procedures involve a degree of difficulty. Depending on which procedure is done, it can involve taking drugs to prevent infection and pain. It may involve some sort of anesthesia that the patient might have an allergic reaction to or may not be administered or managed safely, which in the worst case, can kill the patient. Cosmetic surgery also involves cutting into the flesh, where there are blood vessels and nerves to which irreversible damage can occur. It may involve breaking, cutting, chiseling, sawing, shaving or drilling of bone and cartilage. It may involve suctioning of fat or amputation of part of the flesh, muscle, cartilage or bone, which cannot be put back once it is taken away. It usually involves blotting or suctioning blood and stitching flesh and sometimes muscles, and setting bones and cartilage back into place. And it involves disposing of removed tissue into a hazardous waste bin.

Even after surgery, any number of known and unknown complications may arise that can endanger the patient's physical and mental health for the sake of a goal that is not always met in operations that cannot be reversed. During the recovery period that starts immediately after the surgery is completed, the patient might experience bleeding, severe swelling, intense bruising and infections. There is always a risk of improper healing, along with the question of how the surgery site will age. Depending on what procedure is done and how it is done, the altered body part may age in undesirable ways.

The Origin of Cosmetic Surgery

Certainly there were some operations being done in centuries previous to World War I that could be considered cosmetic surgery, but the biggest boost to developing techniques for altering a person's appearance took place during that war, when doctors developed surgical procedures to repair damage done to the faces and bodies of injured people. A British doctor named Sir Harold Gillies is often credited with advancing the profession by way of the work he did on the war victims. Since World War I there have been many developments in the field of surgically altering bodies and faces to change their appearance.

Among the other pioneers of the cosmetic surgery industry was a Berlin orthopedic surgeon named Jacques Joseph, who developed techniques in 1898 that led to what is called "rhinoplasty" when he performed an operation to reduce the size of a patient's nose. Just a dozen or so years ago a French doctor who performed abortions started using a suction tube to remove fat tissue in a procedure that is now known as "liposuction" surgery.

Along the plastic surgery history time-line there are other doctors who named so-called revolutionary techniques after themselves.

Presently there are questionable doctors who seek out business by advertising in the classified sections of vanity magazines to get patients to travel to foreign countries for surgery performed at low cost.

The United States Census Bureau estimates that 22% of the population will be 55 or older by the turn of the century. In 1996 there will be one American turning 50 every 8.4 seconds. By 2001 this will increase to every 6.8 seconds. The proportion of elderly in the world's population will nearly double by 2030. This age change will be reflected in an increase in the number of businesses that cater to the needs and wants of older individuals.

Women make up about 80% to 85% of the cosmetic surgery patients in general, but some doctors say that over 40% of their patients are men.

Before plastic surgery became popular, it was performed on victims of accidents, diseases and infections; people with birth defects; and criminals wanting to completely change their appearance. Now that the oldest of the baby boom generation is nearing 50, the number of people with aging skin and graying hair has increased. Because of this and the accessibility of the growing number of doctors selling themselves as plastic surgeons, cosmetic surgery has turned into a multibillion dollar industry. This has made the specialty of plastic surgery one of the top-paying areas of medicine and has fostered some unscrupulous doctors who are so caught up in trying to cash in on this lucrative business that they are willing to perform practically any surgery on anyone.

The Doctors Who Perform Cosmetic Surgery

In the past centuries most people who became doctors learned the trade by working with an established doctor in an apprentice system (it is still done this way in some parts of the world). Many of these old-time doctors never held a degree, were not supervised by anyone, were governed by few laws, and were not subject to certification boards or insurance company guidelines. Primitive treatments were practiced, surgery was performed without anesthesia by doctors who wore no special sanitary surgical clothing and dangerous procedures were the norm, while improvements were few and far between and opportunities for quackery were broad and common. This contrasts quite dramatically with the standards of today's medical community, but the quackery element still exists and is probably more prevalent in the area of cosmetic surgery than in any other area of medicine. (That is, if the kind of cosmetic surgery we are talking about here can be called "medicine.")

Many doctors disagree on what training is necessary to perform cosmetic surgery. Cosmetic surgery is performed by doctors who may or may not have received training specific to plastic surgery and may be assisted by a staff who may have insufficient medical knowledge. Anyone who has a medical license can legally perform surgery in their office. Clearly many surgeons who are now performing cosmetic surgery are drawn to the field because of financial interests found in this area of medicine. Many of them are performing newly learned procedures on uninformed patients. The result is that people are sometimes left maimed, psychologically distraught, financially burdened and sometimes dead.

One type of doctor who often performs plastic and cosmetic surgery is an otolaryngologist. This specialist has received his training in the physiology of the head and neck area and is often referred to as an "ear, nose and throat doctor." When otolaryngologists practice plastic surgery they usually limit themselves to the head and neck. Other otolaryngologists, though they may not be trained to do so, also perform plastic surgery procedures on areas below the neck. Additionally there are ophthalmologists doing eyelid lifts, gynecologists doing liposuction, dermatologists doing face-lifts, general practitioners doing breast operations, and so forth.

Surgical procedures that can be performed in a doctor's office can be done to high standards by caring doctors but also attract doctors who would not be able to meet the standards of a hospital peer review committees, which limit what procedures a doctor can and cannot do in the hospital on the basis of experience. The surgeon operating outside the hospital setting can also hire anesthesiologists, surgical assistants and nurses who might not be accepted into a hospital based on their own professional histories. Some of these physicians have not had any formal training in the area of medicine they practice. Many of them are performing newly learned procedures on patients who believe the doctors are well trained and experienced.

Why People Undergo Plastic Surgery

Basically, there are two reasons why people undergo plastic surgery:
- To alter a birth defect or repair a body part that has been changed by trauma, a disease or an infection. This reason for having plastic surgery is more accepted by society.

    — Or —

- To change a body part for cosmetic reasons. This reason is thought by many to be a narcissistic, stubborn and silly indulgence of the wealthy and/or vain.

Plastic surgery is a way of altering what nature, heredity and life have drawn on the body. The reasons to have plastic surgery and the effects of having plastic surgery are nearly always more than skin deep. Usually the patient has a belief that, if one of their body parts resembled some ideal image, the patient would be happier.

In the case of a patient who has a birth defect or who has suffered some sort of damage to a body part and is seeking to repair that damage, if the surgery is done correctly, the patient may function better and have an improved self-image, and, if there is a good result, the surgery may improve the patient's physical and mental health.

In the case of a person who is seeking surgery simply for cosmetic reasons, the surgery may also, if it is done correctly and for the right reasons, make the person happier and improve their confidence. However, if the person has emotional problems, is seeking to improve a relationship, or has unrealistic life goals and expectations, cosmetic surgery may be of no benefit and the person's best interests may best be served by, before ever seriously considering any type of cosmetic surgery, seeking professional counseling and finding ways of improving self-esteem and body image.

Anyone looking to be transformed to physical perfection through cosmetic surgery has unrealistic expectations. Your problems will not disappear because you happen to look different. You will be the same person with the same problems but with less money and a body part that looks different. Your same life will be waiting for you just as soon as you recover from the surgery.

Elements that will increase the chance of unexpected surgical results or injury are

- Putting too much trust in the doctor and his staff
- Letting the doctor and his staff's knowledge and authority intimidate you
- Having a doctor who does not have enough training
- Having a doctor who works too fast
- Having a doctor who does not have enough help or is assisted by a staff that lacks thorough training
- Having a doctor who tries to cut costs in the office and the operating room

Being a Cosmetic Surgery Patient

It should always be remembered that the medical subspecialty of cosmetic surgery is a money-making enterprise. Because you are the patient — or a potential patient — you are the target for the revenue source. Just as in any other business, profit is the bottom line. As is too often the case with other professions, a cosmetic can judge his success by his financial status and the quest for luxury can become more important than the safety and health of the patients who seek his services.

The advertising that cosmetic surgeons put out, the doctors themselves, and their office staff may speak of cosmetic surgery as almost glamorous. They may downplay the recovery period while overlooking the details that the patient should know about, pertaining to the risks, the extent of the injuries inflicted by the surgery, the information needed for postoperative care, and the length of the recovery time. They may also place promises where promises cannot truthfully exist. Some of the patients who get caught up in these titanic promises of cosmetic surgery are the same as that big boat: disasters waiting to happen.

As with any other surgery, cosmetic surgery has risks. Not everyone looks or feels better after cosmetic surgery. If you are considering cosmetic surgery, do not be too eager about hopping up on that operating table. Prepare yourself with knowledge. Spend some time doing research before you spend money on a doctor. Take caution with each step you take in this area of the medical industry that is filled with the purest forms of greed and vanity.

Do not automatically trust someone because that person has a doctorate degree in medicine. When no immediate health threat exists, do not let a doctor or his staff set a date for an operation, get you to pay for the operation or get you anywhere near the operating room before you are ready and informed and have made your own decision as to whether cosmetic surgery is for you.

> *Not some, not most, but all doctors, at one time or another, make errors. This is the nature of medicine; it isn't an exact science. It's not simply a matter of adding up the symptoms, as you would a column of figures, and get the total, or diagnosis, then feed the result into a computer out of which comes the answer, the treatment. It's not at all like that.*
> — from the book *The Making of a Surgeon,* by William A. Nolen, MD; Random House, 1968

It should be remembered that somewhere along the line in his practice, every cosmetic surgeon makes mistakes or has performed surgeries that did not turn out right. Many cosmetic surgery procedures now available have become popular within the last few years. This was after most of the doctors performing the procedures completed their training.

There can be no guarantee on the final results of cosmetic surgery. The surgery can result in a final appearance that is opposite to what the patient expected. It may turn out better than the patient thought it would or may leave the patient deformed. A negative result can send the patient into seclusion with a mind-wrenching obsessive depression and on a search a for a doctor who may or may not be able to fix what the patient dislikes about the altered body part.

Whereas a certain number of mistakes are to be expected in any profession, all too often it is not an injury or sickness that does the most harm to the patient, but the medical treatment the patient receives that causes injury or death. Although the number of fatalities in operating rooms has dropped dramatically over the last few decades, the current estimates of the number of patients who die each year because of operations that have gone bad are still uncomfortably high.

There is no accurate record of how many people have died as the result of complications associated with cosmetic surgery. Many of these deaths are untraceable because of the way medical records are kept. Deaths in surgery centers away from hospitals, where many cosmetic surgeries are performed, are not always recorded accurately. The death certificate may simply state that the person died from heart failure or respiratory failure and not list the consequences or the disease that led to the death. Doctors and others whose careers can be harmed if they are involved with a patient death may also take actions to keep the death quiet. This can hide product fault, criminal activity and medical malpractice. This also results in inaccurate health statistics and makes it difficult to trace diseases and inherited health problems.

Questions to answer before undergoing cosmetic surgery:
- What are the likely benefits of the surgery?
- What are the reasons you are basing your decision on to have the surgery?
- Do you know what your body's response to the surgical wound will be?
- Do you know the length of time you will need to recover and what type of care you will need?
- Are the doctor and the surgical team qualified to do the surgery?
- Are the doctor and his staff going to do what is best for *you*?

2 • THE INDUSTRY

The American Healthcare Environment

In America, healthcare represents 13.9% of the country's gross domestic product. The average of $3,299 per person spent on healthcare is the highest of any developed nation, and the 7.8% growth rate in 1993 for health spending in America was higher than the national inflation rate of 2.7% and greater than the growth of the gross domestic product. Healthcare is the number one profit industry in the country and employs more workers than any other industry. According to the Department of Health and Human Services, the federal government paid 31.7% of the nation's healthcare bill in 1993, and spending in the federal Medicare program grew more rapidly than private insurance in 1992 and 1993. In 1994, Medicare, which is available to Social Security recipients 65 and older and some disabled persons, spent roughly $164 billion.

America is also where the most up-to-date and advanced forms of medical science and technology are found. It is the home of the Cleveland Clinic, the Mayo Clinic and all of the world's top medical schools and hospitals. These facilities are used by world leaders and the wealthy citizens of the planet who jet to America whenever they are in need of serious healthcare.

The healthcare world is not a perfect place where everyone does what is right and everyone wins. It revolves around big money and career advancements; therefore, people do not always do what they are supposed to do. Many of the actions of doctors and hospitals these days are motivated by financial gain, and they too often judge their success by it. Many surgeries and other treatments are financially driven rather than symptom driven, and the financial and legal interests of today's medical industry are clouding over the real needs of the patients, while healthcare providers are conducting business within a system that has a flagrant disregard for consumers' right to know. It is also a healthcare system where the accessibility to quality healthcare declines and the chances of mistreatment increase the lower the individual's financial status and the darker their skin color (during the Clinton healthcare campaign it was noted by White House officials that only 40% of Latinos are covered by employer health insurance in comparison with 70% of the American average).

As the talk of restructuring the healthcare industry blew through the mass media, many Americans were made aware of the problems facing medical consumers. Some attention was given to the abuses that occur within the medical industry and the fact that doctors do not always know or do what is best as they work in an industry where patients and government health plans are regularly overcharged.

The healthcare industry is an industry just like any other — driven by profits. The well-financed people at the top hire lobbyists who influence lawmakers to pass laws that protect key players and help them make more money. The result is that doctors do not live by the same standards and rules that govern the rest of America; some abuse the power they have been given and at times some quite literally get away with murder.

Hundreds of billions of dollars are spent every year on medicine and medical care in the United States — more than in any other country. Lobbying groups spend millions of dollars to pump out their propaganda as persuasive, and often confusing, TV, radio and newspaper advertising to incite the American public to support their special interests. Lobbyists also successfully encourage, entice and manipulate lawmakers to pass laws in favor of the act of making money in medicine — laws that protect doctors, medical insurance companies and other healthcare interests — and these laws are not always best for consumers.

Many bills introduced to protect medical consumers and improve medical standards have been stifled by medical lobbies, whereas laws that do get passed may protect and improve some standards, but usually protect only doctors' standard of living. Just as candidates for office win because they have the most amount of money backing their campaigns (in 1992, the candidate who spent the most amount of money won in 388 of 435 House races), the bills with the most money backing them often pass into law.

The California Medical Board

Currently the governing bodies that are set up to enforce standards, such as state medical boards and peer review groups, do not do their job. Very often when these governing bodies investigate bad medical care, they seem to protect the negligent practitioners more than the consumers who register the complaints.

> . . . last year, California took less than two disciplinary actions per thousand physicians. In Florida, it was almost 10 disciplinary actions per thousand physicians and about 8.3 in Maryland. It would take a leap of faith, I think, to imply that California doctors are seven per thousand better than those practicing in Florida or Maryland.
> — Congressman Pete Stark during subcommittee hearing on issues relating to malpractice, May 20, 1993

> . . . there is an obstetrician-gynecologist in Los Angeles, an extremely litigious person who wound up already suing seven or eight different doctors who testified against her, so I will confine my comments to what is in the public record. She was accused of charging between up to as much as $40,000 for hysterectomies, that is not an error in my reporting. It is an error in what she did, obviously.
> The medical board held a hearing for a variety of reasons including which she had been kicked off the staff of more than one hospital and they concluded there were at least six reasons, any one of which would result in her losing her license and for all six of those reasons, they ordered her license revoked.
> By playing various games with the courts, which are beyond my ability to understand the detail of, 3 1/2 years later, she still is practicing in a little dinky hospital that I wouldn't let my dog go to, but she is still practicing, including going on television and TV talk shows and so on.
> — Dr. Richard F. Corlin, American Medical Association during Congressional subcommittee hearing on issues relating to medical malpractice, May 20, 1993

An internal report that was released in August of 1993 by the California Medical Board questioned the quality of the medical expertise used by the state in its disciplinary cases concerning doctors. The report stated that, in too many instances, the doctors the state used as experts against other doctors were themselves not qualified for their roles. It stated that investigating physicians were sloppy in the way they reviewed cases, or lacked up-to-date medical knowledge or expertise in the specialty of the physician they were examining. The report was a serious blow to the medical board, which had repeatedly been criticized by consumer groups, prosecutors and legislators for failure to take timely or adequate action against bad doctors.

In the spring of 1989, a lengthy report criticizing the California Medical Board was released by the University of San Diego's Center for Public Interest Law, which monitors state licensing boards. The report rebuked every step of the system that was supposed to process consumer complaints against bad doctors and claimed that the people paid to run the system were not properly trained and lacked medical or legal expertise. The report, which recommended substantial structural and administrative changes, concluded that the board was ineffective, had not been protecting consumers for a number of years and was letting bad doctors, including ones who had killed patients, continue practicing medicine. As an example the CPIL cited the case of one Los Angles-area obstetrician who killed nine babies and was charged with 45 felony counts, including nine counts of second-degree murder, before the Board took action against him.

In 1990, the assistant director of the Board told state legislatures that there was a backlog of 600 uninvestigated cases of public complaints against doctors even though he knew the actual figure was about 800. Investigators with the Board witnessed top officials destroying hundreds of files containing these consumer complaints. Outraged investigators complained to their union and the CPIL, who in turn filed complaints with the state governor. An investigation by the state was called for. Since the attorney general's office declared a conflict of interest because it represented the Medical Board in actions against doctors, the California Highway Patrol was brought in to do an investigation.

The investigative report, which was released by the CHP in January 1993, accused the Board of lax administration, misconduct, corruption and appalling mismanagement. The report detailed the destruction by the Board of the files containing inadequately investigated consumer complaints against doctors. Several of the cases involved a string of patient deaths in a Los Angeles hospital. Among the deaths was one patient whose colon was ruptured during surgery to remove an ovarian cyst. In a subsequent operation performed to repair damage from the first, the patient's heart was punctured and she died. In another case, an accident victim was given an over-the-counter painkiller and discharged, only to die later from fractured ribs and a lacerated liver.

The CHP report also alleged that a diversion program created to rehabilitate doctors with drug, alcohol or psychological problems had been improperly used as an alternative to disciplining unfit physicians. One administrator accepted gifts from a doctor he was overseeing in the rehabilitation program. The program was accused of lax monitoring of doctors and was described by some critics as a money-making scheme that benefited clinics connected with the program's staff.

All of these allegations have brought lawmakers to introduce legislation that would strip the Board of the power to investigate, prosecute and discipline their own profession. They believe that, as a way of making the state physician disciplinary system more responsive to consumer complaints, the power should be given to an independent unit of the attorney general's office.

Knowing Your Rights as a Patient

Whenever a person subjects themself to treatment by a medical professional, that person should never assume that the professional is going to do what is best or is even properly qualified. Doctors are not all-knowing and do not always possess good judgment.

Consumers entering the medical world need to be aware of what is and is not acceptable and what is and is not good medicine. They need to know what to look for so they can prevent situations where they can be taken advantage of and harmed by the negligent acts of caregivers who may be nothing other than opportunists interested in self-promotion.

Often, boards use the term "acceptable standards of practice" to describe actions that border on malpractice, or that at least amount to treatment that is not in the best interest of the patient. Often the only way bad doctors are held accountable for incompetence and patient abuse is when they lose a malpractice lawsuit — but doctors win most of the lawsuits brought against them and laws are being passed that limit the monetary awards that courts grant to malpractice victims.

The less a person knows about a medical treatment, the more susceptible they are to mistreatment. Some of the operations being done may be of no benefit to the patients. The x-rays that the patients are subjected to, the tests that are performed on them, and the drugs that are prescribed may also be damaging to a patient's health. In the long run, some forms of treatment may cause problems and diseases that will show up years later in the patient or in the patient's children. Some people who go into the hospital with the goal of getting medical care end up getting post-mortem care as their body is prepared for its trip to the cold hospital morgue. Situations like this are particularly tragic when a complication is the result of such unnecessary procedures as those done to satisfy vanity.

Doctors

People who become doctors are not derived from some unique human pedigree. They are simply people who have gone through years of specific schooling and learned certain things to obtain a degree in medicine. There are some very good doctors who have an up-to-date knowledge in their area of medicine, are experienced in the treatments they prescribe, possess a keen understanding of how the body works and always try to do what is best for their patients. Some doctors have performed medically miraculous operations. There are doctors who spend their careers in distressed areas of the world with limited medical supplies working against the odds to try to improve the health of people who otherwise would not have had the chance to get proper healthcare. There are doctors who form teams and fly to war-torn countries to perform free operations on people who have been injured and doctors of mercy who remain in war zones to save the lives of innocent victims.

However, there are also selfish, arrogant and manipulative doctors who show more interest in making money than in guarding the welfare of their patients as they prescribe therapies and procedures that are done for no reason other than to get money from the patients and insurance companies. Many doctors have been sued, many have had their licenses taken away and some have been sent to jail for many kinds of unprofessional, deceitful, injurious and life-threatening actions. There are unskilled doctors, doctors who do more harm than good and doctors who perform operations that, for one reason or another, should not be done.

There are doctors who have been sent to jail for raping their patients while the patients were under anesthesia. There are doctors who misuse their accessibility to drugs and regularly abuse them. Some doctors are so addicted that they perform surgery while under the influence.

Steps taken in the United States to become a conventional medical doctor

- Obtain Bachelor of Science degree
- Take either the Graduate Medical Aptitude Test or the Medical College Admissions Test
- Attend (usually) four years of medical school
- Two years before graduation from medical school and at the end of the fourth year, take the standardized US Medical Licensing Examination that is administered by the National Board of Medical Examiners to determine placement in residencies and whether the student should remain in medical school
- Serve (usually) one year of internship
- Obtain a state medical license. If they practice in a town that is near a state border, they may elect to also get a license in the neighboring state
- Get a Drug Enforcement Agency registration number so they can legally prescribe drugs
- Complete a residency program. The residency system was developed several decades ago at Johns Hopkins University in Baltimore, Maryland. The Resident Matching System assigns residents to the hospital where they will serve their residency. The residency can last for two or more years depending on the specialization. During the residency program the residents work long hours and are exposed to a wide selection of cases. Residents are paid but the pay varies from hospital to hospital.
- Go into private practice or join an existing practice or organization
- Pass specialty board exams and present a portfolio that details cases of patients they have treated
- Sometimes continue on with fellowship training in a subspecialty area
- Attend continuing education programs to keep updated

According the Washington-based Association of American Medical Colleges, a record 42,500 people applied for 15,975 slots at America's 126 medical schools for the 1993-94 school year.

If a doctor who has been educated in another country wishes to practice medicine in America, they must complete an equivalency exam in order to obtain a medical license in America. They also may be required to complete an internship in America.

In past centuries it was common for a doctor to have little, if any, formal training, and even those who were considered to be the best doctors prescribed barbaric treatments, such as trying to bleed the sickness out of a patient. Since then the standardization of medical schools combined with the advancements seen in medical science have led to the modern-day doctor's training that is rigorous, pressured, stressful, time-consuming, expensive, and involves committing a large amount of information to memory.

However, it is hard to ignore the great financial incentive for all of the time, money and energy that a person spends to become a doctor. Doctors make many times the income of an average American; currently a doctor in America makes an average income of just over $170,000 (cardiosurgeons, orthopedic surgeons, cosmetic surgeons, radiologists, anesthesiologists and some other specialists make much more than this, on average).

Doctors' standing in society is promoted to a high level of respect by commercials that use wording such as, "In clinical studies doctors agree that . . ," or, "Nine out of ten doctors." Many people take these testimonies as truth without questioning who the doctors are, what kind of doctors they are, who paid for the study and what it is that is being considered "clinical." The studies may also be biased, flawed or based on out-of-date or falsified information.

One early radio personality, Henry Morgan, made fun of medical advertising lingo when he spoke about the fictional town of More, Utah. Morgan said that the town of More had two doctors and those doctors were who the commercials were referring to when they claimed that "More doctors recommend . . ."

The authority figure they represent can be and is used by some doctors to their advantage. Some patients expect their doctor to wear the white "authority" jacket or they do not feel as if they are talking to a doctor. Some people are intimidated by any sign of authority, and many people automatically become more reverent and respectful toward the appearance of authority. Within medical facilities some people experience what is called "white coat hypertension." This is when a patient who becomes nervous around medical authority experiences an elevation in their blood pressure when they are around doctors. Some doctors are so caught up in being an authority figure that they use their title everywhere they go and are so uptight they are offended when anyone refers to them on a first-name basis.

Some people have learned the hard way that doctors sometimes make mistakes. There was a man in Europe who went in to have a cancerous leg removed but woke up after the operation to find the medical team had amputated the wrong leg. A similar error occurred when a man in Florida underwent surgery to amputate an infected foot. There was a man in California who underwent surgery to have a cancerous kidney removed. When he awoke he found the surgical team had removed the wrong kidney. There was also a California woman who went in for an appendectomy (an operation where the appendix is removed) and was accidentally given a partial hysterectomy (an operation where the reproductive organs are removed). Every once in a while there is a person who is misdiagnosed with a terminal illness and, after experiencing the mental anguish of thinking they are going to die, later find they had been misdiagnosed. Other people have gone through operations and later found that the operations were not at all necessary and sometimes were done only so the doctor could make money or be eligible for board certification.

Because a doctor in private practice is his own boss, the people who work in his office orbit around him, no one supervises him, and there is no one to fire him if he does bad work. He simply opens the door to let the next patient in.

> *I think it is important to note here that getting involved in the medical delivery system is a risky business. It is as risky as driving on the freeway. Simply by the luck of the draw, you can get hurt and need additional care. That is costly, and not necessarily the kind of malpractice that one would associate with negligence, despite the number of patients who suffer from injury.*

Here is another problem. Despite the number of patients who suffer an injury from negligence, few of the nation's 600,000 practicing physicians have had any disciplinary measures taken against them. For example, in 1991, State medical boards took only 2,800 disciplinary actions against physicians and they ranged from mere reprimands to a paltry few license revocations.

— Congressman Pete Stark during subcommittee hearing on issues relating to medical malpractice, May 20, 1993

Some areas of medicine evolve so rapidly that some medications and surgeries quickly become outdated. Some of this is due to the fact that some treatments are found to be dangerous, damaging or useless. Other changes occur after better treatments are found. Many surgical procedures now available have become popular within the last few years. This was after most of the doctors performing the procedures completed their training. Many of these procedures are taught at weekend getaways or are taught during day-long seminars.

Just because a doctor says he is *qualified* to do the operation does not mean that he has *experience* in doing the operation. Someone has to be the very first patient for the doctor to perform a newly learned technique on.

Licensing of Doctors

I think that many Americans are going to be surprised and frankly quite alarmed to hear that any doctor with a medical degree and State license can go out and do everything from brain surgery to cosmetic surgery. So we have a situation today where dermatologists, obstetricians, gynecologists, otolaryngologists, osteopaths and others are doing cosmetic surgery — literally everything from face-lifts and nose jobs, to breast enlargements and tummy tucks.

— Congressman Ron Wyden, during Congressional subcommittee hearings on plastic surgery industry, 1989

A state medical license can be obtained by taking examinations given by a state board or by mutual exchange of privileges if a doctor is licensed in another state, or by meeting the requirements of the National Board of Medical Examiners.

Each state has its own board with its own set of rules, and boards do not always implement established procedures (doctors who are in the military are federally licensed and play in a league separate from doctors who are not in the military). The state licensing boards have also organized their own umbrella organization called the Federation of State Medical Boards.

State medical boards, many of which operate on very limited budgets, are composed largely of doctors and are meant to monitor and discipline or weed out bad doctors to protect the health and safety of the public. Before a state board can impose sanctions against a doctor, negligent actions or impaired performance must be reported to the board. Even when a doctor who is guilty of the most atrocious mistreatment is reported to the proper authorities, it can take years for any disciplinary action to take place.

One gynecologist who lost his license in California in 1991 was accused by the Medical Board of sexually abusing 69 patients over a ten-year period. Many more patients later called the Medical Board with complaints about sexual misconduct. The doctor was subsequently connected to over 100 complaints of sexual abuse by former patients. The county district attorney's office and the state attorney general decided not to press sexual abuse charges against the doctor because many of the alleged abuses dated to the late 1970s and early 1980s and could not be prosecuted because of a one-year statute of limitations on such crimes. This doctor lost his medical license in California and eventually declared bankruptcy.

Some people think that if a doctor were dangerous he would not be allowed to be a doctor. This is not true. Many states fail to take disciplinary actions against doctors even after the Drug Enforcement Administration has revoked or put limits on their federal narcotics license and after they have lost Medicare privileges. Because of laws, regulations, glitches in the system, and corruption in governing boards, bad doctors are not being cleaned out of the system the way many people think they should be. In California, doctors do not have to even report malpractice settlements under $30,000 to the state medical board. To protect the doctors' careers, the awards over $30,000 that were reported to the California state medical board before January 1, 1993 (when a new law went into effect) are kept secret from consumers — another result of lobbying by the doctor's political group: the California Medical Association.

In reality these boards that are meant to protect patients from dangerous doctors continue to inadequately investigate claims against doctors who are incompetent or impaired by debilitating conditions such as alcoholism, drug abuse or mental illness. Few of the bad medical professionals are ever disciplined, and therefore they continue with their careers. Many times the ones who are protected by the system of the state medical boards are the bad doctors, not the patients subjected to malpractice, who are left to fight against the doctors in the battlefields of the courts.

> *Negligent and incompetent doctors are rarely disciplined or removed from practice. At most, about 0.5 percent of the nation's doctors face any action from their state medical boards each year. On average, only 3.44 serious disciplinary actions are taken for every 1,000 doctors.*
>
> *State medical boards may take more than two years to even investigate complaints of doctor incompetence or misconduct, allowing the doctor to continue to treat other patients all during this time.*
>
> — excerpt from news release by Public Citizen Health Research Group, Washington, DC, 1993

After a doctor is convicted of a crime, the state medical board may take no action or may suspend the doctor's license pending an appeal on the conviction. After the conviction is upheld, the state may revoke the doctor's license after the sentencing. Even after all of this the doctor may appeal his case, and the court can overturn any actions taken against the doctor.

> One Los Angeles-area cosmetic surgeon is still in business even after losing several well-publicized malpractice lawsuits. One woman who won a lawsuit against the doctor went to him for breast reconstruction after a mastectomy. While operating on the healthy breast he botched the operation and the woman was left without a nipple. Another suit was filed by a woman who lost an eye after having an operation to lift an eyelid. Another patient went to him for a partial face-lift and ended up having a heart attack. The doctor claims he operated within acceptable standards of practice.

It is difficult for consumers to find out who the bad doctors are because many of the records detailing bad doctors are for use only by state medical boards, licensing agencies, hospitals, insurance companies and other professionals and are not available to the public. If a doctor is recognized as being incompetent or negligent and is brought before a medical review board in one state and eventually loses his medical license there, he can move to another state and continue ruining lives in his "practice of medicine."

It is not unusual for a very bad doctor to have practiced in two or more states (or even other countries) where he has been disciplined by governing bodies for any number of violations, and where he may have left behind a trail of mistreated patients and malpractice lawsuits. Some of these doctors have gone as far as to change their names to avoid any problems their past may cause. The new state may not know of the doctor's history. The doctor's insurance carrier might, but these records are not normally available to consumers. Some hospitals fail to check up on the history of doctors they give privileges to. Even some hospital doctors have been found to be unlicensed.

Specialists

Evidence shows that too many cosmetic surgeons have no formal training. Others using the shield of established professional society logos have little more training in specific cosmetic procedures.

I think that many Americans are going to be surprised and frankly quite alarmed to hear that any doctor with a medical degree and State license can go out and do everything from brain surgery to cosmetic surgery.
— Congressman Ron Wyden during Congressional
subcommittee hearings on plastic surgery industry, 1989

Consumers should beware of doctors who are willing to do anything and everything to unsuspecting patients. When searching for a doctor to perform a particular type of surgery, it is best to hire a doctor who specializes in the surgery that might be performed and is highly familiar with the anatomy of the area of the body that might be operated on.

Any doctor can legally call himself a "specialist" in any area of medicine and start practicing, but among specialists there are some very good ones who have spent extra years studying and researching one area of medicine. There are specialists who limit their practice to the head and neck and subspecialists who limit themselves to an even smaller area such as the hands or eyes or a certain disease.

As of July 1993 there were 39 specialty areas of certification and 71 subspecialty areas in which certification is authorized by the American Board of Medical Specialties (ABMS). About 70% of American doctors are in specialty practice.

The trend among today's medical students is to enter into a specialty area. The discarded Clinton health plan sought to establish a National Council on Graduate Medical Education that would have limited the number of students allowed to enter into specialty areas. The goal of these student regulations was to form a balance between specialists and primary-care, thus widening the accessibility of primary-care doctors while cutting the costs of healthcare by limiting access to high-cost specialty care.

While limiting the number of specialists and patients' access to them may be helpful in cutting healthcare costs, it does not necessarily provide for better healthcare as some diseases and health problems are better treated by specialty doctors. Some people believe the result of limiting access to specialists might be that more patients who need specialty care will find that their health plans limit access to the needed care and the patients' health can deteriorate while trying to cut through the red tape.

The Board Game

Membership in a board is voluntary and is not a requirement to practice medicine. Though the primary goal of board certification seems to be to protect the public, just because a doctor is board certified does not guarantee that he is a good doctor. Nor does it guarantee that everything will go right with operations that the doctor performs — or that he even has had adequate training to perform the surgeries that he does perform. Because more and more consumers are seeking out board-certified doctors, being board certified could mean money in the bank for the board-certified doctors, and a do-anything-to-get-board-certified attitude may be the product of this.

WYDEN: Is it your view that, generally, in the cosmetic surgery field, not to take any one discipline or any one profession, that generally in the field the number of quacks and charlatans is growing and growing along the lines that the subcommittee has been told about?

CALEEL: I believe that there are individuals who abuse the privilege to practice medicine. I believe that in the current setting that there are a significant number of them in the field of cosmetic or plastic surgery.

WYDEN: Doctor, do you believe that with the technological advances that have been made in surgical procedures over the last 30 years, that a person who has a medical degree and a State license should be allowed to simply declare that they are a specific type of surgeon?

CALEEL: I do not believe that an individual with a medical license can declare themselves in any specialty area.

WYDEN: That is what goes on, though, is it not? We have heard widespread testimony that someone with a medical degree and a State license can claim to be a surgeon with a particular specialty. That can take place, can it not?

CALEEL: Yes; it can.

WYDEN: So you said that it does take place. Do you think that this is right, given the technological advances in the last 30 years?

CALEEL: No

— Congressman Ron Wyden questioning Dr. Richard T. Caleel, president, American Academy of Cosmetic Surgery; president, American Society of Liposuction Surgery, Inc., during Congressional subcommittee hearings on the plastic surgery industry, 1989

Legally anyone with a medical license can perform plastic surgery. Others may take the steps to become board certified through the ABMS by going through a program accredited by a Residency Review Committee sponsored by a specialty board. Other doctors can and have formed their own "boards" and sold certificates to these "boards."

The ABMS was incorporated in 1933 and has become recognized as the official medical certifying group. Many professionals believe that only ABMS-approved boards are legitimate.

The ABMS does not certify boards unless they meet the specified criteria of the ABMS. The ABMS certifies only 23 specialties.

If the doctor is a member of the ABMS, this means that the doctor has passed certain difficult comprehensive oral and written exams to evaluate his skills. Before surgeons can take these tests they must have a medical degree, complete years of specialized surgical training, complete a residency, hold a valid registered full and unrestricted license to practice medicine in a possession, territory, or state of the United States or in a

Canadian province, and must have practiced for two years. Before they can take the oral exam they have to submit a twelve-month portfolio case list of operations they were involved with and hold privileges in a hospital approved by the Joint Commission on Accreditation of Healthcare Organizations, or its Canadian equal.

If the doctor says he is board certified, do not assume that he is certified in the area of medicine in which he makes his living. Some doctors who perform cosmetic surgery operations have no specialized training in plastic surgery or are certified in boards unrelated to plastic surgery or boards that are not approved by the ABMS. They may have been certified in another area of medicine and then decided to enter into the cosmetic surgery business. Some doctors are certified by more than one ABMS board. There are also many doctors who are not certified by any board.

There are two main boards representing plastic and cosmetic surgeons. One is the American Board of Plastic Surgery (ABPS), which was organized in 1937, and the other is The American Board of Cosmetic Surgery (ABCS), which was first incorporated in the early 1980s. The "plastics" are certified by the American Board of Medical Specialists (ABMS) and, beside the other requirements to become ABMS certified, they must have completed a residency in plastic surgery and have practiced plastic surgery for two years — altogether the ABPS certification amounts to five to seven years of training after medical school. Once doctors have been granted certification by the ABPS they are known as Diplomates of The American Board of Plastic Surgery.

The ABMS does not certify the ABCS because the ABCS does not meet the specified criteria of the ABMS. The "cosmetics" are surgeons who are certified by the ABMS in one of the other 23 specialties the ABMS certifies and then are certified by the ABCS. The ABMS only recognizes plastic surgeons who have been certified by the ABPS. A bit confusing but maybe it works better for some people that way.

The ABPS and the ABCS are in an ongoing tangled web of finger pointing, one accusing the other of various professional legitimacy problems. When the ABCS was founded, there were doctors included who had failed the ABMS certification process. Caught up in this mess is the problem of doctors who claim to be board certified but are not.

If a plastic surgeon is one who specializes in the head and neck area, he may be a fellow of the American Academy of Facial Plastic and Reconstructive Surgery (AAFPRS). To be so he must be board certified with training and experience in facial plastic surgery and be a fellow of either the American College of Surgeons or the Royal College of Surgeons.

> *Some of these guys are pretty clever. They form boards, and they go to the printer and they have their little certificates made up and hang them on their wall, and these are all impressive.*
> — Joyce Palso of California, (who had heart failure, a stroke, and had to have a valve in her heart replaced because of a tummy tuck that went bad) telling a Congressional subcommittee about her ordeal.

Consumers should not be impressed or intimidated by the fancy certificates, awards, licenses and diplomas hanging on a doctor's office wall. Every doctor has one or more of them, including doctors who have injured, disfigured, raped and killed patients. However, making a note of these papers can be helpful for checking on the background of the doctor.

> *Doctors can have a lot of diplomas and certificates on their waiting room walls, and they can list all kinds of medical societies and organizations after their names, but the public just does not know which doctors are trained and competent in this field.*
> — Congressman Norman Sisisky, from Congressional subcommittee hearings on plastic surgery industry, 1989

It can be easy to get the board certifications confused with other fancy-looking certificates that may simply be documents of membership or awards from societies, associations, academies or groups who have nothing to do with the doctor's education. Memberships in some of these societies have no bearing on professional skill. Some may simply be certificates the doctor received from legitimate professional two-day seminars he attended. Some societies give important continuing education classes, seminars and workshops that increase a doctor's skills and knowledge, but just because a doctor is a member of the group does not mean that the doctor has attended any of the classes given by the group. They may be organizations that any doctor can join simply by paying some money to the group, or the group may be an association that the doctor and some of his buddies started so that they would have one more official-looking certificate. The certificates may look fine as decorative items in the doctor's office, but as a representation of the medical care you might receive from the doctor, they may be meaningless.

There may be times when the proven talents of a particular doctor who lacks board certification can be what it takes to get the surgical result you are looking for, but usually choosing a surgeon who is board-certified by the ABMS (not just board "eligible") is a much better gamble than choosing one who is not.

A person seeking a good doctor should not stop the background check of the doctor once it is found that the doctor is board certified. Being in good standing with his board could simply mean that he has paid his cash dues. It does not mean that all of his operations have wonderful results.

(To check if a doctor is certified, contact the various medical boards listed in the Research Resources section of this book. Find out what the bylaws of the boards are and ask what the requirements are for a doctor to be in good standing.)

The Marketing of Medicine

Estimates of the amount of money Americans spend on surgery every year are in the hundreds of billions of dollars. It is not possible to get accurate figures of the amount of money spent on surgery because there are so many insurance companies, government agencies, hospitals, medical centers and private surgery suites that have their own bookkeeping and record systems that are shut off from statistical analyzers, and because many smaller operations are paid for in cash. Many of the cash payments are untraceable because they are kept quiet for tax reasons.

Hospitals have started giving seminars about back pain, are holding weight loss programs, are offering substance abuse treatment programs, have opened sports medicine clinics and are conducting health classes for the elderly. Many hospitals open their doors and hold seminars to introduce these programs and new elective surgery procedures to the local community. Some people in the surrounding communities may take advantage of these offerings as a sort of social gathering. It may be seen simply as good public relations for the hospital to get people familiar with the hospital as a friendly place. What it boils down to is that the hospital is a business, and businesses need to make money. Hospitals are owned by corporations and must make a profit to satisfy shareholders. If a hospital is operating in the red, has bank loans that must be paid, or is under other financial constraints, the hospital administrators are under pressure to carry the business into financial security, and that translates into advertising, public relations and marketing to bring in business.

American doctors have a history of performing unnecessary operations on unsuspecting patients. A perfect example of this is the number of tonsillectomies that were performed on children during the 1960s that were of no benefit other than the financial gain seen by the doctors and hospitals who were involved with these operations. In the 1970s the overuse of cesarean sections to deliver babies was a bonanza for doctors, while most of the patients were again unsuspecting. Whereas most of the unnecessary surgeries are performed on women, both women and men should keep an eye out for doctors who want to operate too quickly and hospitals that are much too involved in marketing trendy surgeries and procedures.

In recent years the medical industry has been struggling to conform to cuts made by Medicare, intense pressure from insurers and employers to slash medical costs, and negotiations with HMOs to discount fees. Added to this is the current talk about medical industry reform legislation that may change the way healthcare is financed. All of this has forced many independent doctors to join other doctors in group practices, which belong to managed care programs. The economic changes of the 1980s and 1990s combined with the growing popularity of cutting patient costs by letting patients recover at home (outpatient surgery), and with at-home care (where patients are treated at home by traveling therapists and nurses), has brought national hospital vacancy rates up to 35% and more. Several hundred hospitals and medical centers have closed their doors since 1980. Rural hospitals have been among the hardest hit by these changes because they cannot afford to update their equipment to keep up with the technological advances of today's medicine.

To counteract the shortage of patients, the revenue-hungry medical industry has to develop new income sources to get people into operating rooms. This has led hospitals to become more profit-minded and manage their square footage like department stores, open the doors to their employee gyms to the public for a membership fee, treat doctors like commissioned salespeople by offering incentives to doctors for bringing in new or more business, and compete with other hospitals by reaching out to and offering incentives to doctors in the surrounding communities to refer patients.

> *The Federal Trade Commission has made a decision that in effect permits unbridled advertising, and has failed to follow up on some of the really outlandish advertising claims. As a result, consumers find it very difficult in my view to make the best or the most appropriate choices for them.*
> — Congressman Ron Wyden during Congressional subcommittee hearings on plastic surgery industry, 1989

Whether it be done by a kindergarten dropout or someone with a doctorate in medicine, salesmanship is salesmanship and is done with the goal of getting money from someone else. Since the early 1980s when American doctors first started advertising, medical advertising has proliferated and saturated all forms of advertising media as doctors and hospitals clamor for a share of the market and plead consumers for business. Every possible angle is being used to get the attention of potential medical consumers as hospital administrators and doctors use the tactics learned at seminars on how to advertise and market themselves. Just as people waste hard-earned dollars when they fall for any other sales pitch to buy a product that they do not really need, it is an increasingly common practice for consumers to waste money on medical procedures that are not necessary, carry serious risks and are often advertised in misleading and deceptive advertisements that lack factual substance.

In recent years the marketing of medicine has intensified. On any given day, medical advertising can be found in newspapers and magazines and on billboards, on radio and television, in junk mail, on door-to-door fliers, and through telemarketing. There are also "health" fairs held at malls and stands set up in supermarkets to give "free" tests to find people willing to spend their money on medical services. In the area of cosmetic surgery there are doctors who network with local hair stylists and makeup artists to refer clients to the doctors. In a business sense this is all done for good reason. According to the United States Department of Health and Human Services, Americans currently spend more than $900 billion a year on medicine-related products and services. At current levels of growth that figure is expected to exceed $1.7 trillion by the year 2000.

To earn money in their professions, mechanics need cars to fix, cooks need people to feed, painters need houses to paint, and surgeons need people to operate on. The surgeon, like everyone else, has bills to pay and has to make a certain amount of money every month. He has to feed his family, maintain his home and a certain lifestyle that he has become accustomed to. He also has an office to run, taxes and rent to pay, office supplies and machinery to purchase, staff wages to meet and medical supplies to purchase. On top of all this, he has to cover one of his largest expenses — malpractice insurance (if he has it), and this may cost anywhere from about $10,000 to $50,000 a year. He may also be making payments on student loans or payments to a bank, his family or the local hospital to pay for loans that he used to open his practice. (Laws state that when hospitals loan money to doctors they are to be charged fair market value interest rates similar to what the doctor would pay to a lending institution.) He may be overspending for one or more of these things and may have allowed himself to get into more debt than he is able to meet. To make the money to cover these expenses, there needs to be a continuous flow of patients paying him for his services. Similar to people in other professions, if these financial burdens are hard to bear, the doctor may be working harder to make the money to pay for the bills. He may also be prescribing treatments that are not needed and performing unnecessary surgeries in an attempt to lighten his financial burdens.

Medical centers that are blatantly driven by profit have become a common sight throughout American cities. These surgery boutiques are usually located in highly trafficked commercial districts with well-placed designer signs letting every passerby know what surgical procedures are performed there. Their newspaper ads are mixed in with ads for health clubs and dress shops. Their offices blend in with hair salons and restaurants and do everything short of hiring mascots to stand out front to wave customers into the parking lots. Some of the doctors who run these surgery boutiques had to settle for opening their own medical centers after no hospital would grant them privileges or after their privileges had been revoked. Their appointment books stack the patients one on top of another and the staff seem to have been hired on the basis of physical appearance and their sales ability to get the patients to sign the insurance and consent forms.

Two men chatting on a park bench got on the subject of their health and doctors. One was especially proud of his doctor.

"He never operated on you unless it was necessary. He wouldn't lay a hand on you unless he really needed the money."

Many people believe that medical advertising is screened by a government agency and that, therefore, all claims about health products, procedures and services must be truthful. This is not the case with most healthcare advertising. There is no federal, state or local government agency that approves or verifies claims in advertisements before they are printed. There is no government regulator watching over the shoulders of every doctor and medical facility to direct the advertising and marketing materials these businesses put out. Authorities can take action only after untruthful or misleading advertisements have appeared, but such actions are very rare.

Plastic Surgery Pushers

> . . . *All of the people who are coming out of residency in the New York area will tell you flat out that what they are going to need besides the money to set up their practice is an extra $25,000 to $50,000 for their first year public relations and advertising or they are not going to survive.*
> — Dr. Mark Gorney, past president, American Society of Plastic and Reconstructive Surgeons during Congressional subcommittee hearings on the plastic surgery industry, 1989

Plastic surgery is the fastest growing medical specialty. From the mid-1960s to the late 1980s, the total number of US physicians more than doubled. The number of physicians entering the field of plastic surgery quadrupled in the same amount of time, whereas the US population increased by less than one third. There are now many associations for plastic surgeons — some hold conventions in resort locations such as Cannes, France, where the International Symposium on Plastic Surgery was held in 1994.

Every year there is more cosmetic surgery being done than the year before. After First Lady Betty Ford publicly admitted to having had a face-lift in the 1970s, the jungle seemed to have been let out of the closet and the popularity of cosmetic surgery exploded. The number of cosmetic surgeries being done increased more than 60% during the 1980s. The American Academy of Facial Plastic and Reconstructive Surgeons reported that its members performed 58,000 face-lifts in 1993. That is more than a

170% increase in five years. There was a 90% increase in eyelid-lifts in the same amount of time.

The cosmetic surgery market has spread so widely to all income levels and ages that one plastic surgeon's society has even gone so far as to publish a guide to surgery for teenagers. Cosmetic surgery is becoming so accepted that with some people it is not a matter of *whether* they will have cosmetic surgery, but *when*. Some people spend their life savings to undergo cosmetic surgery. There are also people who have special savings accounts set up for cosmetic surgery. In the 21st century, going to a cosmetic surgeon may become as common among some people as a visit to the dentist.

> *Many are hucksters who misrepresent their inadequate training to make a fast buck.*
> — Congressman Ron Wyden, during Congressional subcommittee hearings on plastic surgery industry, 1989

The cosmetic surgery industry has become so lucrative that there are increasing numbers of entrepreneurial doctors switching their focus of business from other areas of medicine and advertising themselves as cosmetic surgeons. The doctor switching into cosmetic surgery may have gotten tired of dealing with ailing patients and the process of filling out the insurance and government paperwork found in other areas of medicine. Because cosmetic surgery patients are usually healthy, and oftentimes have the cash or the credit to pay for the operations, there are few insurance or government forms to fill out. This can make the cosmetic surgery field financially more desirable for the doctor.

The instant cash flow that doctors find by performing cosmetic surgery has provided many of them with generic wealth where they do their paperwork with gold-coated pens, scoot about in European automobiles, live in high priced homes, maintain country club memberships, rendezvous at parties filled with the rustle of designer clothing, enjoy expensive vacations and join in on the accusations by other doctors who say that the government will ruin the healthcare industry through healthcare reform legislation.

> *He's booked solid, months in advance. Whenever someone cancels out on an operation there is always someone else wanting to get operated on. Every day he is in town he is either operating or seeing patients. We're so glad when he's*

out of town or does his day at the hospital so we can relax around here.
> — receptionist who works for a cosmetic surgeon in Santa Monica, California

Because of the large number of new doctors entering the cosmetic surgery field, the amount of advertising being placed by cosmetic surgeons has also increased. This has increased the consumer's odds of choosing the wrong doctor if he or she is not careful. A doctor can take a weekend seminar on liposuction or other area of surgery, purchase some new equipment and be in business the following week, advertising himself as a specialist in the field. Because cosmetic surgery patients usually pay for their procedures cash-up-front, a few operations will cover the cost of the new equipment and the surgeon can start making a profit within a week. The potential of making large amounts of money in the field of cosmetic surgery can also obscure a doctors' focus on ethics.

Some of these pseudosurgeons have realized huge profits in recent years thanks to a laissez-faire FTC. The agency became an unwitting accomplice to the physical and emotional scarring of too many patients by failing to protect Americans from misleading advertising and cosmetic surgery hype.

Untold numbers of patients seeking the fountain of youth through a face-lift, a tummy tuck or an acid peel sometimes get more than they bargain for, suffering infection, stroke, and occasionally death following procedures that are advertised as safe, easy, and painless.
> — Congressman Ron Wyden during Congressional subcommittee hearings on plastic surgery industry, 1989

Deceptive advertising runs rampant in the cosmetic surgery industry, where advertisements by shysters vastly overestimate the benefits the surgery can have on a person's life. There are also untrained surgeons who take advantage of trusting patients and doctors operating on patients in unlicensed and uninspected operating centers. Surgeries are often sold as simple, low risk and pain free, when they often are not. As a result, patients are being maimed and having their lives endangered by doctors who do not have enough training or experience to provide the results the patients desire. Some of the operations do nothing but introduce struggles into the patients' lives. The disappointment rate is so high and there are so many bad operations being done with unsatisfactory results that some plastic surgeons spend the better part of their time in the operating room performing surgery to try and correct the mistakes and shoddy work of other surgeons.

A doctor who practiced cosmetic surgery in New York reportedly spent over a million and a half dollars a year on advertising. He had plans to open surgery centers in various parts of the country, where he could provide affordable cosmetic surgery to many people.

He drove a Rolls Royce and provided a chauffeured limousine to bring patients in and send patients home. His operating rooms were so busy that sanitation was overlooked to keep up with the quantity of patients. Reportedly the office staff, and even his chauffeur, gave injections and removed stitches.

He used fake diagnoses so that insurance would cover some of the operations. Hernia diagnosis was used to cover tummy tuck operations. Deviated septum diagnosis was used to cover nose jobs. Anything to get insurance to pay the bills.

Along with the assembly line-type operations came faulty surgery. Eyelid-lifts were not done well, nose jobs were botched, and women who went in for breast surgery ended up with lopsided breasts or with their nipples misplaced or removed.

Many malpractice claims were filed against him, and in 1987 he pleaded guilty to charges brought against him that stemmed from the way he "practiced medicine." He was sentenced to three months in jail, five years' probation, and he lost his medical license.

From hair care to pedicures, there is money to be made in trying to make people look the way they want. Some of this money has been made by companies selling such items as dimple clips and face-lift tape through mail-order ads in the back of magazines. Even companies that manufacture products that were not meant for cosmetic use have made millions from people who use the products in unconventional ways, such as people who use Preparation H to reduce wrinkle lines (not a suggestion). Presently the American retail cosmetic products business is a multi-trillion dollar industry. The prescription treatment for hair loss, Rogaine, had worldwide sales of $110 million in 1993.

In late 1993, a product containing an asthma medication (aminophylline, a diuretic) was introduced onto the market and immediately received a lot of media attention because the manufacturers claimed it was effective in reducing the size of women's thighs. At the time this book was being written, this ointment, known as "thigh cream," was being manufactured by dozens of companies that were selling tubes and jars of the stuff for anywhere from $10 to $50 dollars. This product alone was expected to pour nearly $100 million into cosmetic counter cash registers in 1994, even though there was no solid evidence that it even worked.

Estimates of the amount of money Americans spend on cosmetic surgery every year range from one to five billion dollars. It is not possible to get accurate figures of the amount of money spent on cosmetic surgery because many operations are disguised as "functional" or "corrective" surgery so that insurance will cover the operation and many cosmetic surgery patients pay doctors in cash.

In the fashionable Place Mall located in Santa Monica, California, several cosmetic surgeons got together in 1991 and opened what could probably best be described as a cosmetic surgery marketing center. The storefront was located in the center of the mall and was set up so mall browsers could stop by and view large before-and-after photos on the walls and in binders of people who had undergone cosmetic surgery. Visitors could also watch a video, be given pamphlets, and schedule an appointment to see one of the doctors at the their office. The staff was very pleasant, ready to answer any question or provide a way for inquiring mall shoppers to find answers to their questions. What made the staff different from the salespeople who worked in other stores at the three-story mall was that the staff did not sell books, dinnerware, trendy gifts or clothes; what they sold was cosmetic surgery.

Cosmetic surgeons whose main focus is on cosmetic work do not have a natural market. They do not cure any diseases and, with the exception of their occasional patients who are cancer survivors, accident or abuse victims or persons with birth defects, cosmetic surgeons have to appeal to a market of people who generally do not need surgery and are not experiencing any health crisis. It is the goal of cosmetic surgeons' advertising and marketing to convince people to undergo unnecessary operations. Like salon workers who offer a woman a deal on a facial when the woman has her hair styled, some of today's cosmetic surgeons try to sell their patients an extra nip and tuck, implant or sculpting and reshaping when the patient shows up for something less.

> *These unqualified physicians are not offering their services in remote areas where there are not trained surgeons. Curiously, they congregate in the high density wealthy areas where trained surgeons are readily accessible. These physicians are not attempting to offer a service to the community, but they are impaired physicians, not by alcohol or drugs but by greed.*
> — Dr. Harvey Zarem, past director and senior examiner, American Board of Plastic Surgery, from Congressional subcommittee hearings on plastic surgery industry, 1989

> *...elective cosmetic surgery has moved from the plush salons of Southern California to Main Street, USA. Riding a promotional wave of unbridled, often misleading, and sometimes false advertising.*
> — Congressman Ron Wyden, from Congressional subcommittee hearings on plastic surgery industry, 1989

> *The media is often a magnet for criticism for the way it represents and objectifies women, and for the unrealistic standards of physical appearance it sets for women. What the critics seldom mention, however, are thousands of research studies exist which confirm that physical attractiveness is a highly valued and highly sought after quality in our society. And particularly where women are concerned. Like it or not, looks matter a lot in our culture. Even in 1994, there is a double standard of appearance in American society, and women face greater pressure than men to be good looking.*
> — From research study titled: *Men's Magazines: the Facts and the Fantasies*, by Dr. Debbie Then, Social Psychologist and Research Scholar, August, 1994

The cosmetic surgery industry has long been considered to be exploitative of women as it plays off a society that is obsessed with appearance and that purchases practically any item that holds the slimmest potential for making a person more attractive. Most of the cosmetic surgery advertising is aimed toward women and pushes a narrow-minded assumption of what constitutes beauty with a tone suggesting that a certain appearance is best — thin, tall, sexually available, hair like that, lips like this, nose like so, hairline there, nipples here, taught chin, tight butt . . . . The tides have recently turned as there are now advertisements popping up in newspapers and magazines encouraging men to undergo cosmetic facial, scalp, liposuction and penis surgery.

Men and physical appearance enhancement
Q: Will you ever consider physical appearance enhancement techniques to improve your looks?
24% Yes
76% No
Of the men who replied YES, they plan to improve their looks using the following procedures:
50% hair transplant
25% color hair to remove gray
14% teeth bleached/bonded
4% each: face-lift, nose reshaping, penis enlargement
— From research study titled: *Men's Magazines: the Facts and the Fantasies*, by Dr. Debbie Then, Social Psychologist and Research Scholar, August, 1994. Study was based on 58 responses received to confidential questionnaires mailed to 215 Stanford Business School Masters of Business Administration students.

In America cosmetic surgery is most common in California, where 631 ABPS-certified plastic surgeons reside and many uncertified plastic surgeons practice (1993 figure). According to the California Medical Association, about one in 12 of America's plastic surgeons reside in Southern California. There were 137 plastic surgeons listed in just one of the dozens of 1993-issue phone books in Los Angeles, which is considered to be the cosmetic surgery capital of the world. People there seem to flock to cosmetic surgeon's offices as if the state constitution declares "And plastic surgery for all!" and some spiritual guru announced that only people who resemble Ken and Barbie will inherit the earth. It is also where many posh mansions are owned by these surgeons who have hit the medical jackpot. Even in Salt Lake City, Utah, which is a very conservative city, plastic surgery advertising took up three pages in a 1993 phone book.

According to the American Academy of Facial Plastic and Reconstructive Surgery the most popular plastic surgery operations in 1992 were:

1)   eye lifts
2)   nose jobs
3)   liposuction
4)   collagen injections
5)   face-lifts
6)   breast enlargements
7)   Retin-A treatments
8)   chemical peels
9)   tummy tucks
10) dermabrasion treatments
11) forehead lifts
12) breast lifts
13) fat injections
14) ear surgeries
15) male breast reductions

The negative publicity in the media about breast implants has made the popularity of breast enlargement operations fluctuate in recent years.

They may have went through years of hellish medical school and passed all the tests, but you still have to question the mind and morals of someone who makes money by operating on people who have nothing wrong with them other than maybe low self-esteem.
> — A woman who had to have her nose rebuilt using ear cartilage after a doctor went too far when giving her a nose job.

GORNEY: At every house in the Long Beach area there arrived a bunch of coupons with 50 cents off on salami, $1 off on shoes, and a discount on a plastic surgery consultation. That is the level at which we have arrived.

WYDEN: Are we at the point now where a significant amount of cosmetic surgery is just being sold like a bar of soap, or a tube of toothpaste, or a used car?

GORNEY: Very much so. I showed you those ads where people are soliciting by direct mail. It is being touted as totally harmless and very risk free.
> — Dr. Mark Gorney, past president, American Society of Plastic and Reconstructive Surgeons and Congressman Ron

Wyden, during Congressional subcommittee hearings on plastic surgery industry, 1989

I am now on several mailing lists of plastic surgeons and their groups. They have sent me videos, follow-up letters, questionnaires, postcards, newsletters, invitations to attend free seminars, and Christmas cards. One surgeon has sent me numerous letters inviting me to come in for a free hair transplant consultation. Another offered free limousine service to and from his office and another (I am not making this stuff up) offered a to serve a free three-course gourmet meal after the transplant surgery. And my mail carrier must think I am an incredibly vain and insecure person.

The manufacturer of collagen, Collagen Biomedical, sent me several coupons for $25 off collagen treatment injections at any participating surgeon's office, an offer for a free collagen skin test and, to help me look my best, an offer to join the "Collagen Replacement Therapy Savings Plan Program" by purchasing a Collagen Replacement Therapy Savings Plan Membership Card from a participating doctor. The savings plan works just like the discount card that you can get at a Subway Sandwich Shop where you get a hole punched in your card every time you buy a sandwich and you get a free sandwich when there are no more spaces left. But with the Collagen Replacement Therapy Savings Plan Program Membership Card, the doctor validates your card every time you let him inject collagen into your face and when it is fully validated, he injects collagen into your face on the next visit for free. Of course, as the invitation they sent me mentioned, the savings will vary based on the retail price of the Collagen Replacement Therapy Savings Plan Membership Card. It differs from the sandwich shop though because the gloves the doctor wears when he is injecting collagen into your face are more expensive than the cheap vinyl gloves they wear at the sandwich shop when they are preparing your sandwich, the doctor also wears a face mask and you are still hungry when the injections are over. Maybe if they offered a free three-course gourmet meal and some snacks and stuff after the collagen injections, such as the offer from the hair replacement doctor, we could start talking business here.

One particular cosmetic surgeon must spend a fortune on marketing and advertising every year. I attended one of his crowded seminars that was given at a fancy hotel. The seminar reminded me of some kind of religious revival meeting and included appearances by several people who claimed to be satisfied patients of the doctor. Along with these patient's testimonies there was an upbeat presentation by the happy doctor that included a slide show and a question and answer period. The seminar ended with encouraging words to come visit the doctor. As we exited the conference room we had to walk past the doctor, who was smiling and shaking the hands of the attendees. Just outside the conference room we walked past tables set up where consultation appointments were being scheduled and a book the doctor wrote was being sold by smiling women who worked for the doctor.

The marketing letters I have received from this doctor are filled with encouraging words. The letters say that if I desire to "improve my appearance and experience the happiness that I will see in his patients," then I should schedule a consultation with him. The letters mention his computer imaging system that will let me see the new me. The letters say that he and his staff have helped many people just like me. Furthermore, I would receive a 20% courtesy discount on the price of the consultation if I brought the letter to the consultation. It did not mention anything about a three-course gourmet meal.

Along with his letters, this doctor has sent questionnaires; fliers telling about the rather upbeat, vague and pro-surgery book he has written on cosmetic surgery; a video; a lengthy list of his credentials; copies of articles that have mentioned him or that he has written; and postage-paid return postcards for me to fill out my name and address to request further information from him.

I do not know what else he could possibly send me — maybe videos of him actually performing surgery (two doctors did do this), or maybe he could send some of his former patients armed with copies of his book to come knock on my door and tell me how plastic surgery has changed their lives. Or, maybe he can offer discount cards that he validates every time I let him perform surgery on me and then offer some free procedure when the card is all validated. Just think, eleven plastic surgery procedures for the price of just ten!

The latest postcard I received from this doctor was an announcement for another one of his free seminars. At the seminar, which the postcard noted would have a "capacity crowd," this doctor offered a free drawing for a $2500 gift *certificate for cosmetic facial surgery — to be performed by guess who?!*

After all of this marketing material he has sent me, I took particular notice that one of his letters contains the following sentence:

"It is my intent to be of genuine, thorough help to each person — and NEVER to 'pressure' or 'sell.'"

I'm glad he included that sentence because, for a while there, I was beginning to think that he was trying to sell me something.
— The author

Some cosmetic surgery advertising borders on being a parody of itself. One Los Angeles cosmetic surgeon who runs advertorials (advertisements designed to appear like an article) in the Los Angeles Times has sold himself like an appliance store by promising to match any other surgeon's advertised prices. Most cosmetic surgeon advertisements reflect the male-dominated industry by playing off the inadequacies that our sexist society projects onto women. One ad in a newspaper laid it right on the line with bold letters stating, "Sagging breasts can be restored to a pleasing conical shape." It is a wonder how men would feel if the same prominent ad stated, "Withered penises can be restored to a pleasing trunk-like shape." One California cosmetic surgeon calls himself a "facial architect." Others claim to be artists who work on the "ultimate art form": the human body. As if everyone should have a designer theme to their face such as the mansions where these cosmetic surgeons live. The only art many of them practice is the art of persuasion by using all the right words in coaxing patients onto operating tables.

"Compare the Difference"
— actual words in bold typeface that appeared in ads placed in the *Los Angeles Times* newspaper by a doctor who does penile enlargement procedures

In Los Angeles there is a doctor who is known as the "penis enlargement doctor" who reportedly spends $200,000 a month on marketing and advertising, employs a marketing expert and sales personnel who work off an 800 number. This setup runs 26 sales offices that net the doctor and his colleagues 150 operations a month at a cost of nearly $6,000 each. His patients can pay for the operation by using a signature loan agreement through a finance company. All of this brings the doctor a reported $1 million a month.

In September 1994, in the classified section of the Cleveland, Ohio, *Plain Dealer*, an ad appeared under the heading of "sales." The ad read: "Internationally recognized Beverly Hills elective cosmetic surgery group seeks a reliable, experienced sales professional for in-office presentations at its new office in downtown Cleveland. Prior one-on-one presentation experience is mandatory. Experience in self-improvement programs, franchise activity, real estate, enrollment counseling, high-end apparel or insurance is preferred. We have a rewarding compensation package."

The marketing of cosmetic surgery has become a mini-industry all its own as various cosmetic surgeons fiercely compete for a share of the market. One Sunday edition of a California newspaper had 24 advertisements placed by cosmetic surgeons enticing readers to get this or that cosmetic surgery procedure. Toll-free telephone numbers are becoming a common offering by doctors who are also now marketing themselves with videos and high-quality varnished full-color photo brochures. Free seminars are offered at hospitals and hotels. Some doctors have gone to the extent of hiring publicists and marketing experts to increase business by arranging interviews, sending out press releases and placing articles in newspapers and magazines, all with the goal of getting the doctor's name mentioned in the right areas, as if some type of fame will prove he is a good doctor.

Some cosmetic surgery ads seem to be competing for the most appealing names to use for the various surgery procedures by using soft terms to describe the surgeries such as "facial rejuvenation," "nose contouring," "nose refinement," "nose beautification," "eyelid enhancement," "perma brows," and "breast enhancement." Many ads include horribly lit "before" photos next to pleasantly lit "after" photos which may have been taken without any surgery actually being performed. (One California doctor was found to have used before and after photos that had been altered with a computer.) Some ads feature photos of perky, smiling models who probably did not undergo the cosmetic surgery procedure that they are pitching. Some of the ads are so uppity that you are sure cosmetic surgery must be one of the most fun and entertaining experiences that anyone could ever go through. Do not delay, call now, operators are standing by!

Millions of people undergo plastic surgery every year.
Chin implants, dental implants, nasal implants, cheekbone

implants — a dozen different facial implants. Don't you think you're carrying the Mr. Potato Head game a little too far?

What do plastic surgeons really do? They diagnose ugliness? They charge 75 bucks for a consultation to tell you if you're ugly. If you're thinking about going to a plastic surgeon, call me first. I'll tell you you're ugly for half the price.
— Danny Woodburn, Los Angeles comic

One of the marketing techniques used by cosmetic surgeons is to make potential patients feel like they need surgery to "correct" what some of the cosmetic surgeons refer to as "diseases" and "deformities." Anything they can say to make you feel ugly and like something is wrong with you so you come to the conclusion that cosmetic surgery is more of a need than a want. People may *want* cosmetic surgery, but it is rarely a *need*. Still, some people are convinced that they will never be fully happy or a success in business or romance until they appear a certain way. These people are the ones the cosmetic surgeons are trying to lure into their offices. These are the people who have built the business of cosmetic surgery into a multibillion dollar industry.

One of the marketing tools cosmetic surgeons are known to use are offers for free consultations. This consultation involves going into the doctor's office and filling out papers handed to you by a receptionist who will probably robotically mention the "good work" the doctor does. You will then wait your turn to visit with the doctor who, sure as the moon, will find some part of you that can be "accentuated," "enhanced" or "improved upon" to bring about your "self-improvement" or "self-beautification." Surely there is some "service," "technique," or "procedure" that you can trust the doctor to "perform" on you after you have listened to his comments regarding how much better you will look or feel. This is, of course, if you hand the doctor or the staff person who handles the "financial arrangement" some thousands of dollars, get scheduled for a surgery sometime in the days or weeks to come, sign a consent form, and let him cut away at your flesh. Such a deal.

3 • THE CUT UPS

Surgical Chameleons

One of the issues unique to cosmetic surgery that separates it from other areas of the cosmetic world is that it permanently changes a person's image. Whatever plastic surgery operation someone is getting, it is as a result of their refusal or inability to accept their appearance as it is. Somehow the person is trying to resemble some personal ideal and this has driven them to the point where they are willing to pay money and to take certain risks to get a surgery that may simply be a passing fancy.

The availability of cosmetic surgery is producing cosmetic surgery mavens, or addicts, who go in for one operation after another. One 24-year-old Los Angeles man interviewed for this book had 11 cosmetic surgery procedures, which included four nose jobs, chin and cheek implants, ear pinning, breast reduction surgery and liposuction of the neck, hips and waist.

Among the people in the news who have had cosmetic surgery are people who have carried movie star worship to the extreme in attempts to become like their favorite star through surgery. Among the people who have made the rounds of the talk shows are people who have undergone surgery to appear like Dolly, Elvis, Liz, and Michael and one woman who had tens of thousands of dollars worth of surgery performed on her face and body in an attempt to look like her ideal, a Barbie doll. It is as if cosmetic surgery will allow them to share the fame of the people they try to imitate. In Europe there is a performance artist who has had several operations to transform her face and body so that they conform to what she claims were the Renaissance ideals of feminine beauty.

It is not uncommon in Los Angeles to meet or hear of people who have had two, three and four operations to correct what a cosmetic surgeon did to them. One woman, after having one botched nose job, went on to undergo eight additional operations that cost thousands of dollars each to correct what the first doctor did to her. Some women with breast implants have had half a dozen or more operations in attempts to correct or remove crooked, leaking, hard, deflated or misplaced implants. Each operation costs thousands of dollars, with its attendant risks of not turning out well and with the always present possibility of complications and risks of surgery.

Some of the doctors who perform these operations on these sorts of people with bizarre requests argue that they are operating on a person who is an adult and is capable of making an adult decision and that everyone has the right to do what they want with their body. On the other hand, if that adult does not have the mental stability or maturity to make a responsible and safe decision, then what reason is there to do the operation other than for that of financial gain on the doctor's side?

Plastic Surgery Nightmares

Unfortunately, we know that countless patients are being injured. They are being physically and emotionally scarred and they are being financially drained.

According to the American Society of Plastic and Reconstructive Surgeons, 11 deaths have resulted from one procedure alone, liposuction, since 1982.*
— Congressman Ron Wyden. Presenting information at Congressional subcommittee hearings on plastic surgery industry that were conducted in 1989*

It was like, "Let's try this, try that, oops! That didn't work. Hey! Maybe this will work. Oh. But, then again, maybe not. Sorry. Maybe you should find another doctor." Meanwhile I'm having to wait a year or more between each surgery.
— a woman who had numerous nose jobs to try to get a nose she liked

Medical procedures are subject to mistakes, and not all mistakes are the result of doctor error. A patient's dissatisfaction with the outcome of a cosmetic operation is always a possibility. A patient may be dissatisfied with the results of the surgery even when the doctor considers it to be a good result.

Some surgeries do not turn out right because the surgeon did sloppy work, and for various other unforeseen reasons, many surgeries do not result in what the patient was expecting. A small but unwanted change can mean a lot when the person is going to be looking at it in the mirror and in photos for the rest of their life.

There is a cosmetic surgeon in Los Angeles who has garnered a reputation for doing more surgical changes than his patients desire. I have talked to several of his former patients. Upon being confronted about why he does more than the patient wants, he always responds with the same explanation. He acts as if he thought the patient wanted the additional work and says there was a misunderstanding. This has brought him a humorous nickname that unfortunately cannot be mentioned here because it would identify him and he is so lawsuit-happy that the author of this book would likely become one of his targets.

A bad cosmetic surgery result can have a very negative effect on every area of the patient's life, cause public embarrassment, be a drain on the patient's emotions and relationships and lead to financial difficulties as the patient spends time and money trying to correct, or at least improve the unsatisfactory results.

A patient who undergoes surgery with the goal of becoming happier with their appearance can become angry, irrational, depressed and even suicidal if the operation does not turn out the way they expected. These emotions can be amplified if the change brings criticisms instead of compliments and especially if it causes a physical condition that alters a movement or function of the body such as eyelids that will not close or causes breathing problems in a nose that was narrowed too much. They may experience coping problems similar to, or more intense than, those of people who have been raped or likewise violated. These symptoms, which can emotionally cripple a person, include feelings of helplessness and of being deceived, revolving thoughts of the predicament, nightmares, sleepwalking, insomnia, loss of appetite, loss of concentration and an overabundance of anger. They may also entertain thoughts of violent revenge against the doctor.

Those who have had botched cosmetic surgery may, in addition to living their own nightmare, find the doctor and his staff very unsympathetic. The doctor and his staff may simply ignore the patient and the patient's phone calls, hoping that the patient will "get over it."

Probably for as long as there has been surgery, there have been dissatisfied patients who have gone to the extreme of murdering their surgeons, and some dissatisfied patients have committed suicide. People who are thinking these types of thoughts should promptly seek some type of psychological therapy.

In America there have been several cosmetic surgeons murdered by dissatisfied patients, and some dissatisfied patients have committed suicide. At least two cosmetic surgeons have committed suicide after performing botched operations that left their patients deformed.

Among the dissatisfied cosmetic surgery patients who have killed their surgeons was a Washington state woman named Beryl Challis, 60, who had several cosmetic surgeries performed on her by Dr. Selwyn Cohen. These surgeries included a secondary nose job to redo an earlier nose job, liposuction on her abdomen and thighs, which was also done twice, and eventually, without her husband's knowledge, a face-lift in March of 1990.

After the face-lift surgery, Challis started complaining that she thought her face was too tight and caused a choking feeling on her neck, discomfort, pain and hair loss along the incision sites. After numerous follow-up appointments with Cohen, the doctor suggested facial massage and sent Challis to consult with other surgeons and eventually to a psychologist.

On April 15, 1991, a year after her face-lift surgery and three weeks after purchasing a gun, Beryl Challis went to Dr. Cohen's office one last time. That is when she found him alone and shot him five times — then returned home and committed suicide.

Many thousands of people who have bad surgical results go in for additional surgery to try to correct it. Some of the originating doctors offer to do operations over for free or at a discount price. It is probably a bad idea to trust a doctor and let him operate on you again if he has already botched one operation. You may find it hard to find a doctor who will give you a second operation. A patient who was dissatisfied once is likely to be dissatisfied again. Why should a doctor spend time on you when he can take on other less complicated jobs?

Sometimes the second surgery does not correct the problem and leads to further disappointment. Other dissatisfied patients cannot afford to get a second surgery that may cost more than the original surgery, they may not be able to handle the trauma of going through another surgery, may find that there is no way to correct their problem or feel they cannot trust another doctor. People caught in this situation who were interviewed for this book repeatedly said the same thing: They would give anything to have their original body back.

The doctor who performed the surgery may become rude, and his compassion for the patient may quickly disappear when he hears the patient criticizing his work. There have been patients in this situation who have been physically pushed out of the doctor's office and told to never return. The doctor knows that it may be in his best interest to say as little as possible. This silence comes into play because any admission of negligence or malpractice may become part of a lawsuit and interfere with his malpractice insurance and career.

As when you go to the grocery store, when you go to the cosmetic surgeon you should want to know what you are getting for your money and should make sure you get what is best for you. Giving the surgeon too much power is like going to the grocery store, handing the cashier your money and telling them to get the amount of food that can be purchased for that amount of money. The cashier may have very different tastes in food and buy you all sorts of things that you do not like. When you go to the cosmetic surgeon you have to make sure you get what you like; if you do not do this, it will be too late to realize you made a mistake and, unlike the grocery store scenario, you cannot return the item for a new one.

If you are one who is trying to find a doctor to make a bad cosmetic surgery result more agreeable to you, try to separate your emotional reaction from the analysis of what can be done to make you happier with that part of your body or face. What you may think is best for you during a crisis period in your life may not be what is best for you in the long run. Talking your situation out with someone such as a therapist may help you make safe decisions about your personal crisis.

Plastic surgeons and surgery in the news:

A cosmetic surgeon in Miami who was known as "Doctor Lips" because of the frequent operations he performed to enlarge the lips of his women patients, was convicted of manslaughter in the death of a male patient who bled to death during an operation to tighten his tummy and enlarge his penis. Prosecutors said the doctor, 37, was negligent in taking the 47-year-old lounge singer as a patient because the victim had an enlarged heart, wore a pacemaker and was on blood-thinning medication.

One California woman who had a tummy tuck complained of ongoing sharp pains in her abdomen. Her doctor told her that it was typical to have discomfort after such a surgery and she needed to be patient while her body healed itself. Months went by and the woman still felt that she was having more pain than she thought should be expected. A relative took her to see another doctor, who ordered x-rays. What they found was that the doctor had left surgical scissors inside the woman's tummy. This required another surgery to remove the scissors. (A similar situation occurred in Kentucky when a doctor left a surgical glove in one woman's tummy. In another operation a towel was left in a man's torso and in South America one woman underwent surgery to remove two pairs of scissors that were left in her abdomen during an earlier surgery.)

An unfortunate twist of circumstance placed a Chicago-area cosmetic surgeon in the news when he was murdered in August, 1993, by Jonathan Preston Haynes, a former government chemist who subscribed to the beliefs of white supremacy and who described himself as a neo-Nazi supporter. Haynes intended to kill hairdressers, manufacturers of tinted contact lenses and cosmetic surgeons because they provided ways for people to obtain what he called "fake Aryan beauty." Haynes, who later confessed to killing a well-known San Francisco hairdresser in 1987, originally intended to kill a contact-lens manufacturer in Chicago but dropped the idea because the manufacturer was out of town. He then picked the cosmetic surgeon because the Wilmette, Illinois, doctor's advertisement in the phone book was the biggest one on the page. Haynes was charged with murder and at his trial he acted as his own attorney, called no witnesses and presented no evidence. In April, 1994 he reportedly showed no reaction when the judge sentenced him to death.

Probably the most bizarre case involving cosmetic surgery that I found while researching this book did not have anything to do with the surgery itself, but with the way one woman obtained money, part of which she reportedly spent on a face-lift.

Dorothea Puente was arrested in 1988 in Southern California, where she fled after the decomposed bodies of seven of her tenants were unearthed from the backyard garden of her Victorian-style Sacramento home. She buried her dead tenants in the yard because she did not want to alert authorities to the fact that she was running a boardinghouse in violation of her parole. At the time, she was on parole after having completed a prison sentence for drugging elderly people and cashing their disability and Social Security checks. She was charged with cashing over $80,000 in disability and Social Security checks of her victims, who were elderly alcoholics and homeless people. She admitted that she may have forged checks sent to her deceased tenants but contended that she never murdered anyone. She was eventually convicted of three murders and was sentenced to life in prison without the possibility of parole.

Ilich Ramirez Sanchez, better known as "Carlos the Jackal," who was wanted in connection with a 1976 hijacking of an Air France jet to Uganda and at least 83 deaths worldwide, including the 1972 massacre of 11 Israeli athletes at the Munich Olympics, was arrested in August, 1994, in Sudan. He was handed over to Interpol, the international police agency, and extradited to France where he will stand trial for his crimes. Carlos, who became one of the world's most notorious and elusive terrorists and who had been on the run for over 20 years was taken into custody in a private hospital in Khartoum after he was put under anesthesia so he could undergo liposuction to remove fat from around his waist (At least that is what was widely reported. Other sources claim he was undergoing surgery to remove varicose veins from his scrotum).

In July, 1994, a forty-eight-year-old woman who worked in the administration department of the Catholic Diocese of Arlington, Virginia, was convicted of two counts of embezzlement after she put fake employees on the payroll and issued their paychecks to herself. She traveled with her sister to Utah where they posed as nuns and spent the money on dental work and tummy tucks.

In April 1988 a Harvard-educated neurosurgeon called 911 to report that one of his patients had died in his Los Angeles office. The doctor falsely reported the name of the dead person as that of another man. This was the year after two business partners, who did not want to remain in a business and did want to collect on a $1.5 million life insurance policy, had offered the doctor $25,000 up front and $25,000 on delivery of a body they could use to complete the paperwork needed to collect on the insurance policy. The autopsy report was completed and the "living" business partner had the body cremated. Several months later, after $1 million had been collected, fingerprints showed that the dead person was not the person listed on the autopsy report. In 1991, the "surviving" business partner was arrested on his catamaran by the Italian government after his Dutch girlfriend turned him in after seeing an Oprah television show mentioning the story. The "dead" business partner was arrested that same year at the Dallas-Ft. Worth Airport. He had been living in Miami and had undergone cosmetic surgery and hair transplants.

Women with Breast Implants

> *Every period of history has had its own standards of what is beautiful and what is not. . . in the nineteenth century, attaining the beautiful female body required wearing a corset, which led to difficulty in breathing, constipation, weakness, and a tendency to violent indigestion. Women's bodies have always and everywhere been perceived as unfinished in want of carving, perforating, incising, refining, and realignment to make them a thing of beauty and joy to individual and society alike.*
> — from the book *Body Traps,* by Dr. Judith Rodin, William Morrow and Company, 1992

During World War II, Japanese women who worked as dancers in adult clubs injected silicone directly into their breasts to enlarge them. Some of these women found that the injected silicone migrated to other parts of their body, which caused lumps to form beneath their skin. Some of these women died when the injected silicone interfered with their blood flow or prevented an organ from working properly. This led to the development and manufacture of silicone-gel-filled sacs called "breast implants," which were introduced onto the market in 1962.

Breast implants are basically round, sealed silicone sacs, filled with silicone gel or saline (a saltwater solution). In some cases they can help relieve the personal tragedy of losing a breast to cancer.

No one knows how many women have had breast implants nor does anyone know how many of these women experienced problems with their implants. Since the 1960s, more than two million women around the world have had breast implant operations. Many were told the implants would not only increase their breast size but would keep their breasts looking fabulous into their old age. Many women were told by doctors that because implants are not living tissue, they could not grow cancer, and therefore the breast implant material was safer than breast tissue. Some doctors were marketing breast implant surgery for what they foolishly referred to as "a cure" for small breasts (micromastia), which literature from one doctor's association referred to as a "deformity" and a "disease." Some American women traveled to countries in Central America to get their implants because the operations were done there at bargain prices but under what were usually chancy conditions.

It has been reported that an estimated 20% of the breast implant surgeries done in the United States have been performed on women who had breasts removed (mastectomy) because of cancer or cancer risk. The other approximately 80% of the operations have been done for "cosmetic" reasons. Most of these enlargements or "augmentations" were done using silicone gel-filled breast implants that were advertised as "safe" and "problem-free." Because there was little or no testing done by the companies that made the implants, the women who received them were, basically, guinea pigs.

Though articles detailing complications of breast implants first started to appear in medical journals in the 1970s, typically this material was read by doctors and did not make its way into the mainstream media. What most women were told was that there were no problems with these implants, that they were perfectly safe and that the benefits to an implant patient's self-image would outweigh the health risks.

Some of the women who received implants eventually found that their implants had ruptured, which required another surgery to replace. Other women had implants that were not placed in the right position or that moved to another position toward the tummy, under the arm or near the collarbone after a number of weeks, months or years. This also required another surgery to reposition or replace the implants.

Some of the women with implants experienced shrinkage of the membrane of fibrous scar tissue (made up of collagen strands and fibrocytes formed by fiber-forming cells called "fibroblasts") that envelops the implant (eventually referred to as "fibrous capsular contracture"), which caused the breast to become hard, oftentimes causing pain and changes in the appearance of the breast. Many women who experienced this were told to come into the doctor's office, where they were given either a closed capsulotomy (the FDA now advises women with breast implants and their doctors not to perform closed capsulotomy procedures), where the breast is squeezed to break the scar capsule (which often also ruptured the implant); or if that was too painful (which it often was), the women would undergo surgery to remove the scar tissue. This surgery, called an "open capsulotomy," sometimes also required the replacement of the implant. The surgery also caused another incision scar and more damage to the breast tissue, as well as damage to the women's finances — but not to the doctors'.

Until the middle 1970s, the manufacturers of medical devices were left alone to research the safety of their products. This changed with the slew of injuries being reported that were the result of the use of a birth control device called the Dalkon Shield. In 1976, Congress passed the Medical Device Amendments to the Food, Drug, and Cosmetic Act, giving the FDA regulatory authority over the testing and use of medical devices. Many of the devices that were already on the market, such as breast implants and penile implants, were allowed to remain on the market, with the understanding that the FDA would later go back and require the various manufacturers to submit scientific evidence of safety and effectiveness.

By 1990 the mass media were filled with conflicting stories about breast implants. A fingerpointing frenzy erupted among the doctors, implant manufacturers and patients. This threw many women who had breast implants into a panic as they tried to decipher their way through a growing maze of conflicting information. Anyone who followed these news stories can understand how confusing the situation was — and continues to be.

Many doctors who made money from performing the implant operations appeared in the media saying that the implants were safe and cautioned that some women may be rushing to get their implants removed for reasons not entirely reasonable and that the explant surgeries may create more health risks than leaving the implants in. One cosmetic surgeon appeared on television saying that he had given his own daughter her implants and would have never done so if he did not believe they were safe. Women whose breasts were destroyed by breast implants were seen on talk shows and in news reports telling nightmare stories and discouraging women from getting breast implants. Other women who were interviewed said they had never had problems with their breast implants. One news report showed implants being hit and twisted to prove their strength. Yet other news programs showed implants that had been removed that were leaking, deflated, and moldy. Implants were shown with disintegrated shells so sticky to the touch that the surgeons had to change gloves several times during the explant operations. Although the implants were clear when they were put in, when they were removed they were various shades of black and brown.

Studies funded by cosmetic surgeons found breast implants to be safe. One of the companies that made the silicone gel-filled breast implants admitted that some of their implant manufacturing records had been altered by employees. Studies were released that showed evidence of silicone degrading the immune systems of laboratory rats. Another study, by the Maylor College of Medicine, showed that women with breast implants may develop severe central nervous system disorders similar to multiple sclerosis and develop lesions of the brain and spinal cord.

Some doctors have said that once the gel leaks out of the silicone sac, it stays in the location of the breast implant. This is not true. Although it is believed that most women do not experience serious problems with their implants, women with silicone-gel breast implants have free-flowing silicone in their systems that travels by way of the vascular and lymphatic systems. This gel can settle in the eyes, uterus, muscles, kidneys, lungs, ovaries and any other area of the body, including the brain. Researchers at Massachusetts General Hospital used magnetic resonance spectroscopy — a technique that analyzes the chemical composition of tissues — to find that silicone from breast implants travels to the liver. Because the gel slowly seeps or "sweats" through the semipermeable silicone sac where it is contained, the implant does not have to break for there to be silicone-related health problems. It was proved that even unruptured implants leak gel into women's bodies when it was found that implants that were removed from women's chests weighed less than when they were put in.

Liquid silicone that has bled out of silicone-gel implants is blamed for what is being called "silicone poisoning" or "human adjuvant disease." The silicone travels with the body's blood and other liquids, leaving behind scar tissue and clogging the body's systems. This is believed to be the cause of the varieties of health problems that women with these implants are experiencing. These problems can include restricted blood flow, heart irregularities, blurred vision, chronic headaches, shortness of breath, bronchial asthma, insomnia, general anxiety, disorientation, chronic fatigue, cramps, pain in the muscles and tendons, swelling and pain of the joints, spasms, twitches, burning and tightness sensations and swelling of the skin, dry eyes and mouth, rashes, fever, sweating, chills, sensitivity to heat and cold, nausea, vomiting, fungal infections, loss of libido, groin pains, menstrual problems, infertility, miscarriages, stillbirths, malformed fetuses, swollen and tender lymph nodes, swelling of the hands and feet, carpal-tunnel problems, unusual hair loss, rheumatoid arthritis, thyroid and other hormone abnormalities, lupus, scleroderma (a rare connective tissue disorder that, among other things, can lead to a sometimes life-threatening buildup of fibrous tissue in the lungs) and cancer. Some doctors argue that women with breast implants who have developed some of these diseases may have done so regardless of their breast implants.

Some women with these symptoms who sought medical attention for these problems were told that the sicknesses were unrelated to their breast implants, and they were told to take pain relievers or antibiotics or were sent to psychiatrists. The women were taking medication to treat their illnesses and were getting little or no results. They found few medical resources available to them for help with the problems the implants had caused. This triggered the formation of silicone-implant support groups such as The Coalition of Silicone Survivors, The American Silicone Implant Survivors and others (they are listed in the back of this book in the Research Resources section).

On May 16, 1992, a dermatologist on the east coast was found dead of a drug overdose in a fashionable hotel room. Along with his dead body were suicide notes scattered throughout the room. He had apparently grown despondent after several women on whom he had performed breast implant surgery had filed lawsuits against him. He left behind a wife and two small children.

When there is "gel bleed," scar tissue can form around the leaked gel. The scar tissue can calcify and leave the surrounding breast tissue marbleized with this mix of scar tissue, calcification and gel. This can hide the potentially cancerous lumps that form in some women's breasts. This scar tissue entwined with the silicone can become rock hard and lead to what is called "rock breasts." Hardened breast implants can cause continuous pain and changes in the breast and nipple sensation and can prevent the women from being able to sleep face down or on their side.

Some of the silicone gel-filled implants had a special coating of polyurethane foam. This textured coating was intended to reduce the risk of capsular contracture. These types of implants were taken off the market after it had been found under laboratory conditions that the polyurethane coating could chemically break down to release very small amounts of a substance called 2-toluene-diamine (TDA), which has been shown to cause cancer in lab animals. Women with these types of implants have had this chemical detected in their urine. Concerns have been raised about whether the TDA could find its way into breast milk and whether this might pose short-term or long-term risks to nursing infants. Removal of these implants is more complicated than removal of uncoated implants because the tissue surrounding the implants grows into the polyurethane sponge covering.

Because the problems with silicone implants are caused partly by the silicone gel flowing through the body in the blood system and this foreign body can play with the immune system as well as cause other problems, some people involved with the issue have questioned whether women with silicone-gel-filled implants can safely donate blood.

Many thousands of these women with breast implants filed lawsuits against both the doctors and the manufacturers of the implants. In March and April 1994, there was an agreement reached between some of the implant material manufacturers, including 3M Company, Union Carbide, McGhan Medical Corporation, Wilshire Foam, Baxter International, Bristol-Myers Squibb, and Dow Corning — a company that supplied other implant manufacturers with silicone gel. The $4.23 billion class-action settlement was agreed to, but the details were to be worked out on how women were to be reimbursed on the basis of severity of claimed inflictions, what those afflictions actually are, and the age of the women. Not all women with problems caused by the implants were expected to join in on the settlement, but more than 410,000 woman did seek compensation under the terms of the settlement, including 137,000 who claimed to already have experienced health problems caused by the settlement proposed by implant makers. The companies still deny any link between the health problems the women are claiming and the implants they received. The companies agreed to the settlement to avoid hundreds of millions and possibly billions of dollars in accumulative costs of fighting thousands of individual implant cases. If the settlement is carried out, it will be the largest single product-liability settlement in US history.

On March 28, 1995, a Texas state judge, Michael Schneider, overturned a jury verdict that found Dow Chemical Company liable for injuries believed to be caused by silicone-gel filled breast implants that were made by its Dow Corning Corporation affiliate. Instead, the judge upheld the verdict against Dow Corning and found it liable for the entire $5.2 million in damages awarded to a woman.

The jury verdict, which was the first that found Dow Chemical liable for health problems believed to be caused by breast implants, was important because it held a parent company responsible for the actions of a joint venture subsidiary that it does not directly manage. It declared that Dow Corning and its 50% shareholder Dow Chemical were responsible for the injuries allegedly caused by the breast implants. Under the jury verdict settlement, Dow Corning was to pay 80% of the award and Dow Chemical was to pay the balance.

On May 10, 1995, Dow Corning placed a full-page advertisement in about a dozen major newspapers including the Los Angeles Times, the New York Times and the Wall Street Journal. The headline of the ad read "Here's what some people don't want you to know about breast implants:" The ad said that several studies that were done by prestigious organizations concluded that breast implants were not scientifically proven to cause the health risks that many implant recipients were claiming. The ad did not say who funded the studies. The ad said that lawsuits filed by lawyers representing women claiming to have been injured by breast implants are interfering with the development of medical products. The ad said that lawyers were "standing to collect hundreds of millions and even billions of dollars from breast implant lawsuits."

The ad appeared on the same day that a breast implant trial in Texas was involved in the jury selection process. Claiming that the ad may have an influence on potential jury members, the judge overseeing the case declared a mistrial after plaintiff's attorneys accused Dow Corning of jury tampering. The trial involved the breast implant manufacturer Baxter Health Care Corp., and not Dow Corning.

On Monday, May 15, 1994, just as this book was being prepared for the printers, Dow Corning Corporation filed for federal bankruptcy protection. Dow Corning was to be the biggest contributor to the global breast implant settlement. The company had pledged to contribute $2.02 billion over 30 years to the $4.23 billion settlement. This maneuver effectively froze 19,000 implant lawsuits, halted an implant trial in Sacramento and put an Orange County, California trial on hold. Company officials put some blame for the bankruptcy filing on the large number of woman who opted out of the breast implant settlement and sought to sue the firm separately. The slow actions of Dow Corning's liability insurers were also given as a reason for the bankruptcy filing. The company chairman and chief executive, Richard Hazleton, was quoted in the Los Angeles Times as saying that "Attorneys with lawsuits outside of the global settlement have not reduced their exorbitant demands," and that the lawsuits represented "a potentially enormous financial and management drain which threatened our business."

Breast implants in the news:
A Tampa, Florida, woman was shot in the chest while arguing with a man outside of the nightclub where she worked as a nude dancer. The medical team that treated the woman credited the woman's breast implants with saving her life. The bullet was reported to have been deflected by the

implants, which prevented the bullet from entering the woman's chest cavity.

An Indiana woman who makes her living as an exotic dancer fought the IRS and won after she claimed a $2,088 deduction from her taxes for surgery she underwent to enlarge her breasts. The woman, who goes by the professional name of "Chesty Love," won her claim when the judge ruled that the implants, which increased her bust size to 56FF (that is about ten pounds each) and which she considers to be a stage prop, are a business asset.

In 1994, when the Popeye's Chicken and Biscuits fast-food franchise opened up several dozen new restaurants in Southern California, they purchased billboard space throughout the region to announce their new prominence in the area. Their VP of marketing thought they had chosen a humorous phrase that would draw attention. When the company received complaints from breast cancer victims, the company decided to take down the billboards that held the claim: "The best breasts in L.A. without plastic surgery. Popeye's New Orleans style chicken." To counteract the bad publicity, the company offered free billboard space to the Central Los Angeles Chapter of the American Cancer Society to be installed in sequence with National Breast Cancer Month (October).

A 51-year-old woman with breast implants went to an emergency room in Frisco, Colorado, concerned about a swishing sound in her breasts. A doctor attributed the sound to the trapped air in her breast implants, which expands at high altitudes because the outside pressure is lower than the sea level pressure that the implants are normally exposed to.

And the story of the quest for the perfect breasts continues . . . In July of 1994, when a company announced that they had received approval from the FDA to begin implanting a new type of breast implant with a soy-based liquid filler in a limited number of American women, thousands of women contacted the company wanting to know if they could get in on the study.

Explanting Breast Implants

Doctors who made money inserting implants now make money taking them out. Explant surgeries became more in demand after thousands of women who heard the bad news about silicone gel started to ask doctors to remove their silicone gel-filled breast implants. An estimated 25,000 women had implants removed in 1992. Approximately 60% of these women had their implants replaced with saline implants, while the rest decided against implants or proceeded with operations to reconstruct their breasts with tissue from other parts of their body.

Capsule: Scar tissue that has formed around a breast implant. The body's natural reaction is to seal itself off from foreign material. It has been described as an eggshell-like formation around the breast implant.

Capsulectomy: Removing the capsule around the implant. Usually done at the same time as the implant removal while keeping it intact with the breast implant. Many professionals say that the capsule should always be removed to avoid irritation and possible health problems.

Explant surgery is done through a larger incision than the implant surgery incision, and the surgery is also more invasive that implant surgery as the tissue that surrounded the implant often needs to be cut away. This tissue may include muscle that has marbleized with silicone that has leaked from the breast implants. There will still be some residual of the silicone left in the breast area and throughout the body.

In 1991, a California woman had an operation to have her implants removed. Shortly after the operation she developed serious infections. She went to another surgeon who operated on her and found that the last surgeon had only burst the implants and left the silicone sacs in the woman's breasts. The second surgeon removed the implants, the infections cleared up and the woman sued the negligent doctor for malpractice.

Anyone planning explant surgery should make arrangements days before the surgery to have the implants saved for them for lab testing and legal records. (For information on how the explanted breast implants should be preserved, see the Breast Implant heading in the Research Resources section of this book.)

If the doctor or medical facility refuses to give you your implants, contact a lawyer and one of the implant survivor groups listed in the Research Resources section of this book.

Insurance companies have been reluctant to pay for implant removal (a factor that motivated one woman to remove her own breast implants — not something that anyone should ever attempt). Explant operations start at a price of about $3,500, and complicated explant surgeries can cost as much as $15,000. Many women find that the implant-related illnesses improve after the implants are removed. The women are often left with scarred and disfigured breasts. The amount of nerve damage and scar tissue caused by the surgeries can leave the breasts temporarily or permanently numb.

RICHARD'S LONELINESS ONLY DEEPENED AFTER SYLVIA'S HELIUM BREAST IMPLANTS.

CALLAHAN

4 • JUSTIFYING THE WANT

Ethnicity

One common complaint heard in cosmetic surgeons' offices is that noses are too wide or too big and it is embarrassing for the person with the feature. What it is to be embarrassed about? Embarrassed to be identified by their ancestry? Too big for what? Too big to be considered to be in an elite race? Too big to be identified in what prejudiced society promotes as a more significant group of people? Where is the tolerance and appreciation for diversity? What message is the acceptance of these surgeries sending out?

Part of why cosmetic surgery is criticized so strongly by some people is that it erases people's ethnic identification as if there is something wrong with one group of people who look a certain way or who have descended from certain areas of the world. African people having their lips made thinner and their noses narrowed, Asian people having their eyes changed to appear more Western or having implants to make the bridge of their nose more pronounced, and people of Mediterranean and Persian ancestry having their noses made smaller are some of the types of cosmetic surgery that have come under the criticism of people who consider these practices to be a form of ethnic cleansing. Placing the value of a person or making assumptions about a person based on their physical structures and natural appearance rather than respecting the person as an individual based on the content of their character contributes to intolerance and prejudice. Though they may simply be giving in to the dominant culture that places value on a certain kind of beauty, people who have gone through with surgeries that change ethnic features have been accused of rejecting their culture.

During my research for this book, I came across several medical books about cosmetic surgery and a few beauty books that mention the "perfectly proportioned face" or "well-proportioned face," which, these books mention, conform to the "accepted standards of beauty." Every one of the books speaks of certain precise measurements where the features of the so-called perfectly proportioned face are distributed at specific angles, widths and lengths. A few of the cosmetic surgery books and one of the beauty books mention that a person with a face that does not match up to these measurements may want to "correct" the characteristic by undergoing cosmetic surgery. The photos and illustrations in every one of these books use a certain type of face — that of a person with what could be described as white, Western European features.

What makes some people like and other people dislike various facial features is personal taste and sometimes prejudice. The increased popularity of operations that change the structure of the face shows shades of one of the human race's darker aspects. It has always been one of the more common practices of racist people to comment about the features of what they consider to be the unsuperior race. During Hitler's regime it was taught that certain facial characteristics of the Jews were ugly and unacceptable and that the features of Hitler's race were superior.

Somewhere along the line, some plastic surgeons, being influenced by the thought patterns that define a particular kind of appearance as ideal, have decided that features which deviate from this ideal are socially unacceptable and have branded them as medical concerns. Some of the literature published by the plastic surgery organizations and some of the plastic surgery manuals and brochures written by these doctors describe certain features as "deformities" that can be "fixed." If the doctors can convince people that these are *deformities*, the doctors can then make money to *fix* them.

There is nothing wrong with having a wide or large nose or large lips. They are ethnic qualities and are also natural and normal features of the people who have them. It is not something that *needs* to be corrected because there is *nothing* to correct and the features are *not* deformities.

The bearers of these kinds of facial features may not like those characteristics of their faces and *want* them changed and have the right to have them surgically changed, but it is not a *need*. What the surgery may do is leave the person with an odd appearance as the altered feature does not match the ethnic qualities drawn on the rest of their face.

A person's ethnic heritage is represented on their face. Surgically altering these characteristics will alter the person's facial definition of ancestral origin. Anyone going in for cosmetic surgery to alter the features of their face should consider what meaning the ethnic identification of their face means to them. They should ask themselves if the motivation to change their feature is because of thought patterns constructed by prejudices and if the feature is something that they have come to feel is *wrong* with them because of racial slurs. Studying their ancestry and culture might teach them to value their ethnic qualities, install pride relating to their ancestral history and bring them to a different conclusion. They may end up welcoming comments that they once thought of as insults.

As with any operation that changes a person's appearance, a person who is considering surgical alterations to their face should keep in mind that they will look different from their parents and siblings, their children will not be born with the new look and the person also may not always like the change that was made.

Vanity Surgery for Teenagers

> . . . the masters of the miracle make-over prey on the insecurities of Americans of all ages.
> — Congressman Ron Wyden, from Congressional subcommittee hearings on the plastic surgery industry, 1989

Today's teenagers are bombarded with appearance ideals thrown at them by the clothing and makeup manufacturers who try to instill brand names into their impressionable young minds. It is these companies' goal to hook the youth in their formative years because marketing survey statistics show that consumers often remain loyal to specific brands. It is also these companies' goal to get their hands on part of the $30 to $50 billion that the teenager and college-age population controls.

75 female college students at Stanford University were asked what they thought about the typical ads in women's magazines that feature stylized photos of female models. Here are some of their responses:
- The ads make me feel fat and ugly because compared to the models, I am fat and ugly
- The ads make me feel fat and ugly, that is why I do not read them

- The ads make me feel insecure and ugly. They make me feel that I need to lose weight to be beautiful.
- They make me want to be thinner
- They make be feel yucky and unsatisfied with my body proportions
- The ads make be feel fat, especially because I know men look at the pictures and think the models are perfect. The ads make me feel that I will never be someone a man will notice
- The ads make me feel fat and ugly, which I'm not. They make me want to constantly improve and change physically, which just isn't my top priority
- The ads always make me feel fat and ugly. They make me feel like being 100 lbs. is the norm, and thus I am way above what I am supposed to be
- I'm comfortable with my looks but I hate how the ads influence other people's perspectives, especially males
- I wonder if the models in the ads are all anorexic to look that way. I think I feel this way because I was very thin naturally as a girl, and when I started gaining weight in late adolescence, I started dieting. I developed an eating disorder and looked just about like the women in the magazines
- The women are often intimidating and make me feel like I should starve myself in order to look like them. I think I feel this way because magazines reinforce a certain body type which not many women can conform to
- I hate the way the ads make me feel. Maybe not when I look at them, but later, when I look at myself in the mirror. I feel depressed because I don't live up to the societal standard of beauty
- The ads are generally sexist, and push for the passive, perfect woman who wants/needs a man
- I'm thin, athletic, and reasonably attractive. For about six years I compared myself to these supermodels and came up severely inadequate. They lower my self-esteem and self-confidence
- The ads don't make me feel fat or ugly, because I am pretty and thin, and ads reinforce that ideal
- The ads are frustrating and inspiring
- The ads make me jealous, but they inspire me to take care of myself

- I feel fat and ugly, but the ads usually just motivate me to improvement

The study was done using a small group of women at a top college, therefore, no sweeping conclusions generalizing the whole population of American women can be made from the results. However, these findings are important as they represent the opinions, perceptions, attitudes, and beliefs of a group of intelligent and well-educated young women who comprise the target group to which fashion and beauty magazines are marketed.

— Study was conducted during the spring of 1992 by Debbie Then, PhD, Social Psychologist

Teenage vanity magazines fight for advertisers who want to market their wares to the youth market. Cosmetic firms give away samples of their products at high school sporting events and sponsor cheerleading teams. Clothing designers and makeup companies work with TV shows aimed at the young population by coordinating their seasonal lines to appear on the bodies and faces of young TV show stars during the right months. With all of this action it is no wonder that today's youth are more aware of their appearance than any past generation.

As the popularity of cosmetic surgery expands, the average age of those seeking cosmetic surgery is becoming younger every year. An estimated 4% of cosmetic surgery patients in the United States are teenagers. In Los Angeles it is estimated that more than 20% of cosmetic surgery patients are teenagers. Some cosmetic surgeons say that teenagers make up over 25% of their practice. The most common cosmetic surgery procedures performed on these young people are nose jobs, chin implants, breast implants, liposuction and surgery to position wide-set ears closer to the head (otoplasty).

Some doctors say that it is surgically safe to perform alterations on teenagers as soon as they are physically mature. One of the pamphlets distributed by one plastic surgery organization mentioned that, in some instances, cosmetic surgery can be performed on children younger than 14 years old. It is doubtful that any child so young is capable of making a responsible decision to make a permanent change to their body at such a mentally immature age, before their body has finished growing.

Teenagers, who are known for overreacting to the slightest facial blemish and fixating on what they consider to be physical flaws, may be going through a stage where one of their features is developing slower than others. Sometimes the body does not finish growing until a person has reached the middle 20s. It is best to wait a few years for the teenager to grow up rather than do something they will regret later in life or that, when the risks and rate of dissatisfaction are taken into account, could introduce complications into the young person's life. Beyond those procedures to align teeth or bind ears, any surgical changes to the appearance of the body should be looked at very cautiously when the potential patient is a teenager or young adult.

Teenagers have not developed or learned to accept their individuality, they also may not realize that it is okay to have a unique look and that attractiveness comes in many varieties. More than likely they have not learned the value of their personality, talents and appearance. They also may not have had anyone encourage them to find their best qualities.

Adolescence is a time of growth, learning and adjustment. Nearly everyone goes through a phase of awkwardness with their growing body. Being unhappy with some feature is part of growing up and might be more about what the teen plans to do with the rest of their life than with a concern for the present. This stage in life can be more awkward than usual if the teenager already has self-esteem problems and if some insensitive person is making negative comments about a teenager's appearance or physical structure. This may have brought the teenager to constantly compare themself with the next person and may create a desire to look like someone else.

Children may distort their actual image as relatives continue to point out from what side of the family the child inherited their traits. As the family continues to mention these characteristics, the child may begin to think that everyone is judging them by physical attributes. This can bring about crippling shyness. Teenagers' happiness can revolve around their appearance and this may be instigated by the portrayal of beauty in the media and the media dictating what look is and is not "in." They are likely to be associating their happiness with their appearance and any kind of negative comment regarding this can seem monumental to them. Teenagers have even committed suicide after getting caught up in the appearance game.

From early on people are taught how appearance influences a person's status in life. In fairy tales the character the child is supposed to like is always described in physically complimentary terms while the character who is supposed to be hated is always described as ugly or with physical ailments or characteristics. This practice of type-casting characters is further carried out on television and in films. This pattern of judgment can germinate, and by the time the child grows into their teen years they can place too much value on physical appearance.

As with anyone seeking to surgically alter their appearance, special attention should be paid to teenagers to try and pinpoint what their motivations are, find out if their likes and dislikes are consistent, and find out who first suggested the operation or who is motivating the teen to undergo the surgery, and what the teenager wants as a final result of the surgery.

> Some men feel worse about their bodies after looking at perfectly sculpted male models. Others say a comparison motivates and inspires them to work out.
> — From research study titled: *Men's Magazines: the Facts and the Fantasies,* by Dr. Debbie Then, Social Psychologist and Research Scholar, August, 1994

No one should undergo cosmetic surgery because of the influences of peers, friends, or relatives; a doctor who plays on the teenager's insecurities; or a parent's anxiousness to satisfy a child's desire.

When parents push a teen to undergo cosmetic surgery, it should be looked at with even more caution and possibly as a form of mistreatment. The parent may have some growing up to do. The parent may be trying to compensate for disappointments in his/her own life. If this teenager–parent team goes to the wrong doctor, the doctor may not take enough care to detect problematic motives and perform the surgery simply for the money.

Your Well-Being

Some people go along with a thought pattern that they will never be accepted by people who they think matter, and they will never accept themselves, nor be happy, unless they appear a certain way. An individual may have to deal with some prejudices of the people they communicate with, but if they have a negative image of themself and they think they are going to be a failure, then they may very well become one. The trail to success starts in the mind. If an individual thinks they are going to be a success, then they have a much greater chance of being a success. People of all shapes and sizes succeed in every area of life. The recipe for success is based more on the way a person thinks and conducts himself than on the way he looks.

Some people think they should resemble the impossible images slathered throughout advertisements and fashion magazines. What they may not realize is that many photos of commercial models have been altered with computer graphics and retouched with airbrushing even after the models have spent hours getting their hair, makeup and clothing just right and the photographers have spent equal amounts of time arranging and adjusting the photographic lighting, screens, and camera lenses.

Even if a cosmetic surgery procedure does have a pleasing result, it probably will not change the person's life. All they will be is the same person but with any number of surgically altered body parts. Although it might improve their self-confidence, it generally will not change the way they think. At best they may like the change in their appearance and this might help their self-image. But, they also might not — and the results can be disastrous. Someone who was not happy before surgery can become extremely unhappy and even suicidal if the surgery does not turn out the way they envisioned it.

Some cosmetic surgeons will spend one or two hours talking to prospective patients to get to know the patient's motives and expectations and find what is generating the desire to take on the gamble of cosmetic surgery. Other doctors will spend a minimal amount of time with the patient, schedule them for an operation, do a quick slice, cut and stitch and be done with it. No need for that doctor to worry what the outcome will be. Whether or not one patient is dissatisfied there is always another with cash in hand waiting at the door.

Though psychology is not a plastic surgeon's area of expertise, many cosmetic surgeons claim that they put their patients through a psychological review before the surgery. A psychological review by a cosmetic surgeon could be limited to one simple question such as "Have you ever been under psychological care?" If the person wants the surgery bad enough, they can simply lie to get around any possible hurdle that would ruin the goal of getting the surgery. The magic words that many cosmetic surgeons look for is when the patient says: "I'm doing it for myself."

An important question that might be asked of anyone
considering cosmetic surgery is:

What is the person expecting out of the surgery in the
way of the surgical result providing for a want that
currently is not being satisfied?

The motives, expectations, and mental state of the patient
play a large role in cosmetic surgery. Before a person decides to
undergo appearance-altering surgery the operation should be put
in perspective. There are a number of factors that can determine
whether proceeding with cosmetic surgery is a reasonable
decision. Any personal difficulties or life changes the patient is
currently experiencing should be put into consideration. The
patient's true motives should be pinpointed and analyzed. Any
kind of unrealistic expectations should be recognized.

What may be most beneficial to any person who wants to
surgically alter their appearance is to visit with a therapist
who will not benefit from the patient's choice to have the surgery
and discuss the possible benefits from such a surgery. This
protection measure may be done to assure that the person is
making a decision that is in their best interest.

Recognizing Your Motives

Following are some questions that might help to demonstrate
a person's motive to undergo cosmetic surgery. These questions
were developed by interviewing persons who have had cosmetic
surgery and by questioning psychologists and counselors. They
also read the text of this book. Many of their comments and
alterations to the text have been included throughout the book.

A) Do you follow other people's standards of beauty?

Though it may not be easy to do, given societal influences,
rather than basing your desired appearance on the features of
another person, it may be healthier, fair and more realistic
to allow yourself to look like a healthy you and not like
someone else who physically impresses you.

**B) Are you undergoing surgery because you know someone else who
had it and you like that person's results?**

Just because a cosmetic surgery had a satisfactory result on
one person does not mean it will turn out well on another.

C) Will the body part look better or just different?
Are you going to replace something you do not like with something else you are not happy with?

It should be remembered that cosmetic surgery can leave scarring, tissue and nerve damage, and damage to organs and the structure of the body — all of which can be much worse than what was bothering the person in the first place.

If the patient was upset by a small detail, the patient may be much more upset if something goes wrong with the surgery and the final outcome is not what the patient had in mind.

Going through surgery to try and gain more confidence and getting a bad result can destroy a great deal of the confidence the patient had to begin with.

If you are some type of celebrity, you may want to take into account that people know you by your appearance and that this appearance has been established in the minds of the public or your fans. Tampering with any of your features may bring you the kind of publicity you do not want.

D) Are you about to hit a decade birthday mark?

It is not a good idea to rush into important decisions, such as the decision to undergo cosmetic surgery, on the basis of a major event in your life, especially on the basis of a major age change. This can be a time when a person is overly aware of their age with illusionary thoughts about body changes and mortality. It may be helpful to delay making the decision until the crisis or life transition has passed.

Cosmetic surgery will not stop aging. It can sometimes, if it is done right, make a person look rested and younger. What it sometimes ends up doing is making the person look unnatural — with obvious surgically tightened skin and altered structures that do not move normally.

E) Are you seeking cosmetic surgery for career reasons, citing that the younger, more attractive workers in your field are promoted and receive a better income?

Are you seeking to remove features which you believe make you an ineffective person or that you believe make you inferior?

Do you think the operation is some type of detour to success and your career will take off after you recover?

Undergoing cosmetic surgery will not guarantee anything. It especially will not guarantee a promotion, and there is no solid promise that it will enhance your career.

Appearance is important in the workplace. This can especially hold true when a person has a lot of contact with people and particularly in sales or another area where a person has to influence clientele to commit to something.

Studies have shown that better looking people get attention, have an easier time finding a job, and get paid more than less attractive people. At the same time there are also professions in which having a face with character can be beneficial. Large aristocratic features can be a sign of authority, wisdom and dominance. Having surgery to remove these features can leave the face looking delicate and unnatural.

Women may be considered less intelligent, less wise, and sexually provoking if they present what can be considered a sensually based image. This can interfere with income.

Grooming and clothes also have a strong influence on career advancement. Though it is giving in to the distorted standards set by commercial society, what may provide some satisfaction to a person who is seeking to change their appearance is a wardrobe change, new hairstyle, or new hair color and, for those who wear makeup, learning new ways of applying and switching to a different color spectrum of makeup. Makeovers provide a significant change to a person's appearance and cost a lot less than, and do not carry the risks of, surgery.

F) Are you seeking to fill a void left by unsatisfied desires in other areas of your life?
Do you think your life will change after an appearance-altering operation?

Cosmetic surgery probably will not make you more productive in any area of your life, will not catapult you into happiness, will not make you more articulate and absolutely will not change your intellect.

Cosmetic surgery can, within reason, if it is a successful operation that is done on the right person for the right reasons, have a satisfactory result that can make a person more secure with their physical image.

No matter what the doctor — or any person who has undergone the same procedure — claims, realistically and truthfully there can be no promises of how the surgery will turn out, how it will affect various areas of your life or whether it will satisfy any wants or needs.

G) Are you trying to bring more attraction to a current relationship?

Cosmetic surgery will not cure an unhealthy or dead romance and should never be done out of desperation for romance, love or attention.

Although looking good can fan the flames of romance, a relationship based on appearance is about as solid and deep as the person's beautiful skin.

Physically imperfect people are just as important as everyone else and many of them get married every day.

H) Are you seeking the operation to look better as revenge to someone who stole your romantic interest or to try to attract a certain individual?

The cosmetic surgeon's scalpel is not a magical wand capable of turning you into a spectacle of desire.

Cosmetic surgery does not hold any promise as a tool to regain a lost love.

I) How is your social life?
Are you seeking to change your appearance because you think it will help get you out of loneliness and boredom?

If a patient does not have the social life that they are satisfied with now, they should not expect to have it after cosmetic surgery. They should also not expect the surgery to place them in what they may consider to be a more privileged social arena.

Even if a person is surrounded by people, they can still be lonely. Good looking people get lonely and bored too. A person's loneliness is often caused by a lack of being able to relate to their surroundings. What may bring more satisfaction to a person suffering from loneliness is to change that which can be changed easily. Realize that as a member of a community you are part of a much larger system than that which you may have become accustomed to in your life.

Rather than seeking to "fit in" by undergoing some cosmetic surgery procedure that may not turn out right, there are things you can do that are more likely to improve social life. Becoming familiar and getting involved with what is going on in your community may give you more of a sense of belonging. Hanging out at a bar does not count.

Not everyone likes to be socially active but, a person who is seeking to change the way they spend their time may want to consider the following:

- Do not always spend your free time with the same group of people
- Do not expect other people to entertain you and make you happy
- Get involved in activities that get you away from your phone and television and preferably out of your house (keeping track of the lives of characters on television who do not actually exist is not a way to learn to relate to real humans or the real world)
- Take a class on a subject that interests you
- Join a gym and go a few times a week
- Join a dance team or take dancing lessons
- Get involved in an outside sport or sporting club
- Take a self-defense class
- Grow a garden or learn how to bake and randomly share some of the results with various people without expecting anything in return
- Go for a walk in a safe park or neighborhood a few times a week
- Walk or ride your bike to the store instead of driving
- Find a hobby or craft group or get involved in some form of art and be patient with yourself as you develop artistic talents (art supply stores sometimes provide art classes or are knowledgeable of local art teachers and classes)
- Volunteer at your local playhouse or with a local live theater group to help build sets, gather or make costumes and sell tickets
- Attend concerts, visit museums and attend local sporting team games
- Exercise your mind. Get a library card and read one or two books (not always fiction and not always non-fiction) a month to keep yourself interesting (librarians and bookstore managers may help you find a book that will interest you) or join a library reading club
- Do volunteer work for a charity group or perform other community service such as working at an animal shelter or getting involved with a local environmental group (there are plenty of non-profit organizations that need volunteer

workers - your library or city hall can refer you to local
organizations that use volunteers)
- Attend a support group that deals with a personal issue
  that affects you
- Take assertiveness training
- Find a church that has activities or find a church that
  will lift your spirits but that will not consume your life by
  taking up all of your free time
- Join a professional or trade organization
- Find a job — even a weekend job — where you will have
  constant contact with many people
- Find any activity that enlarges your group of respectable
  and trustworthy acquaintances

J) Who are you trying to please?

**Are you trying to gain friends and influence people or trying to
blend in with a certain group of people by surgically changing
your appearance?**

**Did someone make the comment that your are embarrassing to
be with because of your physical appearance?**

**Do you feel you are ostracized because your appearance
deviates from what you think is acceptable?**

**Are you dependent on one person to determine how you feel
about yourself?**

If you are going to the extreme measure of undergoing
surgery to change your appearance as a means of getting a
certain group of people to accept you that you believe is not
giving you the attention that you desire, then maybe you
should ask yourself why these people are so important to you.
What do they represent to you? Why do they matter to you?
Why are you seeking their approval? What if they still do
not accept you after you have had the operation? What have
these people done to earn such a friend? How far will you go
to get their attention?

You can change everything about yourself as a way to get
other people to appreciate you, but until you figure out a way
to change what is inside the mind of other individuals, what
makes them tick and their prejudices, you will not succeed in
getting everyone to like you. Not everyone likes everybody.
That is part of life. Realize it. Get used to it.

Learn to like yourself first and foremost. Unless you care
about yourself, others may have a difficult time caring about

you — and, though you may not know it, you may not allow them to.

K) Are you pursuing a change because someone made a negative comment about your appearance?

Who are the people in your life who may be knowingly or unknowingly doing or saying things that can break down your self-esteem and self-respect?

A disrespectful and insensitive person who makes negative comments about others' physical attributes may not be happy with their own situation. Someone in their past may have mistreated them in the same manner and they may be more familiar with "mean" than they are with "nice." They may have been raised in a home where they were not taught to be considerate of others' feelings and where it may have been thought of as funny to insult other people. The person may not know how to direct their anger and, as they lack healthy communication skills and healthy ways of expressing themselves, they take their frustrations out on the people around them. Irrational anger and petty criticism are signs of insecurity.

Being around people who continuously make negative comments about you eventually can cause you to repeat their comments in your mind. It can play with your self-esteem to the point that you take over where they left off. At that point you are the one who is nourishing the abuse that has been shoveled onto you. Going in for cosmetic surgery can be an act driven by the guilt that you are not the person who you think you should be based on the comments you have received about yourself from others.

Whether you realize it or not, having come from a dilapidated past where people were abusive to you in some way has altered your sense of being and made an impact on the way you conduct yourself. More than likely you have developed traits and tendencies in your mannerisms, composure and thought patterns that testify to this and they may be recognizable to other people. Sometimes these can evolve into debilitating psychological patterns of behavior, be evident in your posture and ultimately contribute to physical ailments.

Often people who have been subjected to some type of physical or psychological domination in their own home are passive, are easily taken advantage of and are not aggressive when it comes time to defend themselves. They may hook up with the same type of dysfunctional people because dysfunctional is their familiar form of communication. Any change to something that is unfamiliar may also be uncomfortable even when the change is more healthy.

People's pasts always continue to effect them and it is never too late to learn how your past has effected you. You can learn how to recognize and handle the unacceptable behavior of the people who surround you so that their abusive comments do not direct your actions and alter your life. Visiting with the right therapist can help you learn why a person is mistreating you and why you continue to allow it. (Organizations that counsel people who are in abusive relationships and that can refer them to sources of help are listed in the Research Resources section of this book.)

L) Who is planting the thoughts in your mind to undergo cosmetic surgery?
Is someone encouraging you to undergo the surgery?

Investigate the possibility that your perception of your appearance may be distorted or may have been constructed over time by listening to people who made negative comments about you.

What some people need to be told is that they look fine, should forget about having the surgery, and go live their lives and stop concerning themselves with distorted worries about their appearance. They are likely to benefit from spending some of that money they saved for the operation on ways to build their self-worth. If they have learned to hate themselves they can learn to like themselves. This process might include reading self-help books, getting professional counseling, attending a support group, taking other measures to deal with issues that affect them and becoming more satisfied with their appearance through better diet, exercise, grooming and dress.

Cosmetic surgery should be done only for the person who undergoes it. The person will be the one who will be living inside of that body for the rest of their life.

M) Are you trying to improve a bad body image?
Are you pre-occupied with your appearance?

Do you often think and talk about your appearance so much that people have commented about your being self-indulgent?

You may have distorted your true image in your mind to the point that you often do not quickly recognize your reflection. You may be repeatedly surprised when you do not immediately recognize your own photograph. You may also be basing your image on one bad photograph and may have blown things out of proportion. This is often the case with both men and women who suffer from bulimia and anorexia.

A person's appearance does affect the mind, but too much of the time people who hate the way they look are judging their existence by their physical appearance. In their mind, life problems can be directly related to the level of concern they have with their appearance. This negative vision can navigate them to make irrational decisions.

A person with a bad body image may be thinking that the cosmetic surgery will transform them into a drop-dead beauty and solve what they consider to be their problem. They usually expect too much from the cosmetic surgery.

If you suffer from a bad self-image, it probably will not be cured with cosmetic surgery. You will be the same person, but you will look different. There is no guarantee that you will look better, only different — and maybe not how you would like to look.

Therapists have developed ways to counsel people on how to build realistic visions of themselves, and some therapists specialize in this area. Anyone with a negative self-image may benefit from visiting with one of these specialists or should read some books on building self-esteem before undergoing any type of appearance-altering surgery.

N) Are you involved in an abusive relationship?
Are you frustrated with someone in your life?

If a person is surrounded by people who treat them badly, this will likely have a negative impact on the person's self-worth.

Some people have been led to cosmetic surgeons after having been told by insensitive people around them that it is their fault their body looks the way it does. It may have led to the person developing a distorted image of how they really look. They may feel guilty about the way the process of aging has changed their body as if they are at fault. They may feel they should have been taking better care of themselves. They may not have let themselves accept the fact that, beyond normal upkeep and some preventative measures, aging is a natural event out of their control and therefore they do not need to hide signs of aging as if they did something wrong.

Abuse is a pattern of behavior and is about one person exerting control over another and not about how the other person appears or acts. The abuser has the problem and not the recipient of the abuse. Cosmetic surgery should not be used as a tool to try and change this type of situation.

Abuse can affect a person for many years as the person may be easy to manipulate and continues to feel like they do not have any power even after having gotten away from the abuser. This can also lead to the victim abusing others who are more vulnerable than themselves such as children, younger siblings and even animals.

Allowing yourself to be controlled by the directive remarks of another person enables the abuse to continue. The recipient of the abuse should take action to learn how to deal with abusive people and become assertive. Therapy may help them avoid becoming a repetitive victim of abuse or a victimizer trying to regain power by treating other people badly.

Physical Abuse

If you are seeking plastic surgery to repair damage that was inflicted in an abusive relationship and you have not left that relationship, be aware that if you are planning on getting out of a relationship in which you were physically abused by someone who lives in your household, you need to protect yourself during this transition period. Statistics show that you are more likely to be harmed at this time of leaving than at any other time. This is why it is important that you get help from the right sources.

Contact a local domestic abuse hotline or women's shelter for assistance. Groups that can help you are listed in the Research Resources section of this book under the heading of Abuse.

O) **Are you pursuing the operation out of rebellion?**

Underlying matters of bitter family relations are sometimes the motive to undergo cosmetic surgery. This is more common in younger patients. Teenagers or young adults may be trying to change their appearance so as not to look like a certain member of the family whom they do not care for at this time of their life.

This matter of family characteristics may also be a factor in a parent guiding or urging a child to undergo cosmetic surgery because the child's appearance reflects that of a relative the parent does not like. The parent also may be seeking ways to create what they think are perfect-looking children. In either of these situations, it is the parent who has the problem and not the child. If it has come to the point where the parent has brought the child in for cosmetic surgery, it has already developed into an unhealthy situation. The parent should come to terms with reality and should seek professional help in doing so.

P) How do you express yourself?

It is human to experience a wide range of feelings. It is generally healthy to express feelings in a suitable way because, when pent up, they can result in inappropriate responses and irrational actions. Being around people who do not let you express yourself can make you feel trapped. Under these circumstances you may choose unhealthy forms of expression to escape from your life situation.

Q) How is your self-esteem?

If you have low self-esteem, you may always feel inadequate. Your feelings may be the product of some form of abuse or neglect. You may feel the need to alter something in your life to try and make yourself feel better or to try and get people to notice you or treat you nicer. When you come to the conclusion that you need to change something about yourself, the choice you make can be out of desperation. Your actions may be made too quickly and probably will be inconsistent with what your real needs are.

Many of the problems people experience through life stem from self-esteem problems that were constructed as they were growing up. If a child is subject to mistreatment in the home with people they are supposed to trust or among their peers, any type of abuse can lay the framework for a weak self-image.

A person who suffers from low self-esteem can be caught up in people-pleasing actions and may seek out approval from the people around them. Sometimes people with low self-esteem become "rescuers" by spending more time and energy on helping other people than they realistically should. They may not feel valued by the people at home or at work who may not be treating them right or giving them the attention that they want. As they seek out reassurance from others, they can be especially vulnerable to suggestions and easy to take advantage of. They may think that they will be valued and accepted if they act a certain way, if they talk a certain way, if they look a certain way or if they do certain things for other people. They can get caught up in constantly redesigning things in their mind. Oftentimes they end up redesigning themselves irrationally. In their situation everything can turn into a facade. They can be quite good at putting on a false or superficial appearance that may look good from the outside but is only a cover-up of deeper problems.

When a person in this situation chooses cosmetic surgery as the answer, it can magnify their problems. Even if the surgery is successful, the patient will not be cured of the deeper problem. The feeling that the person needs to change something about themselves does not go away. The person may then try and figure out what can be changed next. They may be unable to pinpoint the real problem and may seek additional cosmetic surgery. This can turn into what some people call "plastic surgery addiction," where the person disregards or does not consider what the real problem may be and by making the choice to undergo additional cosmetic surgery procedures displays their inability to realize, or inability to accept, what their real problem may be.

People with healthy self-esteem do not spend their time concerning themselves with what everyone will think of them or with what they think of other people. They also do not rely on the approval of others to guide their choices in life. Having healthy self-esteem is feeling at peace with yourself. Acting out of low self-esteem is taking drastic and irrational measures to change your life. Two extreme acts that are sometimes driven by low self-esteem are murder and suicide.

R) Have you recently undergone a change in personality?
This may be a display of life transition or a sign of an underlying psychological or physical problem.

S) How will the operation affect you emotionally?

Are you on some sort of medication that can distort your judgment or are there other factors that could be impairing your reasoning?

If you are in psychological counseling, have you discussed your plans to have this surgery with your therapist?

Have you been thinking of going into therapy? Has anyone suggested that you do go into therapy?

Maybe starting therapy will help you make a smarter decision as to whether to have the surgery. It may help to clarify your expectations and how a change in your appearance will impact you emotionally.

T) Are you currently going through a depression or seeking an escape from life problems?

Beware of depression, which can bring about insecurity problems and distort personal concerns by making them appear to be much larger problems than they actually are and as though they are never going to end. Depression strongly affects thinking, feelings and behavior and is considered to be an illness that can be deadly — resulting in suicide (about 30,000 Americans commit suicide every year).

There is a continuous flow of studies being released and debated that show what may lead to depression.

Depression may be caused by decreased amounts of neurotransmitters in the brain or the result of an enzyme defect or other biochemical abnormality, a genetic predisposition or some other factor or combination of factors. Bad nutrition, food allergies, inactivity and lack of exercise could also play a major role in a person's depression.

Low self-esteem is just one sign that the person may be in a depression. Others include an inability to concentrate or think clearly; a loss of energy and drive; a loss of interest in themselves and others; anxiety; irritability; indulging in activities with a high risk of damaging consequences; feelings of worthlessness, inadequacy, shame and guilt; feelings of loneliness; undue pessimism; a change in sleep patterns — especially an inability to stay asleep; overeating or undereating; excessive sleeping; obsessive thought patterns; inappropriate responses to daily experiences; a change in desires and hopes for the future; and suicidal thoughts.

Depression exists in every part of the world in both men and women of all racial, ethnic, educational, income and age groups.

Being pleased with your appearance can be a boost to your emotions but if you think that looking good is paramount to a happy life, you should take a look at the lives of some of the people who are known for their good looks. Hollywood and the modeling industry are full of unhappy life stories among those whom some people consider to be the best looking people alive.

Cosmetic surgery can probably do little if anything to rescue a person from depression or from the grief caused by a divorce, the death of a loved one, or some other personal tragedy or disappointment. This is a time to seek relief through other avenues and not the avenue that leads to the cosmetic surgeon's office.

U) Are you an overly confident person?

This is where the person has already decided, before entering the cosmetic surgeon's office, and before doing any real research and considering the risks involved, that they know everything necessary and will undergo the surgery. They may bristle with enthusiasm and an unrealistic abundance of self-esteem. Altogether, they may refuse to accept that their calculations are incorrect and be unwilling to accept that the decision to undergo cosmetic surgery may not be in their best interest. The latter can drive them to seek out a doctor who will agree with their views.

This enthusiasm may be a form of anxiety and anxiousness brought on by a person who has overestimated the benefits of the cosmetic surgery. It also may be related to hypochondriosis or to bipolar disorder (manic depression) where the person has grandiose visions and is experiencing overly self-assured feelings that they can do anything. These feelings of confidence exist until the person flips back into a depression. Plastic surgery is not a treatment for these states of mind.

No one should be in a hurry to get onto a cosmetic surgeon's table. Cautious steps should be followed to ensure that the patient understands the risks and is making a decision that they will be happy with for the rest of their life. This includes the possibility of deciding against the operation.

V) Are there any other awkward situations or life difficulties that are driving you to make irrational or desperate decisions or impairing your judgment?

If you are desperate to undergo cosmetic surgery, you may be overlooking many things that may be important later. You may have unrealistic visions of how good you are going to look after recovering from the surgery. You may not have paid enough attention to the risks of the operation. You may be placing too much trust in the doctor and have, in your excitement, not done enough of your own research to realistically know what can and cannot be done. You may not have asked for a second and third opinion by two other unrelated doctors, and may not have done enough background checking into the qualifications of the doctor, his operating room staff and the qualities of the operating room.

W) What if cosmetic surgery was not an option?

If cosmetic surgery was not available to you, or had not been invented, what would you do to create the satisfaction that you currently believe cosmetic surgery will bring?

A Better You

Cosmetic surgery that is successful can make some people more happy with their appearance. It can also do the opposite, as operations that are capable of improving appearance can also disfigure. There are limits to beauty and youth. There is only so much you can do to improve the outside. If the person on the inside is unstable, cosmetic surgery probably will not be of much help.

Many patients enter a cosmetic surgeon's office with unrealistic results, wanting to appear similar to a famous model or movie star. If you take a look at the movie stars, you will find that the big stars are not all that perfect looking. Many are defined by recognizable features and sometimes physical imperfections such as gaps between the front teeth, classic noses, scars, moles and other unique markings and shapes. Some movie stars are hard to recognize outside of the controlled environment of a movie set when you see them face-to-face without the makeup spackled on their faces and rugs on their heads and through the Vaseline and burlap coated movie camera lenses. Hollywood lighting, lenses, makeup, prosthetics, custom wigs and clothing can make a big change in anybody's appearance.

> *Sometimes you'll be interviewing actresses, and you can't remember their names . . . is it Julie? Sandy? Because it's the same nose, the same hair. If you just want to be like each other, then why be an actor and play different people? Your physicality, that's what we work with — our voice, gestures and language. I'd rather have a big nose and sit down with somebody I don't know and have them [think], She has a strong nose, than have had plastic surgery and have them think, Gee, that person hates how they looked so much they changed themselves. I can handle people thinking I was unattractive, but not that I was phony. For me, I see [plastic surgery] as an admission of self-hatred and a kind of phoniness.*
>
> — actress Jodie Foster, speaking to Margy Rochin, *US Entertainment Magazine*, June 1994

The way some people talk about movie stars and the amount of cosmetic surgery they undergo, you could get the idea that there are cosmetic surgeons constructing movie stars from scratch. The number of actors who have had cosmetic surgery and the amount that they have had has been highly exaggerated. Very subtle nip-and-tuck operations are the most common. Plastic surgery can rob actors of the quirks and imperfections that define their character and, if the surgery changes the structure or movement of their face, it can interfere with the language of facial emotion that they depend on. If the surgery turns out wrong, it can attract the wrong kind of attention and interfere with their career. Cosmetic surgery does not improve an actors' talent and any one of them who is betting on cosmetic surgery to dramatically improve their career is betting on a false hope.

> *If we don't represent people — particularly women — over the age of 40, well, no wonder we have a whole generation who are frightened of getting older . . . In England, as an actress, it's such a blessing, you never have to think about how you look. You're cast to play a character — in that sense I'm a character actress — and that is so much more interesting. Here, women go off the map at age 28. You're not supposed to look your age. I want to look my age! Where is our love of growing wise?*
>
> — actress Emma Thompson, as quoted in *The Los Angeles Times*, October 31, 1993

One music star, though he has expressed the desire to work in movies, probably will never be given the opportunity to successfully develop that part of his career because multiple plastic surgeries have given him an appearance that is simply too bizarre and would prevent people from concentrating on a movie's storyline.

To avoid dramatic changes that can be obvious, many of the Hollywood people who do undergo cosmetic surgery often elect to undergo a slight change such as an eye-lift and a few years later undergo a chin tuck or some micro-graft hair transplants. These type of subtle changes done over a long period of time gently maintain their appearance and avoid the attention of the gossip tabloids that some stars have experienced after they have undergone a dramatic surgical change.

What men think about their looks and cosmetic surgery

- I am what I am — altering my appearance does not change the fact.
- Why bother if you are married to someone who loves you anyway?
- I hate the idea of unnatural modifications to one's body — male or female. I don't aspire to change my physical appearance to match some ideal.
- Who cares what you look like — it's who you are.
- I like the way I look and I don't plan on entering any beauty contests in the future.
- I'm relatively cute as is, and besides, I wouldn't want to change who I am.
- I am what I am.
- Looks are just not that important.
- I'll play with the hand I was dealt — I worry enough about keeping thin and in shape.
- I am concerned about the side effects of cosmetic surgery.
- It is unnatural and a total waste of money.
- I am happy taking care of myself and letting nature do the rest.
- I suppose I have just as much vanity as the next person, but not enough to get surgery.
- Cosmetic surgery is a waste of money. I'm married.
- It is just plain stupid. I am not interested in fashion.
- I care about my looks and will "work out" to improve them, but since at the same level I feel it is superficial to be overly concerned with my looks, I don't think I could respect myself if I went through with a physical appearance enhancement.

- I believe strongly that we should be happy with ourselves in our "natural" state. Physical fitness and caring for our bodies is great, but altering it is a sign of poor self image. We should love ourselves as we are.
- I am a good looking person and see no reason to change my looks. However, having been a recipient of frequent "special treatment" solely on the basis of looks, if I were an unattractive person (as society defines it) I would definitely consider rearranging my physical appearance. Looks are an important tool, and "looks are skin deep" may be true to a few people, but not the majority.

Study was based on 58 responses received to confidential questionnaires mailed to 215 Stanford Business School Masters of Business Administration students. The study was small, exploratory, and qualitative in nature. Therefore, no sweeping generalizations to the population at large can be drawn.

— From research study titled: *Men's Magazines: the Facts and the Fantasies*, by Dr. Debbie Then, Social Psychologist and Research Scholar, August, 1994

If you place so much importance on the way you look to the point you judge your happiness by your appearance and the approval of others, then it is the way you think that can use some attention.

Comparing yourself with other people is unfair to you because other people have different things such as talents, physical capabilities and interests to work with that you may not posess or have not spent time to develop. Competing with someone who you think is adorable and trying to become more like them can put you in a race that can never be won and that may give you feelings of inferiority and frustration.

Self-improvement is an inside job. All anyone can really ever do is take what they have and do their best with it — and allow others to do the same with themselves. Maybe what you consider to be your faults are actually best for you by positioning you in a course where you can experience the most out of your life. To improve your life, realize what capabilities you have and challenge yourself to improve on these. By doing this, the only person you will be competing with is yourself. By recognizing your own talents, passions and potential strengths and focusing in on these you can make you become a better you.

5 • DECIDING ON SURGERY

Finding a Doctor

If you owned the most expensive diamond in the world you would not let just any jeweler cut it. You would probably look at their background and training and view some of their past work. Likewise a person looking for a cosmetic surgeon should check out more than one surgeon before deciding who will make the cut.

When looking at a doctor's training, think of an athlete. Some athletes train very hard every day and are not so great. Another athlete can train the same amount of time and be world class. Just because a doctor went through the steps to become a doctor does not mean he practices his profession well.

It is all too common for a medical consumer to choose a physician on the basis of his personality and not on the basis of his training, professional history or curative skill. People seeking medical care should concentrate on finding a doctor who is well trained, familiar with the latest information in the field and able to recognize when a patient needs the attention of another doctor. Consumers should also select a doctor who listens to his patient's health concerns.

Basing the choice of a doctor on the appearance of his advertisement is also an inadequate way to select a doctor. Great-looking ads are created by advertising agencies, photographers, graphic artists or some combination of the three. Ads have nothing to do with the capabilities of the doctor other than that they may show the doctor's skill in selecting a good commercial artist.

Signs You've Chosen a Bad Plastic Surgeon
- Your nose is attached with Velcro
- In the operating room, you notice a lot of cans of Play-Doh
- Your new cheek implants feel suspiciously like ketchup packets
- Paper bags with eye holes for sale in the reception area

- His waiting room is crawling with Jacksons
- After several minutes in the sun, your forehead melts
- At first visit, he nervously asks, "You didn't see '60 Minutes' last Sunday, did you?"
- The last thing you hear as you go under anesthesia is, "Sweet dreams, Mr. Face-on-your-ass!"
- You're a guy, you go in for a nose job and you come out a 36 triple D

— from the *Late Show with Dave Letterman*, used with permission from WORLDWIDE PANTS, © 1994 Worldwide Pants Incorporated, All Rights Reserved

Because anyone with a medical license can practice in any area of medicine, including brain surgery, they can advertise themselves in the phone book under any specialty they choose. Many doctors who advertise themselves in the phone book under a specific specialty are not board certified by the American Board of Medical Specialties, are certified in another specialty other than the one they list, or have not received any specialized training in the area of medicine they have chosen to practice. The phone book companies do not have the interest, time or resources to check the accuracy of the information in each advertisement. That is the consumer's job.

In recent years there have been television commercials that advertise 800 phone numbers that people can dial to get a list of specific doctors who practice near to where the consumer lives. These phone numbers are paid for by doctors who join in on marketing costs and pay for this consumer service. This can be one way to initially find a certain type of doctor. However, it should not be used as the only step to find a doctor. Do not wholeheartedly trust that the information the 800 number supplies on a doctor is 100% accurate. Additional background research on the doctor should be done to make sure the doctor is licensed and is someone who has surgical skills that you can trust and depend on.

Consumer access to doctors' professional histories is limited. It took an act of Congress by way of the Healthcare Quality Improvement Act of 1986 and the Medicare and Medicaid Patient and Program Protection Act of 1987 to create the National Practitioner Data Bank (NPDB), which is overseen by the United States Department of Health and Human Services. This data bank contains information about several thousand doctors who have patterns of malpractice. Thanks to the powerful medical lobbies' influence over lawmakers, this data bank, which because of budget cuts was not activated until September 1990, is not accessible to the public, even though it is funded with tax dollars. Releasing information from the data bank is also punishable by a fine.

> *I think it is an effective tool to provide information. Fundamentally, the National Practitioner Data Bank is a tool for collecting data. But a hospital that has to credential and privilege physicians is required to query that data bank when there is an application for referrals and every 2 years at least thereafter.*
>
> *It makes information available, but it fundamentally is not the entity that has the responsibility for excluding an individual from transferring across State lines. For example, it is not a licensing board.*
> — Susan D. Kladiva, Assistant Director, Health Finance Issues, US General Accounting Office, during Congressional subcommittee hearing on issues relating to medical malpractice, May 20, 1993

State licensing boards, hospitals, medical societies, health maintenance organizations and some other professional groups have access to the NPDB. It lists medical malpractice claims paid by insurance companies, professional limitations placed on doctors, actions taken by hospitals and other institutions to deny or revoke clinical privileges of doctors, and disciplinary actions taken by state licensing boards against doctors. The AMA, which works to protect doctors and uphold their standing in society, would like to see the data bank canceled. The consumers' rights organization Public Citizen's Health Research Group would like to change the access rules to the data bank so that the public is given access to it. (For information contact PCHRG at the phone number given in the Research Resources section of this book under the heading of Patients' and Consumers' Rights.)

> *The financial investment industry has a database for itself that is similar to the NPDB. The Central Registration Depository database contains enforcement records against the nation's 460,000 registered brokers and traders, as well as 5,500 securities firms. The records give details on securities law violations, arbitration settlements, fines and lawsuits. It is run by the National Association of Securities Dealers, which is the securities industry's main self-regulatory body. The records have been gathered through the nation's*

commodities and stock exchanges and state regulators. The CRD has been partially accessible to consumers.

In September 1994, the National Association of State Securities Administrators proposed that the CRD be made freely accessible to investors through home computers. Such an action would give investors the ability to research the professional background of investment brokers and firms before making investments with them.

Should not medical consumers be allowed the same privilege with the records now held in the NPDB so that consumers can make sure they are not dealing with some medical professional who has a history of violating patients?

Consumers should demand that they be given access to the NPDB.

— the author

Some of the actions a person can take to find a doctor:
(These are numbered only as a form of reference and not as a grade of importance.)

1. Look in the *Marquis Directory of Medical Specialists.* This reference book is available in many libraries and it lists, by specialty, in alphabetical and geographic order, every surgeon certified by one of the 23 medical examining boards officially sanctioned by the American Board of Medical Specialties. Also, check the *Compendium of Certified Medical Specialists.*

2. Check the *American Medical Association Directory*, which is published by the AMA and is available in many libraries.

3. Write to the AMA to find whether a particular doctor you are interested in checking out is listed in the Physician Master File: AMA, 515 North State Street, Chicago, Illinois 60610.

4. Call your insurance company and find out what doctors are accepted by your plan.

5 . Ask friends or relatives what doctors they go to. Then take measures to check up on the doctors' educations and professional histories.

6. Call the closest university hospital and ask for referrals to doctors who are associated with that hospital. Find out the doctor's name who is head of the surgical department you are seeking treatment in. If he does not have time to perform your surgery, he will likely be able to refer you to another doctor who is familiar with the latest medical procedures.

7. Find a top-rated hospital and ask which doctors are connected with that hospital. Ask for the name of a doctor who is chief of his department in the area of medicine for which you are seeking attention. If that doctor cannot treat you, ask him for two or three names of doctors he thinks are good.

8. Ask for the head nurse at a top-rated hospital and ask them for a referral to a doctor.

Nurses are often aware of the qualifications and curative skills of particular doctors. Nurses are also in the operating rooms while the doctors are performing the operations. They know the doctors who make mistakes and are not so good as well as those doctors who perform successful and responsible operations.

9. Call the doctor's office to ask whether the receptionist will mail you the doctor's resume, or curriculum vitae, which should list where the doctor received his education, where he served his residency, what he considers to be his specialty, the boards he is certified with and where he has practiced.

10. Call the state medical licensing department or medical board to find out whether the doctor is licensed by the state (the phone numbers to every state medical board can be found in the Research Resources section of this book under the heading of State Medical Boards).

A. Find out the doctor's birth date (for searching records).

B. Ask for the address of the doctor to see if he has more than one business address.

C. Ask for the doctor's state license number and ask when it was issued.

D. Find out the status of the license — if it is in good standing, if there are any limits or restraints that the state has placed on the doctor, if the doctor has been put on probation, or if the doctor's license has been suspended or revoked.

E. Ask if there is any information about felony convictions.

F. Ask if there is any information about any disciplinary actions taken against the doctor by another state. Call that state medical board and find out the information it has on the doctor.

G. Ask if the state has any information it can release about lawsuits that have been filed against the doctor. Ask if you can find out if the board has formally taken action against the doctor for misconduct, and if so, find out what the charges were.

If the state has not taken any formal action against a doctor this does not mean that he has never botched any surgeries or violated any patients. It may mean that the victim of the bad medical care did not know how to go about taking action against the doctor or was unsuccessful in getting action taken, or it may mean that the victim was left incapacitated or dead.

In California the state medical board decided in May 1993 to give the public access to information about physicians who have lost malpractice cases in jury trials or who have had disciplinary action taken against them by the board for unprofessional behavior, incompetence or for other reasons. Information is not given about malpractice cases where out-of-court settlements were made, where the award was less than $30,000 or where the malpractice case was heard before an arbitration panel. The available records start at January 1, 1993. The board relies on court clerks in each county to report malpractice judgments over $30,000. State law requires this reporting to be done within 10 days of the judgments. Records show that this is not always done.

11. Many doctors have been sued. This does not mean that the doctor is a bad doctor. You have to look at the situation and decide for yourself. Some areas of medicine attract more malpractice suits than others. If there are a number of lawsuits or criminal charges against a doctor, this is probably not a doctor you should trust with your health.

Pending lawsuits and legal judgments against a doctor are public record. These records and all sorts of other legal action documents, which are available at the district attorney's office at the county courthouse, include information on lawsuits that are currently pending and lawsuits that have gone to verdict in the county and the details of the verdicts.

Using the doctor's birthdate from the state board, search the criminal case index at the county courthouse of the city or county where the doctor practices to see if you can find any criminal information about the doctor. Search the index of civil cases for lawsuits against the doctor. You can also search for the lawsuit by using the type of lawsuit or the type of surgery. Other information might be found in the court's minutes book.

If the doctor was sued along with a hospital, medical center, group practice or other institution, the lawsuit might be filed under the name of the institution and not under the doctor's name. (You might also want to check and see if the doctor is suing someone else and especially if he is suing one of his former patients.)

Some files may have been sealed by court order.

Some lawsuits may have been settled out of court as a way to avoid a lengthy and expensive court case and so that the doctor would not have any record of a court case against him or any recorded admittance of negligence.

If the doctor was sued in an arbitration process, there is no public record, even if the patient won. The arbitration proceedings take place in private, are less formal than the courtroom process and are heard in front of three panelists who are usually retired judges or attorneys as opposed to a jury trial that is heard in court in front of a jury of from 6 to 12 people selected from the local population.

If the actions taken against a doctor were enough to attract attention from the media (a doctor's career nightmare), you may be able to find copies of these newspaper or magazine articles in your local library's periodicals file.

12. Call the state board of medical examiners and have them send you a copy of the file on the doctor.

13. Call the county medical board and society and ask for a list of board-certified doctors who practice in the area of medicine in which you are seeking treatment.

14. Call the professional boards the doctor claims that he is certified with to see if he is in fact certified by them. Ask if he is in good standing (this might only mean that he has paid his dues) and ask what the requirements are for a doctor to be a member of the organization.

If you call 1-800-776-2378, the American Board of Medical Specialties will tell you if a particular doctor is board-certified through them.

15. Contact the Public Citizen's Health Research Group and order their compilation of questionable doctors for the state you live in. The address and phone number of Public Citizen is in the Research Resources Section of this book under the heading of Patients' and Consumers' Rights.

Visiting with the Doctor

The local auto mechanic at the corner garage may have to have more training in his field to get a State license than some of these cosmetic surgeons need to start rearranging a person's appearance.

The public needs to start asking some tough questions about qualifications. The public also needs better information about the types of surgery that are appropriate for their medical needs and who is qualified to perform that surgery.
— Congressman Norman Sisisky during Congressional subcommittee hearings on plastic surgery industry, 1989

When communicating with the doctor:
- Do not take advantage of the doctor's time
- Respect his office hours
- If you are going to call him, make some notes beforehand about what you want to ask
- Be honest and address your concerns
- Know that if you communicate well with the doctor you are more likely to receive the care that is best for you

The consultation with professionals about performing some operation on your one and only body is not a time to be concerned about making new friends and being entertaining, nor is it a time to be unquestioning and docile. This is a time for you to be assertive and do whatever it takes to find out all of your options and have those options explained, get the best information available, seek the best level of communication with the people you speak with, and, if you elect to undergo surgery, seek the best medical care you can get.

Doctors are not mind readers. Do not assume that the doctor knows what you do and do not want. What you tell the doctor will influence his actions. Make sure there are no mixed signals. The more research you do and the more questions you ask and get answers to, the lower your chances are of making the wrong decision and of being surprised by the results if surgery does take place. Any good doctor would not feel attacked by a patient who has made the effort to inform themselves by doing their own research. If anything, it will increase the chances that, if surgery does take place, the doctor will perform a successful operation.

Be wary of a doctor who becomes defensive. A doctor who does not cooperate with you and is unresponsive to your need for information may be hiding something in his history or may be afraid you will find something out that will turn you off to the operation. Remember that the doctor does not make money unless he treats you for something. No sense in divulging the negative things about the surgery, such as the risks, when there is money to be made. If the doctor is offended by your need for information, find another doctor.

You should not settle for a doctor who tries to make surgery look secretive and magical as if only those with a medical education are capable of understanding the procedures. A doctor with this type of attitude may tell you that it is not in your best interest to know the details — that it might upset you or interfere with your rest and healing. If you are going to give your informed consent, he should do his part and inform you. The doctor should be willing to explain the procedures in words you will understand. No surgery is so complicated that it cannot be explained to you. If it would help you understand, have the doctor use medical models, drawings, and photographs to explain the procedure.

Some doctors dance around certain questions and give answers that may be what you want to hear, but may be misleading or are not exactly true. Do not settle for answers that are meant to simply calm you down and pacify your fears. Any doctor who talks to you as if you should not be so concerned about making sure the surgery goes well may not be the doctor you need.

For the money you are paying the doctor, you should get the answers you need and get them in a respectable manner. Do not be afraid to walk out on a doctor if you do not get the service you feel you are paying for. Do not be concerned if the doctor seems disappointed that you chose another doctor. His disappointment may stem from the fact that he, as a person who only makes money when he operates, lost out on a sale (on the other hand, if he is giving you strong warning to stay away from a certain doctor because of that doctor's lack of ethics and skill, you may want to seriously consider his viewpoint).

One should seriously consider backing away from any marketing campaigns put out by cosmetic surgeons promising to transform you into physical perfection. Also avoid newly developed "medical breakthrough" operations as you may find yourself more of a guinea pig than anything else. The doctor to avoid and even walk out on is the one who tries to talk you into additional or unwanted procedures. A doctor with a hard sell tactic is also aiming for that hard cash. If the patient is insecure in the first place, they may end up going for the whole game and be stuck thousands of dollars poorer, leaving the doctor that much richer.

Although some operations can have a very good outcome if they are done correctly and for the right reasons, and many patients have been very pleased with the results of their cosmetic surgeries, any person going in for cosmetic surgery who is counting on a miracle is leaving a gaping hole open for disappointment.

All that matters is that whatever is done is in your best interest and that, if surgery does take place, you are satisfied with the results.

The Consultation

The initial meeting with a doctor is the consultation. This is where the patient talks with the doctor and asks questions while the doctor talks with and asks questions of the patient, considers the patient's health history, examines the area of concern and evaluates the situation.

Plastic surgeons are used to a wide variety of patients, from those who have blown their appearance out of proportion to those who show up with facial injuries inflicted by an abusive spouse and from those who think they know everything to those who think plastic surgeons can do just about anything.

Rather than wear an attitude of distrust when you visit the doctor, it would probably be more productive and beneficial to both you and the doctor if you approached the consultation with the frame of mind that he can provide information that may be beneficial in your making a decision that is in your best interest if you provide the right information and ask the right questions.

Before going to the consultation:
- Find out if there is a charge for the consultation and how much it is.
- Find out what you should bring — paperwork you have from other doctors, a list of medications you are taking, insurance forms, or anything else the doctor may find helpful. (Do not leave your personal medical files that you have brought with you with the doctor or his staff. If they need to keep copies, let them make copies of what they need.)
- Find out how long you should expect to be there (if you know you are going to need more time, let the doctor's office know ahead of time so they can adjust their schedule).
- Write down your symptoms so you do not forget to tell the doctor anything that may be important.

If you expect the doctor to treat you in a professional manner then you should give him the same respect. Be on time or be in contact. If you make an appointment with a doctor and you are going to be late, call his office as soon as you can and let them know you are running late so they can use their time wisely. If you have to cancel the appointment, let the doctor's office know as soon as you can. Do not just not show up.

You should not feel any pressure to undergo cosmetic surgery. It is not the kind of decision that should be made under pressure. It should be your own decision after you have been sufficiently informed rather than a decision you felt you had to make after going through a process of manipulation. Patients who were talked into more cosmetic surgery procedures than they planned on having done are some of the most dissatisfied patients.

Whatever the motivations are for a doctor to be pressuring you into undergoing surgery, those reasons may not line up with your best interests. The doctor may think that he can do a great job on you but his idea of a great job and your idea of how you would want to look may not be in sync.

The doctor is the one you should be communicating with, and all of your concerns and expectations should be very clear with the doctor. Many of the patients who have had a bad experience with surgery later found that they were misinformed, misguided or lied to by the doctor or the doctor's staff. Ignore promises made by the doctor's staff. The staff may be receiving a bonus for bringing in business. The staff might not have any medical training and special training is required for a person to work in the front office of a medical center or doctor's office. At best, the office manager may have attended seminars given by the Medical Group Management Association, but these seminars teach how to manage a medical office, not how to diagnose patients. Any office staffperson who tries to diagnose the doctor's patients is out of place.

You may come across a doctor who wants total control, is not interested enough in what you have to say, thinks he knows the ideal image and gives everyone the same alteration regardless of the patients' heritage, bone structure and personal taste. The features you are looking to change should not end up looking like they do not fit with the rest of your character. If the rest of your features are large, making one of them small can make everything else look larger or off balance.

Your reason for consulting with a cosmetic surgeon may be that you want him to advise you on what you want done. And you may be hoping to find one that has a good idea of what surgical change, if any, will and will not be right for you. But, if a doctor takes control and immediately starts taking snapshots of you and examining you here and there without asking you what your concerns and ideas are, the doctor may have his own ideas of what should be done to you or is in a hurry to get from patient to patient so he can attain his financial goals. This doctor may end up doing things to you other than what you had in mind and may try to talk you into other procedures or a more involved operation than you originally wanted simply so that he can make more money. Suggestions from a doctor that you also have a second procedure done during an operation "while we are in there" can sometimes be translated into, "Hey, I don't have enough experience doing this particular procedure, so why don't you let me try it out on you?" If you realize you are in the presence of this type of doctor, the best thing that can do for yourself is to leave.

When you are consulting with the cosmetic surgeon, you should be in a comfortable position and he should not have you lying on your back on some uncomfortable exam chair or table. An uncomfortable position may make you feel vulnerable.

During the consultation or at any time when they are examining you and you do not understand what it is they are doing, ask them. Not to be rude, but to be sure that nothing is done to you that you do not want done and that you do not want to be billed for. If they seem to be busy or are not interested in answering you, stop them from doing what they are doing; if you have to, tell them to take their hands off of you and remind them that you are paying them and that you want an explanation of what is being done. Their explanation may tell you that they were doing something or planning to do something to you that is not in your best interest.

Some doctors, especially cosmetic surgeons, have autographed "grip 'n grin" (shake hands and smile for the camera) photographs of celebrities hanging on their office walls. This does not mean that the doctor has operated on the celebrity. The doctor may be implying that he operated on the celebrity so that you are brought to believe that if the celebrity has trusted his or her body or face to the surgeon, the surgeon must be good. However, anyone with the right connections can get autographed photos of celebrities. If the photo is of the doctor standing with the celebrity, it may have been taken at some social event and the doctor paid the photographer for a copy of the photograph or the doctor received the photo in appreciation for a donation he made to a charity in which the celebrity is involved. Do not base your decision to employ the doctor on the impressiveness of his connections. Even some celebrities have had sloppy cosmetic surgery performed on them.

Photographs

Most cosmetic surgeons will show you before and after photographs of people who they have operated on. Avoid any doctor who refuses to show you his portfolio of work. Still, when he does show you photos of surgeries he has performed, you can bet that these are photos of his best surgical results and that photos of surgeries that did not turn out right will not be shown.

Keep in mind that the people in the photos may not have the same skin, bone structure, level of healing or other genetic makeup that you possess, and those elements all play a part in the outcome of the surgery.

What may appear to be a good surgery result under photographic lighting and with makeup may appear undesirable to you and have an unnatural operated look under other lighting conditions.

The cosmetic surgeon's office should have a set of 3-angle mirrors, and he should not have to rely on hand-held mirrors and cheap instant snapshots to discuss with you what you want done. You need to look in the mirror and show the doctor exactly what you want done. Instant photographs can distort a person's image because the film often has a green, yellow or blue tint. Even the best-looking people occasionally take bad photographs. You should also not rely on what you think of in your mind to tell the doctor what you want. Mind and memory have a tendency to distort an image. The way you appear in your mind and what you actually look like are usually two different images.

If you do not want the doctor showing your photos to other people or using your name when talking to other patients or professionals, make sure he knows this.

Computer Imaging

Some cosmetic surgeons use computers to show their potential patients a computer-generated image of what may be the final outcome of the surgery. One advertisement referred to this procedure as using a "state-of-the-art imaging computer to preview your improvement." This is done by taking a photo of you with a camera that is connected to a computer. Then the surgeon manipulates the image of your face on the screen to make your face appear the way you would want it to appear after the surgery has healed.

Computer imaging can be helpful but may also mislead people into undergoing cosmetic surgery, and it should be remembered that it is only an image and can give only an idea of the anticipated results. There is no way a computer image is going to tell you much of anything other than how you may appear if things happen in an exact way. You should not believe that the image on the screen is going to be perfectly transferred onto your face.

Some doctors will do a computer image for free. Some charge hundreds of dollars for the use of this high-priced toy. It cannot hurt to have a computer image done. It may be helpful. However, the decision to undergo cosmetic surgery should not be based on a computer image. The computer image is simply one of the marketing tools used by the cosmetic surgeon.

Owning fancy equipment does not mean the doctor is a good doctor. It just means that he can afford fancy equipment.

Face Casting

A few cosmetic surgeons, for a fee, offer potential patients the opportunity to have an assistant to the doctor make a face mold using dental impression material and plaster. The impression can be altered with clay where implants are to be positioned, or by filing where tissue is to be cut away so both the patient and the doctor get to see what kind of change the patient has in mind.

To make a facial mold, the person's hair is tied back and covered firmly with a cloth. A light coat of Vaseline is spread over the face, ears and neck and into the eyelashes, brows and border of the hairline. The face is then coated thinly with dental impression material (that has consistency of a gel but dries quickly) while the person sits in a reclined position. The nostrils are kept open for the person to breathe. Salted plaster is coated over the impression material and left to dry for 20 to 30 minutes. The dry mold is gently removed from the face while the person leans forward, and salted plaster is then poured into the mold. This is left to dry for an hour or more and then the mold is broken away. The result is a perfect impression of the face.

The impression may be painted with water color in the person's skin tone and coated with polyurethane to protect it.

Having two impressions made may be helpful when the person is considering a nose job or any surgery that would change the structure of the face. The second impression may be useful if something goes wrong with the surgery.

Second Opinions

Just because a doctor agrees to operate on you does not always mean that you need an operation or that you will benefit from one.

While physicians usually agree on whether surgery is unwarranted, they do not always agree on whether surgery is the best course of action when there are effective alternative treatments available. In all cases, you, as a patient, are entitled to know the range of choices available to you, to have those choices objectively considered by more than one professional, and to have your own preferences considered before undergoing an elective surgical procedure.

You should feel free to ask . . . questions. Once you have the answers, you will be better prepared to make a decision. Do not be hesitant to seek a second opinion. It is an acceptable medical practice. Most doctors want their patients to be as informed as possible about their condition.

You should consider getting a second opinion whenever the surgery is not required for an emergency condition, and it is up to you to decide when and if you will have it.

A second opinion generally is not appropriate when the surgery is required on an emergency basis and to delay it could be life-threatening. For example, cases of acute appendicitis or injuries from an accident are considered emergencies.
— from the US Department of Health and Human Services Healthcare Financing Administration pamphlet *Medicare: Coverage For Second Surgical Opinions*

A good doctor will not be insulted if you go to another doctor and ask for a second opinion. Getting a second opinion protects both you and the doctor. Some doctors will give you a list of doctors practicing the same specialty. Beware that he may send you to his friend who he has set up to give pre-set advice. It is better to pick the doctor yourself or ask your family physician or insurance plan to refer you to a doctor for a second opinion.

There are at least three sides to every story. Many people recommend that you not only get a second opinion, but also get a third and even a fourth opinion — especially if the first two doctors have disagreed with each other and if you are dealing with a major medical decision. A second opinion can help you feel confident about your final decision.

Many insurance plans will cover second surgical opinions as long as it is for the treatment of a condition covered by the insurance. Your insurance carrier may also require you to get a second surgical opinion. Contact your health insurance representative for details.

Some people do not feel comfortable letting the doctor know that they want a second opinion. However, by informing your doctor that you want to get a second opinion,

*you can then also **ask that your medical records be sent to the
physician providing the second opinion. In this way, you
may be able to avoid the time, costs and discomfort of having
to repeat medical tests.*** [emphasis added]

*When getting a second opinion, you should tell the second
doctor the name of the surgical procedure recommended and
the types of medical tests you have already had. Even if the
second doctor disagrees with the first, you will have
information that will help you make a decision. If you are
confused by different opinions, you may wish to go back to the
first doctor to further discuss your case. Or, you may wish to
talk to a third physician.*

*Second opinions are your right as a patient, and can help
you make a better informed decision about non-emergency
surgery.*
— from the US Department of Health and Human Services
Healthcare Financing Administration pamphlet *Medicare:
Coverage For Second Surgical Opinions*

If it is more timely and convenient, and less costly to transport
your medical records or copies of them from doctor to doctor
yourself, request to do so.

Bring a copy of your medical records from the first doctor
with you when you go for a second opinion.

Talk with Former Patients

It may be helpful to talk with some of the doctor's former
patients who have gone through the same operation that you are
considering. This does not include the office staff, who may have
had surgery performed on them by the doctor. The doctor or one of
his staff may be able to connect you with a few former patients
who are willing to talk freely about their surgery. Meeting a
former patient can give you an idea of what you are in for and an
idea of the possible results. If the surgery was performed on a non-
private area, you can see the type of scar caused by the surgical
wound. (One cosmetic surgeon in Los Angeles was paying his
wife's friends whom he had never operated on to talk to his
potential patients who requested to talk to former patients.)

Before undergoing any cosmetic procedure you might want to
take a look at the photos of cosmetic surgery mistakes in the
medical books found in a university medical library. This can
show you what undesirable outcomes look like and leave you

wondering about the motives of the surgeons who performed the botched surgeries. One bad cosmetic surgery operation can send you on the game of what some people call "plastic surgery hopscotch." Its a game that takes over your life as you run from one surgeon to the next, trying to find one who can fix what was done to you. You may have the misfortune of finding a surgeon who is deceitful enough to take your money and operate on you, knowing that the outcome will not be what you desire and then later blame it on the original doctor — or on you.

Medical Tests

There are thousands of different tests, and new ones are always being developed and becoming available. Doctors and the facilities they own or work for make a lot of money by ordering and performing tests, x-rays, scans, other imaging procedures, and lab tests. Medical testing in the United States is a $430 billion side industry. The RAND Corporation of Santa Monica, a non-profit research group, believes that as many as one in three medical procedures is inappropriate. Many tests are overused. Some are done to prevent lawsuits against doctors or to pay for equipment purchased by the medical group a doctor is a member of.

Many testing facilities are doctor-owned. Even when a doctor refers a patient to a separate medical facility, the doctor may be receiving a commission from the other doctor or facility in a "fee-splitting arrangement" as the referring doctor. A 1991 study by the state of Florida reported that within that state, the number of tests per patient is almost twice as great in doctor-owned labs as in those not owned by doctors.

There are thousands of different medical tests, and new ones are always being developed and becoming available.

Before a test is done you should find out :
- What is the purpose of the test?
- What is the test meant to reveal?
- How accurate is the test?
- Are there other ways to find what the doctor is looking for?
- Will you be giving a specimen, such as body fluid or tissue, for the test?
- Does the test require your presence?

- What type of specimen is needed for the test (urine, blood, mucus or tissue)?
- Where is the lab work performed?

    If the test is performed outside of the doctor's office, do not call the lab to try and find out the test results. They cannot legally give you the results. The only person you should rely on to give you your test results is the doctor.

- If you need to be present for the test, what should you wear, how long does it take and what will you be doing during the test?
- Do you need to avoid a certain type of food or all food before the test is given or before a specimen is taken?
- Will you have to take any medications before the test?
- Are there any injections given before or during the test?
- Will these medications interfere with your ability to drive yourself home from the test?
- Are there any medications that you are currently taking that could interfere with the test results?
- What are the risks of the test?
- How much does the test cost?
- Does your insurance cover the cost of the test?
- Who owns the test equipment?
- Is the test equipment operated by someone who has had special training to operate it properly?

Medical tests are not always accurate even when they are positive. For example, a blood test, developed at the Dana Farber Cancer Institute in Boston, that shows elevated levels of a protein called CA-125 is used to detect ovarian cancer, but endometriosis and pregnancy are also associated with CA-125.

Avoid rushing to get some form of treatment that you know nothing about, that may not be necessary and that may do more harm than good. Unless it would be a health threat to delay treatment, when test results come in that the doctor believes show that you need some form of treatment, take some time to find out what your options are. When possible, especially if the diagnosis shows a serious health problem or the suggested treatment is very invasive, request more tests from a separate lab to lower the chance that the treatment the doctor is suggesting is not based on a false positive (though cosmetic surgery is not something that is done based on the results of a test). Take these test results with you when you have your second opinion.

Whenever you are undergoing a test, avoid talking to the person conducting the test about anything other than the testing procedure being performed. They may be occupied with watching monitors and circuit boards and listening for prompts from the medical machines. If you take their mind away from the procedure they may forget a step and you will end up with an inaccurate test result or the test may have to be repeated.

Whenever you get a test, you should get a copy of the results for your own records.

Medical Records

It has been the general practice in the medical industry to keep medical files on paper, and much of it in handwritten form. One of the problems with this is that some of the written material may be indecipherable because some doctors have unclear handwriting. Another problem is that this paperwork takes up a large part of doctors' and nurses' workday.

Computers are now being introduced into more and more hospitals to store clinical data and other patient records. This is expected to cut down on operating costs as it streamlines menial tasks, does away with illegible handwriting and prevents unnecessary and repetitive testing and medical procedures. It will also make it easier to store medical files in an off-site or out-of-state location in case of a disaster.

Nationally there is a data bank called the Medical Information Bureau (MIB) that is used by hundreds of insurance companies with the belief that it helps guard against fraud. The information is also used to decide whether you are high risk and therefore not financially desirable to insure. Lawyers also can gain access to this information to be used for or against you in a lawsuit. The data bank includes both medical and non-medical information about you that is gathered when you apply for individual life, health or disability insurance or file an insurance claim. The MIB may keep a coded report on each individual who has significant underwriting risks that could affect health or longevity. Depending on the information source and the translation of the records, your MIB file may contain inaccuracies, and this could interfere with your insurance eligibility.

Some information from your MIB report may be obtained free by writing the bureau. If the originating insurance company believes there is sensitive medical information in your file, the company may require the MIB to send your medical file only to your doctor. The MIB has a set process by which you can correct errors or dispute inconsistencies. (The MIB address is in the Research Resources section of this book under the heading of Records.)

> *In my work I have spoken to many, many victims who have brought malpractice cases as well as product liability cases and other lawsuits. I have never heard them complain about the amount of money their lawyer took from their award. I do, however, hear them complain ferociously about the person they are suing and the fact that they delay that case sometimes for years and years and years. Every time they want another document, they have to go back into court to litigate to get that document. It is pulling teeth to go through a lawsuit, generally, against these big corporations or large defense insurance firms.*
> — Pamela Gilbert of Public Citizen's Congress Watch, testifying before subcommittee hearing on issues relating to medical malpractice, May 20, 1993

Because physicians and hospitals do not necessarily keep records indefinitely (in Los Angeles some medical centers sell old medical records to companies that provide props to movie and television sets), and there is always the chance of records being lost during office moves and disasters, anyone wanting a copy of their medical records should seek to get their own copies as soon as possible.

Some doctors might require you to send a letter of request before they will supply you with copies of your files. Although most doctors will provide you with your records, some records can be legally kept from you. Obtaining your records may be difficult because each state has its own set of medical records disclosure laws. Some doctors may tell you that you do not need to keep records and this could be because the doctor is trying to protect himself. Some doctors might delay giving you copies of your records so they have time to alter any information that could be used in a malpractice lawsuit. If you request a copy of your records from a doctor you are disappointed with, the doctor may have his staff tell you they misplaced your file because he may think you are going to sue him.

Contact the file clerk or medical record librarian of each institution (hospital, ambulatory surgery center or doctor's office) where you have received treatment (for good reasons, separate laws govern those records kept for mental health purposes and may not be available to you).

Medical records can include
- Your medical history form
- Consultation forms
- Doctors' notes and order sheets
- Diagnostic images made by various image-producing machinery
- Videos of your tests or actual surgery — fiber optic cameras can film the inside of your body
- Lab results and pathology reports
- Hospital admission and discharge paperwork
- Nursing care records/nursing documentation and flow sheets/progress notes
- Operating room reports
- Prescription records
- Letters among doctors, lawyers and medical facilities

Even if you are successful in obtaining your records, you may not be able to read everything on them. Besides the common abbreviations, the doctor may have his own set of abbreviations that only he and his office staff understand. Some doctors use a variety of colored stickers on patient records. These might be used to protect your privacy. One colored sticker may mean that you are pregnant and you do not want anyone to know. Another colored sticker may mean that the file contains information regarding the sex of your unborn child that you do not want to know. Another colored sticker may signal that you have a contagious disease. Various other stickers, markings, and "office esoterics" may mean that you are a problem patient or that you have a tendency to talk too much. But do not be offended if you see the abbreviation "SOB" on your record. That simply means that you experienced some "shortness of breath."

Keep personal copies of your health records in a safe place where they have little chance of being damaged or misplaced. Keeping track of your health history is good not only for you; it also can be valuable to people who are related to you as there may be a genetic link to your health problems.

(For more on medical records, order the book *Medical Records: Getting Yours*, by Bruce Samuels and Sidney Wolfe, published by

Public Citizen's Health Research Group. See the Records heading
in the Research Resources section of this book for ordering
information.)

Price

The price of each surgery depends on the amount of money the
doctor wants for his time and service (doctors set their own prices
— if the treatment is done in agreement with a health plan, the
insurance company may have a pre-set price agreement with the
doctor), the type of procedure being performed, the amount and
complexity of work being done, the surgical team needed to
perform the surgery, the complexity of the operation, where the
surgery is performed, the type of drugs and anesthesia and other
medical supplies needed and the care needed for the recovery.

Although the doctor who charges the highest price is not
necessarily the best, a patient should be very cautious about
trusting their body to the lowest bidder. The doctor who charges
the least may be cutting corners to offer the lowest price, which
may mean a certain level of the safety and quality are also being
sacrificed. The medical team, if there is one, that works with the
doctor may also lack the quality of education necessary to
provide the care you need. On the other hand, the doctor who
charges the most may be interested in nothing other than making
a profit.

If there is more than one procedure done at once or even at a
different date, the doctor — or the person in his office who
handles the financial arrangements — will usually give you a
lower package price, which is lower than what he would have
charged for two operations that are done separately. Because the
person is already under anesthesia and needs no extra
preparation, two procedures done at the same time are usually
less expensive.

Some doctors will perform additional procedures during an
operation without the patient's consent and then charge the
patient for it.

A Los Angeles woman who went in to have a droopy
eyelid repaired was surprised when she woke up and found
the doctor not only operated on both of her eyelids, but
botched up the eyelid that had nothing wrong with it in the
first place. On confronting the doctor about the situation, the
doctor told her that he thought the other eyelid also needed

a little lift. She was sent a bill that included charges for the additional procedure the doctor performed. She did not pay that bill but ended up having to pay another doctor to repair what the first doctor did to her eyelid. She was left with eyelids that cannot close all the way.

Many doctors would rather have nothing to do with discussing fees with patients and leave financial arrangements up to the office staff. If you have questions about the price you are going to pay for the surgery or other financial matters, talk to the person in the doctor's office who handles the financial arrangements. They may know more about the payments you will make than the doctor does.

(See the Billing Problems heading in the Research Resources section of this book.)

Payment

> STARK: *Can I give you one little bit of testimony we had once not so long ago. Guess who are the biggest users by half, more than all of the other people combined of collection attorneys? Guess who uses collection attorneys more than any other group in the country combined? I don't want to lead you. Just guess. Would you guess it was doctors or hospitals?*
> GILBERT: *Either one.*
> STARK: *More lawsuits for collection are brought by doctors and hospitals than any other group of people combined in this country. So when it comes to suing a patient, to provide the money, they don't wait a minute. But when it comes to the reverse, they are in here pleading poverty and crying all over the place. Very interesting.*
> — dialogue between Congressman Pete Stark and Pamela Gilbert of Public Citizen's Congress Watch during Congressional subcommittee hearing on issues relating to medical malpractice, May 20, 1993

Because cosmetic surgery is not a necessity and is done strictly for cosmetic reasons it is rarely covered by insurance. Payment is nearly always required in advance of the surgery by way of cash, credit, or other payment arrangements with the doctor. Some insurance plans will cover part or all of certain plastic surgery procedures depending on what it is and why it is being done. A phone call to the insurance company to tell them what surgery you are considering will tell you what portion, if any, of the operation they might cover. Depending on the type of operation, the expense might be eligible to be taken as an itemized tax deduction.

Rebuilding breasts or other body parts because they have been damaged by cancer or accident, reducing breasts to relieve back problems, altering a nose to improve breathing, lifting baggy eyelids so they do not interfere with vision, aligning teeth to prevent degenerative problems and repairing a hernia during a tummy tuck are some of the common reasons for surgeries that insurance companies will pay for, and often these reasons for surgery are used by doctors as excuses for cosmetic surgery.

Many cosmetic surgery advertisements mention that there is financing available. In the 1980s a financing program was started that offers 100% financing for people seeking cosmetic surgery. This cosmetic surgery financing plan offers a payback plan in monthly installments at steep interest rates and has so far lent tens of millions of dollars to thousands of patients.

Since the average income of cosmetic surgery patients has dropped to under $30,000 a year, it is a sure sign that most of the operations being done are being financed through some sort of credit plan. Anyone going into debt for a cosmetic operation should question whether it is, in fact, something worth going into debt for, and they should figure how the monthly payments can affect their life. There are many other things a person can do with a few thousand dollars other than spend it on a surgery that may not turn out right.

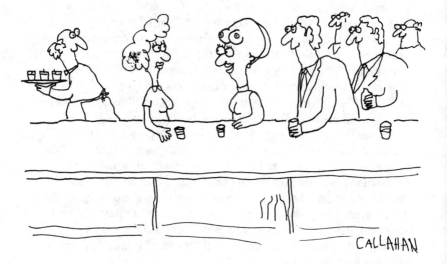

"I'm finally beginning to get some attention for what I have upstairs!"

6 • PROCEEDING WITH SURGERY

Consent Forms

Some cosmetic surgery patients are rudely surprised when they end up with much more done to them than they ever desired and the cosmetic surgeon thinks he did them a "favor." If you are planning to undergo cosmetic surgery, you should make sure you know what the doctor plans to do to you, and everything agreed to and things not agreed to should be detailed in the consent form. Give them an inch and they may take a foot (or too much of your bone, cartilage, organs, or skin).

> *Once they sign those consent forms we can do whatever we want to them. We have all power.*
> — said by a Beverly Hills plastic surgeon when he was asked what he thought of some cosmetic surgeons who do more than the patient wanted done

Consent forms are designed by lawyers to protect doctors. The consent form may have been supplied to the doctor by his malpractice insurance company, the hospital, the HMO he works for or by one of the associations he belongs to. If you are going to be operated on at a medical facility that is not owned by the doctor, the facility will likely have a separate consent form to release the facility from any liability caused by the medical professionals who are treating you.

The forms most doctors use are pretty standard and include spaces for your name and the name of the doctor, the date, the address of the facility where the procedure is being done and the type of procedure being performed. The form may also ask for the patient's permission to let the doctor use any photos or videos taken during the surgery for educational purposes.

You can make alterations to a consent form so that it will also protect you. It is your legal right to cross out anything you wish on any informed consent document you are asked to sign.

If you do not clearly understand what it is the doctor intends to do to you, do not sign the consent form. Never sign a blank consent form. Do not sign anything you are not comfortable with and never sign anything that you do not understand. Always ask questions about what you do not understand. Look for risks listed on the consent form that your doctor did not mention. You are under no obligation to undergo the surgery even if you have already put the money down and signed the consent form. Money can be returned; surgically removed body parts cannot.

Because the use of consent forms has been abused and because elective surgery is planned and scheduled days, weeks or months in advance, a person planning to undergo elective surgery can obtain an unsigned copy of the consent form from the doctor's office days or weeks before the surgery. This will give the patient time to read it over, clear up any questions they have about the wording used on the consent form, and make sure that the operation described on the consent form is in fact the operation that the patient was planning on having and nothing more. It may be helpful to seek the advice of a separate doctor who will not make money if you undergo the operation, or a lawyer can help you compose the consent form to suit your desires. You may want to have the consent form re-typed to include any of the changes you request, and, within reason, you should state what it is you do and do not want done.

Most doctors are nowhere to be found when it is time for you to sign the consent form, as they leave it up to the office staff to get your signature. The office staff is not who you should be talking to when you have questions about the consent form. You should speak to the doctor and have the doctor explain anything and everything on the consent form that you do not understand. The doctor must know about and agree to the modifications before you sign the consent from. Do not settle for a verbal modification to the consent form.

You do not want the doctor to have the freedom to do whatever he feels like doing. Do not sign a consent form that contains any type of wording that gives the doctor and his staff freedom to make additional changes to your body above and beyond what you agreed to.

A model who lived in Los Angeles went to a plastic surgeon to have her breathing improved on one side by having a cartilage bulge removed from the septum. She specified to the doctor that she did not want a rhinoplasty or any outside change to the appearance of her nose. She made her living from modeling her face and she liked her nose, it photographed well and she explained to the doctor that she had no desire to change the appearance of it in any way. The doctor agreed and a surgery was scheduled for two weeks later.

Before she went into the operating room she read through the consent form to make sure it did not mention the word "rhinoplasty." The consent form did not use the word "rhinoplasty" but it did describe the operation as "septoplasty with intranasal reconstruction and bilateral sub mucous resection of the turbinates." It also stated that "I (the patient) also authorize the operating surgeon to perform any other procedures which he may deem necessary or desirable in attempting to improve the condition stated in paragraph #1 or any unhealthy or unforeseen condition that he may encounter during the operation." While the doctor was in the next room getting ready for the operation, the doctor's assistant and the anesthesiologist promised her that the doctor would not do anything that she did not want done. She then signed the consent form.

Basically, as it detailed in the consent form in so many words, she gave the doctor permission to do whatever he wanted — and that is what he did. Not only did he give her a complete rhinoplasty, which she absolutely did not want, he also cut the depressor and nasalis muscles in her upper lip and narrowed her nose so much that the breathing problem she wanted fixed was made worse. The appearance of her nose was dramatically changed and she was emotionally devastated. She had several more surgeries performed on her nose to try to recreate it and that were paid for by her famous actor boyfriend. This all took a toll on her appearance. Her modeling career ended.

The combination of words used on consent forms that give the doctor the freedom to do as he pleases are often in a configuration similar to this:

"I authorize the doctor to employ any assistants, nurses, physicians, anesthetists, and/or anesthesiologists he may feel necessary for the proposed surgery _and for the doctor and his medical team to perform any other procedures in addition to or different from those now_

> *contemplated or described above, whether or not*
> *arising from the unforeseen conditions, which the*
> *doctor or his medical team may, in their*
> *judgment, consider or deem necessary, advisable*
> *or desirable in attempting to improve any*
> *condition that he may encounter during the*
> *operation.*"

If the consent form you are given contains a sentence or paragraph similar to the underlined one, you should cross it out and write that you do not agree to such an arrangement. Many consent forms do contain such a statement and it is designed to protect the doctor from malpractice lawsuits.

The doctor may say that he needs the freedom to include such a blanket statement. The doctor should have the operation well thought out, and it should not be a guessing game where he figures out what he is going to do after he cuts you open in a situation similar to someone opening their refrigerator door and forgetting what they wanted. Although there are surgeries where the doctor needs some freedom, such as when a tumor is unexpectedly found during surgery or some other serious health problem is found that was previously undetected, there are still times when it is safe to demand that the operation be aborted before an unforeseen condition would necessitate a major physical change — such as an amputation of a limb that was not expected. This way you will be able to consider your options and possibly talk to other doctors before proceeding with a change.

Any good doctor would not fight with you regarding any reasonable and smart alteration to the consent form. If the doctor is irrational about the requests you have made, then you have to discuss the disagreements with him, do more studying, and possibly find a different doctor. He may be pushing you into an operation that is not in your best interest.

Under some circumstances the consent form can be specific about what is to be done, the type of anesthesia to be used, the alterations to be done, and within reason, it can specify what is not to be done to the body part that is being operated on. You should state specifically on the consent form who will be the one performing the operation.

The consent form that is given to you will likely mention that you understand there are no guaranteed results. It will may also state that you understand the risks involved with the operation. By signing the consent form, you are saying that you understand these risks and other details of the surgery. You are then giving your informed consent. If you feel that you have not been informed enough, then you should not give your consent, are not ready to sign the consent form and are not ready for the surgery.

It is your body and you are the director of what happens to it. You are hiring the doctor to perform the surgery on you and you are paying for the operation. You are the boss. You want to protect yourself and you want to make sure that nothing is done to you that you do not want done. Do not gamble with your health. Once something goes wrong with it, the rest of your life and the lives of the people around you can be affected. After you have signed the consent form and you enter into the operating room, you will be in the hands of the doctor and the doctor's staff and will have given them the right to do what they will.

Get a copy of the consent form and all of the paperwork for yourself at the time you sign it and keep it in a safe place with the rest of your personal records.

Where the Surgery Is Performed

No hospital review board verifies the quality of these surgeons' work. No one guarantees whether the "operating room" has even basic life support equipment. No one ensures that the doctor has good, qualified staff to give anesthetic, to monitor the patient and to respond quickly should complications arise.

Even normal Government and private audit systems are absent, since in most instances these surgeries are covered neither by Medicare nor private health insurance.
— Congressman Ron Wyden during Congressional subcommittee hearings on plastic surgery industry, speaking about surgery done in doctors' offices, 1989

Surgery is normally performed in one of these three locations:
1. A hospital
2. An ambulatory surgical care center
3. An office surgery room

Cosmetic surgery often takes place outside of hospitals, such as a doctor's office operating room. Therefore, these surgeries are not supervised by anyone other than the doctor and are performed to his standards. This leaves the doctor to determine what will serve as an operating room. There is also no one required to check up on the quality of the doctor's office staff and surgical team and no one to see if the equipment is properly sterilized or if the operating room is a safe place to perform the surgeries.

Some doctors voluntarily pay a fee to have their surgery sites accredited by the Association for Ambulatory Healthcare or the American Association for Accreditation of Ambulatory Plastic Surgery Facilities. This can show that the doctor has taken some steps to protect your safety and that the operating room meets certain standards.

Requirements for standards where surgery takes place vary from state to state. For instance, in California, legislation (Assembly Bill 595) was signed into law on September 30, 1994 that requires accreditation for any setting in that state where surgery is performed with sedation or general anesthesia. The law gives these facilities until July 1, 1996 to comply with the accreditation process. Accreditation certificates will be valid for three years. By calling the state Division of Medical Quality of the Medical Board of California, patients may find out if a surgery setting is accredited, certified, or licensed, or whether the setting's accreditation, certification, or license has been revoked.

Before you decide to undergo elective surgery, check up on the location of the surgery and see if this site has been approved by one of the associations listed above. There should be an emergency transfer agreement with a local hospital in case there is a complication during the surgery. There should also be well-maintained medical equipment including a pulse oximiter to monitor your vital signs during the surgery. Make sure there will be a nurse present during the operation.

If your surgery is to be performed in a teaching hospital, there may be students involved in the procedure and involved in other parts of your care at the hospital. Make sure the doctor you approve of is the one performing the procedure - or at least present and very involved in and closely supervising the procedure (it is your decision as to who treats you). A teaching hospital will likely have the most recent medical equipment and the staff is more likely to have up-to-date medical training. A non-teaching hospital may also have updated equipment, and there you are less likely to have students involved in your care.

Even if the surgery is to be done in the doctor's office or other independent operating facility, make sure the doctor has permission to perform the operation in a nearby hospital. To operate in a hospital, a doctor's credentials are investigated by a credentials committee that limits what a doctor can do on the basis of the doctor's training. A doctor who has gone through the credential and training background check is a safer bet than one who has not.

(Check to see if the hospital has been accredited by Medicare or the Joint Commission on Accreditation of Healthcare Organizations — see the Accrediting Healthcare Facilities listing in the Research Resources section of this book.)

Anesthesia

Although anesthesia mishaps are relatively few in number, when they occur, they generally result in injuries more catastrophic than those experienced in other specialties, and may, therefore, be quite costly in terms of personal and financial loss.
— Lawrence H. Thompson, Assistant Comptroller General, Human Resources Division, US General Accounting Office. Presented at a subcommittee hearing on issues relating to malpractice, May 20, 1993.

The type of anesthesia a patient receives depends on the type of surgery to be performed, the patient's health status and the training and preferences of the anesthesia specialist. Most cosmetic surgeries are performed with local or regional anesthesia. Some operations, such as tummy tucks, are performed under general anesthesia.

- Local anesthetics numb a small area of the body by directly influencing receptors in nerve membranes. Local anesthesia carries significantly less risk than general anesthesia. Local anesthesia with a vasoconstrictor (such as epinephrine) can help prevent fluid loss since it constricts blood vessels and keeps the anesthetic in the desired area much longer.
- Regional anesthesia is administered to numb a specific area of the body. The patient is awake but does not feel any pain in the area where the cutting is being done.
- Sometimes an intravenous medicine such as Valium is given to relax and induce amnesia in a patient who does

not necessarily need general anesthesia. For instance, a patient undergoing facial cosmetic surgery, such as a nose job, under local anesthesia and intravenous medicines may be fully aware of all that goes on around them or may drift in and out of sleep. Sounds may seem to be distant, as if they are coming from another room. The patient may hear what is going on in the operating room but may feel nothing other than a light touching of the area being operated on. There is usually no pain during this time. The intravenous medicine can make the patient lose the ability to track time. The patient may be able to talk a little to the doctor while the operation is being performed or might be unable to formulate words. Memory of the surgical events may be altered or distorted.

- General anesthesia almost always leads to complete unconsciousness. Sensation is suppressed and reflexes are absent.

People who undergo general anesthesia are usually given four types of medications. These include a mild tranquilizer, narcotics to block pain, an anesthetic such as sodium pentothal or propofol to make them unconscious, and another agent to paralyze the muscles. It is rare to have a patient emerge from unconsciousness while under general anesthesia. If a patient who is under general anesthesia does become aware of what is going on, they will almost always drift back into unconsciousness. (If you have had an experience with awareness during general surgery, see the Anesthesia heading in the Research Resources section of this book for the phone number to the AWARE Foundation.)

Invasive procedures necessitate the use of general anesthesia. Some surgeons prefer to use general anesthesia during certain operations so the patient will not hear what is going on and cannot panic, which can elevate the heartbeat, cause shock or other complications. General anesthesia can be used if the patient feels that they would rather not be aware of what is going on or if the surgery requires it.

Many doctors recommend that general anesthesia be used only within the walls of a well-equipped hospital where major surgeries are commonly performed so that if there is a significant complication (such as trouble bringing the patient back out of anesthesia), equipment and an experienced staff will be immediately available.

Before undergoing anesthesia your anesthesiologist or surgeon should be made aware of the following:
* Your past and present drug use. This includes recreational drugs, drugs prescribed by a doctor and over-the-counter medications
* All of your past and present major health problems
* Whether your family members or relatives have had significant unfavorable reactions to anesthesia
* If there is any possibility of pregnancy
* If you have a history of bleeding problems
* If you have recently donated blood
* If you smoke
* How often you consume alcohol and especially if you have within the past 24 hours
* If your have recently lost or gained a significant amount of weight
* If you wear contact lenses or have false teeth
* When you last ate and when you last drank

No anesthesia is totally risk-free. Adverse reactions can include nausea, shivering, low blood pressure and shallow breathing. Anesthesia can cause a patient to vomit, which can cause them to choke, and if any of this food gets into the lungs it can cause an infection. Most patients do not experience any of these reactions and do not remember what went on.

Allergic reactions to anesthesia are possible. These can lead to complications including hives, convulsions, shock and cardiac arrest. If the oxygen level becomes limited the brain can be damaged. In the worst case, death can occur. Serious complications can arise if there is an overdose of anesthesia.

Reactions similar to an overdose can occur when a normal amount of anesthesia is given but the patient's organs are not working in a way that would normally metabolize and eliminate the drug from the body. For instance, if the heart is not working properly, the drug may not travel fast enough to the liver to be metabolized, and this can result in a toxic reaction. An overdose can also occur if the drug is injected too rapidly.

Your Anesthesiologist

One young Los Angeles woman who went in to get a chemical peel on her face was told that an anesthesiologist would be present. She agreed to have the operation after the anesthesiologist did not show up. The doctor administered the anesthetic and placed his office assistant in charge of monitoring the vital signs. The young woman died.

A 41-year-old mother who was in the recovery room after a radical hysterectomy stopped breathing. No one noticed because nurses failed to monitor her vital signs after surgery. She was left severely brain damaged. A court in San Jose, California, awarded her $1.44 million. Under the terms of the settlement, the medical center where the surgery took place did not admit guilt or liability.

Your surgeon should be focusing his full attention on you while someone else administers the anesthesia and monitors your vital signs (including blood pressure, temperature, pulse and respiration) and your oxygen level.

While you are undergoing a surgical procedure, the second most important person in the operating room, next to the doctor, is the person who is administering the anesthesia. Though anesthesia is safer now than it has ever been, a minor mistake can be devastating and even fatal.

The anesthesia will be administered by one of these three people:
- An anesthesiologist: a physician who is trained in the area of anesthesia. He or she administers the anesthesia and monitors your vital signs during and after the surgery.
- An anesthetist: a nurse with some extra training. The anesthetist is often supervised by the anesthesiologist but may also work without an anesthesiologist present.
- The surgeon

There are no laws that require an anesthesiologist or life-saving equipment to be present during an operation. Because anesthesia carries serious risks you should request to have an anesthesiologist or an anesthetist present during the operation. This person should also be with you after the operation until you have safely recovered and your vital signs are stable.

It is best that one anesthesiologist be present for each patient. Many in the medical community believe that a nurse anesthetist has sufficient training to administer anesthesia and monitor the patient. Often when a surgery takes place in a hospital the anesthesiologist is supervising more than one operation at a time as surgeries take place in different operating rooms. In this scenario the anesthesiologist is not always present in the room but is "supervising" the person who is monitoring the patient during the operation — usually a nurse anesthetist. This is called "medically directed anesthesiology."

If you are undergoing a surgery where the anesthesiologist is not always present in the room, you should at least request that they be present when the anesthesia is initially administered and present when you awake from the surgery and until your vital signs have stabilized. You should also request that the anesthesiologist be immediately physically accessible during the operation. This means that they should remain in the general vicinity of the operating room and not on another floor of the facility or outside. If an emergency arises, you will want a specialist near you and not have to depend on the surgeon to handle everything.

The chance of having an emergency during the operation is also the reason you want to have a doctor who has up-to-date emergency equipment immediately available in the operating room and an emergency transfer agreement with a local hospital if the surgery is being done outside of a hospital.

If the anesthesiologist is a member of the American Association of Anesthesiologists, they are supposed to meet with you before the surgery to assess any potential risks and to determine what type of anesthesia is best for you.

In any case, it may be a good idea to meet the person giving the anesthesia before the surgery, either in person or by phone. Get answers to any questions you may have. Find out what school the person administering the anesthesia attended, what year they graduated and what year they were board certified. If you choose a nurse anesthetist, check to see if they are certified by the American Association of Nurse Anesthetists.

If the doctor who is performing the surgery uses the same anesthesia specialist all the time, the doctor's office may have a copy of the anesthetist's or anesthesiologist's resume. Ask for a copy to learn about their education, training and experience.

If you have insurance, find out whether part or all of the cost of the anesthesia specialist is covered. It is possible that you may get a separate bill from the anesthesia department.

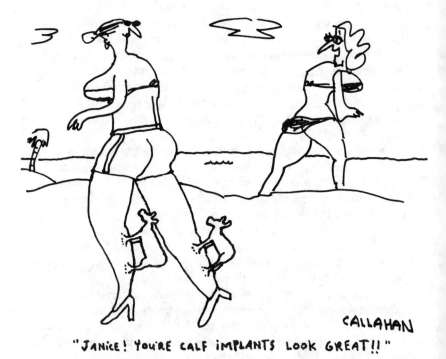

"JANICE! YOU'RE CALF IMPLANTS LOOK GREAT!!"

CALLAHAN, distributed by LEVIN PRESENTS, used with permission.

7 • RECOVERY

Healing

It is not possible to discuss all risks, but this chapter discusses those that are common.

Many cosmetic surgery patients recover at home. If the surgery is more involved, you may spend a day or more in the hospital. It is important for you to know that you may need to take days, weeks or even months off from work to recover. You may also need someone to drive you home from the hospital. You may need rides to and from the doctor's office for checkups, along with a caretaker for days or weeks.

If you have the resources, choose to hire a private duty nurse to care for you while you recover at home. Another option is to use recovery center facilities. These are set up like little hotels staffed by nurses. If you want to be pampered and can afford the extra expense, spend a day or more at a center during the initial stages of recovery. These hideaways usually offer transportation along with room and board at a much lower rate than what a hospital charges. They can also be well worth the extra money to assure that your initial recovery period goes well.

There is no telling how long anyone is going to take to heal until it actually happens. It may take more time or less time than the doctor says. Carefully follow any instruction you are given to guide you through healing. During this period you should let the doctor know whether you have any excess bleeding, fever, pain or any change that concerns you.

Some activities, such as going for walks, may help you recover faster. Find out what you can and cannot do during recovery and how the surgical wound will affect your mobility. Various movements may have to be avoided so there will be no strain to the incisions or the surgical wound — especially during sleep. Any action that would position your head low may need to be avoided — especially if there was surgery performed anywhere on the head or neck. Facial surgery patients may have to avoid foods that require hard chewing and any conversation that would cause any more than very casual facial movements. You may also need help getting dressed. It may be wise to avoid physical contact with animals and small children for a week or more. Bending, heavy lifting and any action that would elevate blood pressure or result in increased body heat might need to be limited for a number of days or weeks. When you sneeze or cough you should do so with your mouth wide open to avoid a pressure burst within your body. You may have stitches or surgical tape and scabbing that cannot get wet, which means you will not be able to shower or bathe for a certain number of days.

Stitches hold the skin and other tissues together so they can adhere to each other and heal.
- When recovering from surgery keep your hands away from the surgical wounds to avoid contamination with bacteria.
- Do not let anyone other than the doctor or nurses touch the sutures, and they should only do so while wearing surgical gloves.
- Do not scratch the sutured area or pull the sutures that seem to be loose.
- Avoid the use of any lotions, creams, oils, cosmetics, medications, cleaning solutions or any type of solution on or near the wound unless you have your doctor's approval.

Smoking of any type should be avoided for at least two weeks before surgery and two weeks after surgery. Nicotine inhibits the healing process because it impairs blood flow to the tissues, increasing the chance of necrosis (skin death). Researchers at the University of Texas Southwestern Medical school found that bones take nearly twice as long to heal in people who smoke. Researchers at Emory University School of Medicine found that nicotine interferes with bone fusion. Nicotine is in all tobacco products. Products such as smoker's gum also contain nicotine and should be avoided by anyone undergoing surgery.

Alcoholic beverages, certain foods and possibly drinks with caffeine, such as coffee, may need to be avoided for a couple of days before surgery and for four to seven days after surgery — or for as long as the doctor advises. Drinks that contain alcohol can interfere with medication and cause you to become lax in caring for yourself during the recovery period.

Products that might need to be avoided or limited befo
after surgery include aspirin and aspirin substitutes, ibuprͮ...,
cough medicine, Alka Seltzer, vitamin B supplements, Darvon
and Darvon-related medications, vitamin E supplements, fish oil
in both pill and liquid form, Pepto Bismol and any other medicine
or diet supplement that your doctor recommends that you avoid.

Water-based cosmetics should be used in place of oil-based
cosmetics around the operation site during the month after
surgery because they are easier to wash off. Oil-based cosmetics
can cause infections. Any makeup used should be new, clean and
hypoallergenic (be cautious when using products labeled
hypoallergenic because not all companies follow the same
standards). Avoid products with dyes that can stain and even
tattoo the fresh scar during the first few weeks after surgery.
Cosmetics with alcohol or perfumes should be worn at a distance
from the operative site, because they can irritate the incisions
and cause dryness.

Limit sun exposure of any surgical wound until the wound has
healed. Apply sunblock and wear protective clothing when you
do go out in the sun.

A list of recovery instructions detailing your specific needs
may be available from your doctor. (See section 7, Strategic
Planning, for more information on caring for yourself after
surgery.)

Bleeding, Bruising and Swelling

Complications from surgery can include hemorrhaging and
hematomas. A hemorrhage occurs when clotting does not proceed
properly. A hematoma is a collection of clotted blood beneath the
skin. A hematoma can also occur inside the body. Both of these
complications may require additional surgery.

Some surgeries can cause intense bruising and swelling. Ask
your doctor about the likelihood of this happening to you. The
doctor may be able to show you photos of someone with surgical
bruises and swelling who has had a similar operation — but
remember that not everyone bruises or swells in the same manner.

Keeping the surgical wound elevated (when the surgery is on
the arms, legs or head) above the heart level for the first 24
hours after surgery can help minimize bruising. Cold constricts
blood vessels. Applying ice and cold compresses after surgery can

help control the swelling. Ask the doctor if applying ice bags or other cold compresses to the surgical site will benefit you.

The swelling and bruising from surgery can last anywhere from a few days to more than a month. Bruising around the eyes can cause persistent dark areas under the eyes. Swelling can sometimes permanently stretch the skin and can result in scarring — especially if the swelling causes stitches to break open or tear the skin.

Bruising that occurs on the upper parts of the body can eventually fall to lower areas as healing progresses. An example of this is when someone undergoes nasal surgery that causes bruising on the eyes and cheeks. This bruising may fall down into the neck over the next several days as the healing takes place.

The body breaks down old coagulated blood and dissolves the dead cells. As the dead cells are diminished, the bruise becomes lighter in color and eventually disappears.

Bruises often appear their worst on the third day. If your bruising keeps increasing beyond what was expected, notify your doctor. A bruise that appears red and feels hot should also be reported because these are signs of infection.

Aspirin (acetylsalicylic acid) can increase bleeding and swelling because it interferes with the normal clotting ability of blood platelets. Some other medications, such as ibuprofen and blood-thinning drugs can also lead to increased bleeding.

Infection

I began to see many, many advertisements . . . and thought well, gee, with all of this advertising this cannot be too unsafe.

The doctor who I chose after checking him out with the American Medical Association and the California Department of Health did the operation in his office.

[After complaining to her doctor that she was short of breath, her doctor told her that she was experiencing the normal aftereffects of surgery. When her bandages were removed they revealed two black patches and a wide-open gap in her lower abdomen that was oozing pus.]

Four weeks after the surgery, I still had an open wound, and I had uncontrollable infections, three kinds of infections. . . . the infections spread through my bloodstream to my lungs and landed in the mitral valve of my heart. The mitral valve was destroyed by infection. I ended up in an emergency room hospital — very, very close to death.

I was in emergency for seven hours. . . . There was this green gel and pus in my incision . . . they removed suture [material] *that the doctor left in my tummy and the infection was clinging to that . . . I was in and out of the hospital six times in a year and a half. Five times I went into heart failure. . . . I had a stroke. The defective valve threw a clot which landed in the right side of my brain . . . I had open heart surgery to replace the destroyed valve in my heart . . . I hear the sound of the fake valve in my heart . . . I will be on blood thinning medication and have to go to the doctor every month for the rest of my life.*

Two months after he operated on me he did the same procedure on a 36-year-old RN. I am the lucky one because I am alive today and she is not. She died.

[She later found that for two years before she had her surgery the state had been trying to take the doctor's license away. The doctor was found murdered several years later in a parking lot of a restaurant.]

— Joyce Palso, testifying in 1989 before Congressional subcommittee hearings on the plastic surgery industry and telling how a botched tummy tuck operation nearly killed her

Infection from surgery is potentially serious and fatal. Any time you undergo surgery, there is a chance of getting an infection. The risk of infection increases if you are a smoker. Infections are one of the leading causes of post-operative death. One of the common causes of infection is improperly sterilized surgical tools or equipment. Infection can also be caused by a surgical site that was not cleaned properly, unsanitary medical workers or unsanitary conditions during recovery. Some studies have shown that patients who receive antibiotics intravenously before certain surgeries will have a smaller chance of infection if the antibiotics are administered no more than two hours before surgery.

GRANDY: Let me ask you this and you might have said this, I didn't pick it up if you did. Did you draw any conclusions in your study as the incidence of negligence and adverse events as relates to age? In other words, are you more inclined to see incidence of negligence and malpractice claims in patients 65 and over?

THOMPSON: *I think in the Harvard study (of New York hospitals) the answer is yes.*

KLADIVA: *What the study suggests is that the individuals who are most likely to sustain injuries in the healthcare system are the older individuals and they are less likely to file claims than are other citizens.*

GRANDY: *But they are also more likely to have accidents wherever they are, right. I mean to some extent the older and frailer and sicker you get, the more likely you are going to be at risk.*

THOMPSON: *Yes. And you should know that if you look at what these incidents are that are being reported out of the Harvard study you will see things like infections that are picked up in the hospital or drug reactions and, especially with infections, older people are probably more prone to pick up an infection.*

— Congressman Fred Grandy, Lawrence H. Thompson, Assistant Comptroller General, Human Resources Division, US General Accounting Office and Susan Kladiva, Assistant Director, Health Financing Issues, US General Accounting Office, during a Congressional subcommittee hearing on issues relating to medical malpractice, May 20, 1993

Depending on what is causing an infection, the type of surgery you had, and your body's ability to fight the infection along with the help of antibiotics, the infection could clear up easily or it could prolong your recovery period and cause unwanted scarring and other complications that might necessitate further surgery.

If you had an implant put in during the surgery and an infection develops, the implant may have to be removed. If the implant cannot be removed right away, antibiotic therapy may be needed for four to six weeks or until the implant can be removed. After the infection has completely cleared, the implant can be replaced, but this requires additional surgery with additional risks. All of these scenarios can take their toll on your health and well-being, and certainly your bank account.

Scars

Whenever an incision is made, damage is done to skin tissue, blood vessels and nerves. All incisions will produce some scarring. No scar is absolutely invisible, but many scars will become less noticeable with time. After several months, the scar may fade to a fine line. Sometimes the scars are larger and thicker than the person would care for. Scars caused by facial surgery can usually be covered by makeup and hair. The most obvious surgical scars are caused by operations done on areas where there are no natural skin folds to hide them.

Your doctor may advise that you use an over-the-counter anti-bacterial lotion on your surgical wound. After the stitches are removed, some people use such things as vitamin-enriched skin lotions, aloe vera and even olive oil to coat the scar. These may aid in healing and result in a less noticeable scar. Oil applied to a wound may cause infection. Ask your doctor before applying any lotion, cream, oil or other product to your surgical wound.

Follow-up Appointments

The follow-up visit schedule will vary depending on what type of surgery you had and how involved it was. There should be daily contact with the doctor or the doctor's office for at least the first few days after any significant surgery. Depending on the surgery, you may have to see the doctor several times within the week following the surgery for operation wound checkups. There might be a follow-up schedule that includes a one-week visit, a two-week visit, a one-month visit, a three-month visit (which is when the "after" photos are usually taken), a six-month visit, and a one-year visit. These are done to make sure there are no problems with healing. The follow-up appointments might be included in the price you pay the doctor for the operation. If you are paying for the surgery out-of-pocket, inquire whether follow-up appointments are included in the surgical fee, or whether they are additional.

8 • QUESTIONS

Questions to Ask the Doctor and Yourself

Many of the following questions are listed to present information so that you will not experience any surprises. Many others may be useful in determining the quality of care you may receive if you decide to undergo surgery.

Find out as many answers as you can that apply to your needs before you see the doctor. Be realistic about the amount of time you require of the doctor, or be prepared to pay extra for an extended consultation.

Turning the consultation into an FBI-type investigation is not the idea here. No doctor should be expected to sit and answer the abundance of questions in the following pages. Any questioning may make a doctor uncomfortable because he is essentially having his strengths and weaknesses evaluated by someone who has walked into his workspace.

Surgery may be beneficial or disastrous. The outcome of surgery depends on the doctor's talents and abilities, techniques used during surgery, and the motives of the medical team performing the operation. It also depends on the motives of the patient, the post-surgical care and the patient's mental and physical response to the surgery.

Because altering a body part can be a major decision, you may feel intimidated during the consultations and forget what to ask. Set the stage to have a successful session with your doctor. Get past the technical terms and medical phrases. Take a notebook and a list of questions — or highlight the questions in this book that you want to find answers to. Some people bring tape recorders to the consultation so they can listen to it later to determine whether there was something they overlooked.

It is good to have a relative, friend or spouse with you when you are talking to the doctor. Your friend may remember what you may forget to ask. They also may ask questions that you did not think of and notice something that the doctor said or did that you did not notice. You are protecting yourself and you have the right to have a third person of your choice in the room with you whenever you are speaking with a doctor. If the doctor refuses your request to have a third person with you, you may want to question this, or simply leave.

Some people are so unfamiliar with and are so intimidated by doctors and lost in the mystique of medicine that they treat medical care with an unquestioning religious reverence. They are passive and submissive rather than active and assertive in their own care, and this is when harm can be done. These are the same people who do not ask enough questions, do not do their own research, are afraid to walk out on a doctor, do not realize that they are hiring the doctor and can end up being, in a sense, used as human guinea pigs in the doctor's "practice" of medicine.

Many people will go to a doctor who is a complete stranger, fill out paperwork that includes very personal questions, go into the examination room, take off their clothes, let the doctor come into the room, be asked more personal questions, let the stranger put his hands on all of their private parts and even let the doctor operate on them — then still feel as if they are being too personal and will refrain from asking the doctor a few questions that will determine whether the doctor is competent and if his prescribed form of treatment is best.

These very same people, if they are in the position to have a home built may, when searching for their architect and builder, do more background checking on these professionals than on the doctor they are trusting with their life. Even after having their house built, they may decide they do not like it. You may live in your house temporarily, but your body is something you will be living in for the rest of your life.

It is important that you make the right choice about whether to have the surgery and if so, how it is to be done and who is to do it. The decision to undergo surgery can sometimes mean the difference between life and death. Because of these risks, the last thing you need when looking into surgery is some clever smarmy doctor whose talk is filled with medical euphemisms and who tosses you vague answers to your questions.

Do not tolerate incompetent medical care. Find the best caregiver you possibly can. You do not want to be one of the thousands of people who find themselves involved with a lawsuit against a doctor while hopping from doctor to doctor to try and find one who can correct messy surgical results.

You have the right to be informed about the operation you are going in for and about the medical staff that is involved in your care. This means checking out the background of the doctor and his staff and may involve researching in books found in bookstores and libraries, reading pamphlets, and possibly watching videotapes that will teach you about your treatment options.

Do not worry about offending the doctor or irritating the staff by asking questions or by letting them know that you are being very cautious. Just remember how offended and irritated you will be if, after you undergo the operation, you find yourself injured, disfigured or handicapped by what the doctor did to you. Besides, if they see that you are serious about getting good medical care, they are more likely to give it to you. But even with all of your precautions there is still no guarantee that everything will go right. Doctors cannot always control everything in the operating room; some of what goes on depends on you and your body's reaction to the surgery, and therefore doctors cannot always be held accountable when things do not go as planned.

Aim to get a complete understanding of the procedure you are considering. Speak frankly with the doctor and do not be afraid to push the doctor to explain things. The doctor went to medical school; you probably did not. It is you and not the doctor who might be getting on that operating table. The doctor may have never been a patient. If the doctor uses a term or phrase you do not understand when he is talking to you or in any literature he or his staff give you, have him explain it to you in words you understand.

If there are questions that you think of after you leave the doctor's office, write them down and ask them later, but before you decide on having the surgery.

The numbers on the following questions are given only as a form of reference and not as a grade of importance.

Not all of the questions listed here will apply to all operations. Additionally, there may be many questions unique to your specific health concern that are not listed here and that you will have to consider.

• EVALUATING THE DOCTOR

Q1: Does the doctor have a resume/professional biography/curriculum vitae that lists his schooling, other training, fellowships and credentials?

Some doctors will freely provide this printed material. Call the doctor's office and see if his staff will send you a copy.

If the resume does not list the insurance company which the doctor gets his malpractice insurance from, ask his office for the name of the insurance company.

Q2: What boards is he certified by and what year did he receive his board certification?

Call the boards and find out if the doctor is certified and how long the certification lasts. If you are having a breast surgery, you probably do not want to go to someone who is board certified in ear, nose and throat surgery.

Q3: Where did he attend medical school?

Q4: What was his degree in?

Q5: What year did he graduate?

Staying current with changes in operative techniques and the increasingly sophisticated medical devices that are now being used requires continuing education. If he graduated decades ago, he should have updated his education to include the modern technological advances in his field of medicine.

Q6: Where did he serve his residency?

Q7: Where did he serve his internship? Was it specialized or general?

Q8: How many years has he been in practice and what other areas of medicine, if any, has he practiced or specialized in?

Q9: Is the doctor a Fellow of the American College of Surgeons?

Beyond residency training, which trains physicians in a specialty, some physicians go on to train in fellowship programs. (The address of the ACS is in the Research Resources section of this book under the heading of Doctors and Surgeons.)

Q10: What does the doctor consider to be his specialty? Does the doctor limit himself to the face and neck or another specific area of the body?

The programs for becoming a specialist include added training and supervised experience. It is best to go with a surgeon who specializes in a few procedures that include the surgery you are interested in and who has received his training in that area.

Q11: When did he last attend a continuing education class, what organization offered the class, and what was the subject of the class?

The Accreditation Council for Continuing Medical Education accredits sponsors of continuing medical education programs and is itself organized under the sponsorship of several organizations: the American Board of Medical Specialists, the American Medical Association, the American Hospital Association, the Association of American Medical Colleges, the Council of Medical Specialty Societies and the Federation of State Medical Boards.

Continuing education classes cost money and take time out of the doctor's schedule but are well worth the investment to his career and curative skills and to the safety of his patients. A doctor may be required to attend a certain class to a requirement of the hospital where he has admitting privileges or the insurance company that insures him. A continuing education class may also be a requirement placed on the doctor by the State Medical Board to meet education purposes of a probation action that the Board took against the doctor because of malpractice.

Simply because a particular doctor says that he attended a continuing education class does not mean that he actually stayed for the class. He may have signed-in and went elsewhere.

Q12: In what other states has he practiced medicine and why did he move from the other state?

Having a doctor who has moved a few times can be a bonus. He may have gained more experience than if he had stayed in the same region because he will have worked with different doctors, learned their techniques and experienced a variety of patients. But if the doctor has had to move because of his involvement in criminal activity or negligent behavior he may be a doctor who you should avoid.

When a doctor loses his licenses in one state he can go to another state and not be subjected to any preclusions when he gets his license in another state. (For various legitimate reasons, some doctors maintain licenses in more than one state.)

Q13: If the doctor was trained and licensed in another country, did he pass the Foreign Medical Graduate Examination?

About 20% of the United States' doctors are immigrants. Some of them received their training in the United States. Some doctors who were born in the United States received their training in other countries. If they have not passed the Foreign Medical Graduate Examination in the Medical Sciences they should not be practicing medicine in the United States.

The Foreign Medical Graduate Examination in the Medical Sciences is a 1,000-question exam that screens the credentials, knowledge in medical matters and English language ability of foreign medical school graduates who wish to practice medicine in the United States. Those who pass these criteria are eligible to apply for residencies in the United States. The exam is given in each state and has been overseen since the 1950s by the Educational Commission for Foreign Medical Graduates. The Commission is a private group that is organized and supported by the nation's major medical associations. The Commission's organizational members are the Federation of State Medical Boards of the United States, the American Medical Association, the American Hospital Association, the American Board of Medical Specialists, the Association of Medical Colleges, the National Medical Association and the Association for Hospital Medical Education.

Q14: What is the doctor's state medical license number and in what year was it first issued?

Call the state medical board to find out this information. The phone numbers of each state medical board are listed in the Research Resource section of this book.

Q15: Does he have a clinical faculty appointment at a medical school? Has he taught or is he currently teaching at any of the local colleges or universities and what does he teach?

Call the college or check the college class directory and see if the doctor does currently teach there. It is a good sign if the doctor is so knowledgeable that he is teaching others to become doctors. Working or taking continuing education courses at a university can give him experience with state-of-the-art equipment and keep him current on the latest advances in medicine.

Do not be fooled into thinking that a doctor is a university professor simply because he has an office on the grounds of a

university. He may simply be renting office space from the
university.

Q16: Does the doctor have an active staff membership at a local
hospital that has been accredited by the Joint Commission on
Accreditation of Healthcare Organizations?

Hospitals have credentials committees that are responsible
for saying which physicians are qualified to practice there and
what they are allowed to do — and for disciplining those who
abuse the privilege.

A hospital credential committee most likely will look for
- Where the doctor completed medical school
- The type of internship the doctor completed
- If the doctor has specialty training
- When and if the doctor passed the national (United States
  Medical Licensing Exam) and state board tests
- If the doctor has malpractice insurance
- The doctor's ability to increase the hospital's profits
- How efficient he is at using the hospital's resources

Before the doctor is granted full privileges in the
hospital he may be subject to a probation period where he is
supervised by another doctor.

A doctor who has been scrutinized by a hospital review board
and is on staff at a local hospital is a safer choice in a doctor than
one who has not. On the other hand, the hospital may not have
checked into the doctor's background as thoroughly as may be
considered safe. This may be because the doctor provided the
hospital with inaccurate information on the application he
submitted to the hospital. Some hospitals also have a history of
accepting doctors who have a record of negligence.

> *THOMPSON: . . . in a hospital today, the care is
> provided not by one physician, but by a whole team and when
> the hospital itself then becomes the focus of responsibility,
> the hospital itself becomes responsible for making sure that
> the team functions as a team.*
> *KLECZKA: But the hospital — I don't know. Who do we
> mean by the hospital, maybe the administrator or some
> overseer is not in every surgical suite where the possibility of
> a malpractice injury could occur. And playing the devil's
> advocate, I would liken that to blaming the car for the*

accident and not the driver and to shift that liability to the hospital where they don't have a direct hands-on overseeing ability for every surgeon who might be working under their roof.

THOMPSON: Well, hospitals are supposed to. Those hospitals are supposed to check what their [the doctors'] credentials are. You [the hospitals administrators] are not supposed to privilege a physician if you [the hospital] are not confident that physician can practice good medicine. You are supposed to have quality assurance systems and risk management systems. This all has to be in place [within the hospital] in order [for the hospital] to be accredited by the Joint Commission.

KLECZKA: I am not sure when you have a situation where a physician is involved in repetitive medical practice-type incidents, but for the one slip of the knife and some examples, the wrong liver being taken out. The hospital just can't comprehend those before they happen, naturally.

THOMPSON: You are not going to reduce to zero the incidence of these things. Indicated in this Harvard study [of hospitals in New York], one percent of the people were victims of negligence and four percent had bad things happen to them. About three quarters of the unfortunate events were accidents — might even be a slip of the scalpel — and only one quarter seemed to involve physicians' negligence.

> — Lawrence H. Thompson, Assistant Comptroller General, Human Resources Division, US General Accounting Office and Congressman Gerald D. Kleckza, during Congressional subcommittee hearings on issues relating to medical malpractice, May 20, 1993

Hospitals in America are run by "allopathic" doctors. These are doctors who have graduated from allopathic schools of medicine. These doctors make up the "traditional" doctors who specialize in such things as cardiology, radiology, urology, emergency medicine, proctology, pulmonology, plastic surgery, anesthesiology, dermatology, rheumatology, endocrinology, gynecology, ophthalmology, hematology, nephrology, otorhinolaringology, pathology, and neurology. Although not all allopathic schools are alike, they require their graduates to have a science background and they all teach the same type of treatments based on drugs and surgery with some lifestyle-based therapies thrown in. This group of individuals largely think of themselves as the "real" doctors.

Locked out of mainstream hospitals are those who practice alternative forms of medicine such as homeopathy, chiropracic care, naturopathy, acupuncture, herbology and hypnotherapy. Though some of these specialists are occasionally allowed into a hospital to treat certain cases and often have patients who are allopathic doctors, in large measure they practice outside of the hospital setting. Some alternative therapies are becoming more accepted by the mainstream gatekeepers because many alternative forms of medicine make patients "feel better" and when patients feel better they heal better.

Q17: Has the doctor ever lost his privileges at any hospital because of unacceptable practices? What were the reasons?

Losing the privileges at the hospital is removing the doctors' ability to treat patients within the hospital and is sometimes done because the doctor did something seriously wrong, has a history of negligence or of being sued for malpractice. The doctor may also lose his hospital privileges because he has failed to stay updated in his field of medicine or because a utilization review showed that the way he practices medicine is too expensive for the hospital — even if his expensive actions were better for the patients he treated. Losing hospital privileges will restrict the doctor's access to medical equipment, severely restrict his ability to practice medicine and have a negative effect on his income. He will then have to try to gain privileges at another hospital or limit the procedures that he can do.

However, a doctor may also may lose privileges if the hospital signed on with a health maintenance organization and for some reason the doctor did not sign a contract with the HMO. If the doctor has a medical specialty in contraception or fertility and was once affiliated with a hospital that was taken over by the Catholic church, the doctor may have lost his privileges at the hospital because the Catholic church is against certain types of medically-induced contraception and fertility procedures.

Q18: Is the doctor involved with any research? What kind of research? What is the purpose of the research? Through what organization? Is he planning on using you as part of a case study or for a research subject? Will there be money made from this study? Does he plan to use your name, personal information or photos of you in the research report?

Ask to see a copy of the information about the research.

Q19: Has a formal accusation ever been filed against the doctor by the county or state attorney general or has any disciplinary action been taken against the doctor?

Doctors can have their licenses revoked, be suspended from practicing for a period of time, be fined or have restrictions placed upon them by the state licensing board. The insurance company through which he gets his malpractice insurance may place restrictions on the amount of money the doctor is insured for or drop the doctor altogether.

You may have to write the state medical board or other governing body to find if a doctor has any record of misconduct, if he has ever been disciplined or to find out what a doctor has been formally accused of by former patients. Thanks to the medical lobbies' ability to influence lawmakers, some state boards are not permitted to tell you if a doctor has lost multi-million dollar lawsuits, has had multiple complaints filed against him, has had a history of drug abuse, has sexually molested a patient or has caused a patient's death.

Q20: Does he carry malpractice insurance?

If he does not, it is time for you to leave the office.

Some doctors say they cannot afford malpractice insurance. Others claim that carrying malpractice insurance increases their chances of being sued, whereas some doctors cannot get insurance because no insurance company will cover them. "Going bare" is the term used to describe doctors who are practicing without malpractice insurance.

Q21: What is the company he has the insurance with and what is the policy number?

The insurance company may be listed on his resume.

Also find out how much he is insured for. You can call the insurance company to confirm this. If he is limited to only $100,000 or so, he may have restrictions put on him by the insurance company because of a history of being sued or a negligent background.

Even if he does have malpractice insurance, it may not cover the operation you are having. Check to see if the insurance plan covers the specific surgery you are considering.

Q22: Has the doctor ever been sued by a former patient? What were the consequences?

Having had a malpractice lawsuit brought against him does not mean a doctor is a poor physician. The determination of whether the doctor is dangerous depends on the consequences of the situation that led to the malpractice suit. He may treat high-risk patients who have a greater chance of complications, or he may specialize in a rare but necessary type of treatment that is also high-risk. About 20% of malpractice suits result in serious settlements and judgments against doctors. About 1 percent of all doctors account for half of the malpractice awards.

Q23: How many times has he performed the operation you are considering, how often does he perform it and when was the last time he performed it?

Remember that the doctors "perform" operations and that some of the performances do not turn out as well as others. Though it is not ethically wrong for a doctor to perform an operation that he has not performed in the past, he should know what his limitations are and refrain from reaching beyond his curative skills. A responsible doctor will admit when it is time to refer a patient to another doctor who has more experience in a particular area. The risks of surgery are reduced if the patient is being operated on by a doctor who is experienced in the type of surgery that is being done.

Q24: Are the doctor, his office, and his staff clean and organized?

Q25: Has the doctor written any articles that have been published in any journals or magazines?

This is also material that his office may freely mail to you along with the resume. Many doctors have written articles for various magazines and have appeared on television. A doctor who has a research article printed in certain professional publications, such as the *New England Journal of Medicine*, exhibits his expertise in a certain area of medicine and can become a medical celebrity and be sought after to give lectures to audiences of medical professionals. Having an article published does not guarantee the doctor is a good doctor.

• COMMUNICATION WITH THE DOCTOR

Q26: Are you difficult to communicate with? Is your own lack of communication skills having a negative influence on your relationship with the doctor?

Is this because you are nervous, or uncomfortable, or is it caused by medication or your health condition?

Having a relative or friend present when you visit the doctor might be of help in this situation.

Q27: Did the doctor give you his undivided attention or was he carrying on unrelated conversations with his employees during the time you were paying him to give you his attention?

Q28: Has the doctor treated you as an individual, or do you feel he is running his office more like a factory where he does the same thing to everyone?

Q29: Do you feel comfortable with the doctor? Do you have doubts about the doctor's abilities? Do you feel the doctor has lied to you or misled you? Did you feel as if you were being manipulated? Has the doctor or the staff made you feel as if you will miss out on something if you do not undergo the surgery?

Often when a person is in a doctors office the doctor is standing while the patient is sitting down. That arrangement invites dominance. If you are talking with the doctor and he is standing and he is not examining you and there is no reason for you to be sitting down and if you are able to stand up, then do so — and vice/versa if the doctor is sitting down. It may improve the way you communicate with the doctor.

Q30: Does the doctor respond to your questions with the attitude that you are out of place in questioning him because he has the medical degree and you do not? Did he react coolly to your questions or speak to you as if he was chastising you for questioning him?

It is your health, body, life and future being discussed. Probably not his. You or someone is paying for the doctor to provide you with his expertise and you should receive it through word or action as your case necessitates.

Q31: Does the doctor show signs of drug or alcohol use? Was there alcohol on his breath? Was he slurring his words? Did he seem level headed?

> *It would be greatly remiss of me to omit the problem of substance abuse among doctors. Doctors have among the highest rates of drug abuse, alcoholism, divorce, depression, suicide, and sundry other forms of social pathology of any professional group. Within the profession those who are drunks or junkies are cryptically referred to as "impaired physicians."*
>
> — from the book *Morphine, Ice Cream, Tears,* by Joseph Sacco, MD; William Morrow and Company, 1989

Q32: Have you spent enough time with the doctor and done enough checking up on his background to make an informed decision in choosing him over another doctor?

Q33: On what merits have you based your decision to allow this particular doctor to perform surgery on you?

Was your decision based on the doctor's charisma, wit or charm? Do you believe he is trustworthy? Does he treat you like he owns you? Is he rude, perverse, or does he act like you are inferior to him? Does he treat you like one of his best buddies? Does he seem too eager to do the operation? Has the doctor spoke of the operation as if it is some kind of secret magical procedure? Has the doctor made inappropriate sexual comments or touched you in a sexual way?

Some doctors will give you a questionnaire that asks your opinion on the doctor, his staff, and their services. Do not fill it out. It might be used against you if for some reason you end up taking the doctor to court.

Q34: Has the doctor answered all of your questions to your satisfaction? Are there still things that are not clear to you?

Get answers.

• OTHER PATIENTS

Q35: Can you see photos of the doctor's former patients who have received operations similar to the one you are looking into? Does the doctor have photos of patients at various stages of healing?

Q36: Could you meet people he has operated on?

Q37: Has the doctor ever had a patient who received the operation you are requesting who was disappointed? Why was the patient disappointed?

Q38: Has one of the doctor's patients ever died as a result of any operation the doctor has performed?

It is a bold question. Depending on what type of doctor he is, a cancer doctor (oncologist) for instance, a history of patient deaths is to be expected. But if he is a doctor who practices a less involved type of medicine — a dentist, cosmetic surgeon, or dermatologist — a patient death is much less acceptable.

Even if the doctor did have a patient die while that patient was undergoing surgery, this still does not mean the doctor was negligent. There may have been an adverse reaction to anesthesia, an underlying health condition, or the patient may have withheld information about their health which led to the death. On the other hand, the doctor may have simply been purely negligent and created a situation that caused a patient to die.

If you do ask the question you may be surprised by the doctor's candid honesty or appalled by his arrogance or distasteful reaction to your question.

• WEIGHING THE BENEFITS AND RISKS

Q39: Are there any pamphlets or other literature that the doctor suggests that you read before you make a decision to have the operation?

Q40: What are the likely benefits of the surgery?

Q41: If you are having this surgery to repair damage, will the surgery itself cause more damage and health risks than the original injury?

Q42: If you are going in for some operation that will supposedly save your life, what are the statistics regarding the surgery's success rate? Do people who have had the operation actually live longer? What is their quality of life?

Q43: What will you be like if you do not have this operation? Will your quality of life be the same, or is this operation, if it turns out correctly, going to improve some area of your life?

Q44: Could being more conscientious about diet and exercise eliminate what is causing you to consider this surgery?

For example, if you are overweight and are planning to undergo liposuction to remove fat that can be lost if you took better care of yourself.

Q45: Are there other ways to treat your condition that could be tried before surgery? Why did you choose this operation instead of another operation or a non-surgical treatment?

Q46: Will the surgery create a long-term problem that does not currently exist?

Q47: What is the chance that more than one surgery will be needed to correct any problem arising from the original surgery?

Q48: Will having this surgery create a situation where you will be more dependent on doctors? For instance, will you need yearly checkups on the surgical site or are you getting some type of implant that may need to be replaced or that cause future problems?

Q49: If you are getting some sort of man-made material put into your body, do you know the risks involved with that implant? Is the implant approved by the Food and Drug Administration?

Does the implant arrive from the manufacturer in a sterilized condition or does it have to be sterilized by someone in the surgical team in the operating room or sometime before it is inserted into your body? How is it sterilized? Is there special equipment involved? Does the sterilization process involve heat or liquids? Is the liquid something that you can have a reaction to?

Is the implant altered in anyway by the doctor or his staff? Is there any glue or other substance involved with these alterations? What type of glue is it? Can your body have a reaction to the glue?

There have been cases where medical supply companies have sold implant devices to unknowing doctors who were told by the supplier that the devices were FDA approved when in fact they had not been.

Do you have the information from the manufacturer of the implant that lists the risks involved with placing the material in the human body? Some implants come with information that is meant to be given to the patient.

Contact some of the implant groups listed in the research section of this book and ask them if they have any information about people having problems with similar implants.

Q50: If something does go wrong with this surgery, how will it affect your family, job, finances, and other areas of your life?

Q51: What kind of burden will your family experience because of your undergoing this surgery?

• YOUR MOTIVES

Q52: Did you plan to have this surgery in the past and then cancel? What was the reason you decided not to have the operation? Does that reason still stand?

Q53: Do you feel uncomfortable letting people know that you are going to undergo cosmetic surgery? What would you think of another person who has had cosmetic surgery?

If you are doing it secretly, how would you feel if you are disappointed with the result and it is on an area where you cannot hide it or it gives you an odd appearance?

If the doctor goes too far with the procedure and you end up with a gross distortion of your desired surgical result, your displeasure may be too overwhelming to ignore. Even if the surgery was performed on an area that is usually covered by clothing, you may not be able to cover up your unhappiness about the ordeal.

Q54: Will the surgery alter a feature that is unique to you and that distinguishes you from the rest of the crowd?

Your unique appearance and imperfections may be what make you noticeable and attractive. They may give you a distinctive appearance and may be a compliment to your personality. In any case, undergoing the surgery might rob you of a quality that is a fixed part of your identity.

Q55: Will the surgery make you look different from the rest of your family and your children? Have you discussed your surgery with your family? How did they respond?

Q56: How will your family, spouse, children and others react to your looking different?

Q57: Has someone tried to talk you out of the surgery or simply told you that you should not have it done? Have you considered their viewpoint?

Q58: Was anyone angry about your plan to undergo cosmetic surgery? Did anyone make any kind of threat against you or threaten to harm the doctor who will operate on you? Have you discussed this with your doctor?

Q59: How do you feel about perhaps not being able to recognize yourself?

Depending on the operation you are having there may be a big change in the way you look to the point that you may look so different that even you will not recognize your reflection right away. This could be what you want. On the other hand, it may be a bad thing if the doctor did more than you wanted done or if you were left deformed or, in your opinion, unattractive.

If you are getting breast implants, breast reduction, liposuction, or some other procedure that will change your bodys' proportions, you may need to purchase new clothes.

Q60: Has your decision to undergo surgery been influenced by the doctor's advertising, his staff or testimonials of former patients of the doctor?

Some doctors will perform cosmetic procedures on his staff because it is good advertising for him.

Q61: Is the doctor or his staff trying to convince you to have more done than you originally intended? Has the doctor responded to you as if he knows what is best for you regardless of what your goals of the surgery are?

Even some people who spend years in art school are incapable of creating a "piece" that anyone else but the artist can appreciate. Just because a person makes his living as a cosmetic surgeon does not mean the work he puts out looks pleasing to anyone other than to him.

Q62: Do you feel the doctor may have convinced you to get treatment for a medical condition that is not serious enough for surgical treatment?

• SECOND AND THIRD OPINIONS

Q63: Have you visited at least one other doctor to get a second opinion about your situation?

Always get a second opinion by a financially unrelated doctor whenever you are told that you need to undergo surgery and when no emergency exists.

Q64: Did the doctor become impatient when you mentioned that you were going to have a second opinion?

Do not submit yourself to surgery based on one doctor's opinion. Your insurance company may cover the cost of the second opinion because it helps to avoid unnecessary surgery.

Q65: If you have a family doctor, did you discuss your plans to have this surgery and ask him about the doctor you are considering for the surgery?

- Ask your family doctor if he knows anything about the surgeon you have chosen.

A doctor may have some insight as to who the really bad doctors are in your city.

- Ask him if he has any advice on the testing that should be done before you have the surgery, preparation you should do, location where the surgery will take place, what safety precautions you should take and any other advice he can give you.

• OUTPATIENT SURGERY

Q66: Does the doctor have hospital privileges to do the operation you are thinking about having?

When the doctor performs the operation in a hospital and the nurse sees him do something wrong, the nurse is obligated to inform quality control at the hospital. The hospital will then be prepared to protect itself by taking actions against the doctor or by preparing for a possible lawsuit. When the doctor performs the operation in his office suite, there is no one higher up than himself. Any actions that can be taken against him because of his negligence will be the result of a malpractice lawsuit or the rare action by the state medical authorities or the Drug Enforcement Administration.

Call the hospital the doctor is associated with and find out if the doctor has privileges at the hospital to perform the specific procedure you are seeking.

Q67: Is the outpatient surgery center licensed by the state? Is it accredited by the Accreditation Association of Ambulatory Healthcare and/or the American Association for Accreditation of Ambulatory Plastic Surgery Facilities?

Surgery centers that are accredited by these Associations have met various standards. Doctors have to pay to have their facilities inspected. A doctor who has gone through the extra effort to have his facility accredited is looking out for the safety of his patients.

Q68: Does the doctor have an emergency transfer agreement with a local hospital?

If you are having the operation in the doctor's office or at an outpatient surgery center and an emergency arises during the operation that requires more attention than he can give you there, he will need to transfer you to the hospital. Therefore, your doctor needs to have an emergency transfer agreement with the local hospital.

Q69: Are the elevators, doorways, and hallways of the doctor's surgical suite big enough to accommodate a surgical table, should an emergency arise that requires you to be moved on it?

Q70: Is there an emergency power supply for the operating room?

Q71: If you are having outpatient surgery and there is a complication that makes it necessary for you to be transferred to a hospital, will your insurance cover the expense?

• THE HOSPITAL

Types of hospitals:
- **Specialty hospital**: usually concentrates on one type of health concern such as cancer or rehabilitation
- **Private hospital**: owned by a corporation, religious group or private individuals. Hospitals owned by insurance companies (such as Kaiser) fall under this category
- **University hospital**: is on the grounds of a university and is used to help teach medical students
- **Private hospital associated with a medical school**: a privately-owned hospital as described above that has an affiliation with a medical school that uses the hospital to help teach its medical students
- **Public hospital**: is owned by either the federal government (veterans hospitals), the state, county or city. Public hospitals are often associated with medical schools. Patient bills are often paid in whole or in part by government agencies
- **Military hospitals**: for military personnel, their spouses and children. They also may be used by politicians, such as those around Washington, DC.

Q72: If you have health insurance, what hospitals are affiliated with your insurance? The hospital will be able to tell you if they are under contract with your insurance company, or you can call the insurance company and ask them for the names of the hospitals in your area that accept your insurance.

Q73: If you are to stay in a hospital after the operation, have you visited and checked out the hospital, its staff, and its resources?

Contact the hospital's public relations or administration office. Ask to see a copy of the hospital's admittance form and other printed material concerning your rights and responsibilities as a patient. The hospital may have a *Patient's Handbook* or a formal *Statement of Patient's Rights* or a *Patient's Bill of Rights* that you can see or obtain a copy of.

The American Hospital Association supplies its member hospitals with its *Patient's Bill of Rights*. To get a copy of this document, call the AHA at the phone number given in the Research Resources section of this book. Compare the document you receive from the AHA with the document you obtained from the hospital and make note of any differences.

Q74: Is the hospital accredited by the American Osteopathic Association, Medicare or the Joint Commission on Accreditation of Healthcare Organizations (or all three)?

Accreditation is a voluntary procedure that the hospitals pay for to show that the facility has passed certain standards.

A hospital that is accredited through the JCAHO goes through an inspection at least every three years. If a hospital has "conditional accreditation" from the JCAHO, this means that the facility did not pass the inspection but has been given a set period of time to correct certain shortcomings. The JCAHO will tell you if a hospital is accredited, conditionally accredited or not accredited. They will also tell you the date of the hospital's last survey and when it is up for renewal. As of October, 1994, the JCAHO began making the detailed facility performance reports available to the public for a cost of $30.

A hospital that has been accredited by the JCAHO is automatically accepted by the federal government as qualified to participate in the Medicare program and by most states as qualifying for state licensure.

The JCAHO is not a government agency and is financed and run by the medical industry. There have been JCAHO-accredited hospitals that have failed government inspections.

(The phone number to the JCAHO is in the Research Resources section of this book under the heading of Accrediting Healthcare Facilities.)

Q75: Is the hospital a teaching hospital? This means that the hospital is associated with a local medical school and students take part in treating the patients. A teaching hospital is more likely to have the latest equipment and a staff who is familiar with the latest developments in their field. The medical students and student nurses are supervised by doctors and hospital staff. The residents and interns often move (rotate) among the various units within the hospital so they get experience in different areas of medicine.

If you are being treated by an intern (a recent medical school graduate) be aware of the presence of the "attending" or "supervising physician." Any crucial medical decisions should be made by the attending physician and not solely by the intern. Also, if there are any invasive procedures that are being performed, the attending physician should be closely supervising the procedure. Regardless, whenever you are being treated by an intern the attending physician should be in the building and not "on call" at home, at church or out playing golf.

Q76: Who will be attending you in the hospital?

New interns and residents arrive in hospitals at the beginning of July to begin a year of their postgraduate medical training. There they will gain experience through their work on the hospital patients. It is "hands-on training" in the purest form and it is part of the way medical students who become doctors learn their profession.

In addition to the doctors, nurses, interns, residents, housecleaning staff, and hospital administrators who may come into your room, there also may be representatives from pharmaceutical companies and medical device manufacturing companies. They may be there on a sales visit or to check up on their companies' products as part of their research and development processes and to see if the equipment is being used properly.

The nurses and others who tend to you in the hospital follow your doctor's orders that are detailed in your chart. This way they will know what drugs you are taking and when to give them to you, what tests to give you and what physical activity and dietary needs you have. Usually a specific nurse will be assigned to you and will coordinate your care as directed by your doctor. The nurse who is caring for you will also have several other patients to take care of. The nurse will be supervised by the head nurse of the hospital unit you are in. If you are having difficulty communicating with the nurse who is caring for you, the head nurse may be able to help settle your concerns.

As in other industries, the medical industry is increasingly dependent on temporary workers. One reason for this is the increased pressure to lower costs. Hospitals no longer have to keep a full staff of nurses and doctors on the payroll. They can use healthcare temp agencies to hire temporary nurses, doctors, therapists and other staff as they are needed. These temporary workers may be used to fill in for vacationing hospital staff or used during the winter season when people tend to get sick more often.

If you are in a hospital that has a religious affiliation there may be a nun or priest or other type of minister stopping by your room to say hello. If you are not associated with that church you should not feel obligated to spend time with this minister unless you would enjoy the company. Otherwise, if you are trying to rest, kindly let the minister know that you would like to be left alone. You are there to receive medical treatment, not to be preached to. Additionally, the hospital may have a small chapel on the premises where you can go to pray or meditate if you are allowed to travel that far from your room.

Q77: How long should you expect to stay in the hospital?

Patients do not stay in the hospital as long as they did just a few years ago. This is due in part to the advances in surgery techniques and surgical instruments that inflict less trauma on the body. Though it is probably in your best interest to remain in the hospital until the doctor says it is safe to go home, no one can stop you from leaving. If you do leave earlier than the doctor advises, you are then leaving "against medical advice." A patient wanting to leave a hospital earlier than the doctor advises could be unsatisfied with the treatment or may have business or family matters that need their attention. Whatever the reason is, checking out of the hospital against medical advice can interfere with your medical insurance coverage. If negligent treatment was what motivated the patient to leave the hospital early, the patient may be wise to consult with another doctor or a lawyer to document the unsatisfactory treatment.

Unless you are a criminal detained in the jail ward of the county hospital or mentally unstable, you cannot be held in a hospital against your will. You have the right to walk out of the hospital without paying your bill and without signing any paperwork.

If you have been told by the nurses that it is time for you to leave the hospital and you feel too sick to leave, ask to speak to your doctor. There may be a complication that the nurses are unable to recognize and that would require that you receive close medical attention and a longer hospital stay.

Q78: If you are going to be traveling from out of town, does the hospital have an arrangement for discount rates at a local hotel?

This hotel arrangement may be helpful to your family if they are traveling with you. You also may not have to check into the hospital until the morning of the surgery and staying in the hotel the night before may be convenient. You may also need to stay in town some days after surgery.

Q79: Will you be on pain medication during your stay in the hospital?

Pain medication can distort your judgment. If there are any major decisions that you need to make during your time in the hospital is there a relative, friend or lawyer who can help you with your decisions?

Q80: Does the hospital keep a doctor on staff who deals specifically with infections?

Q81: Are you allergic to any foods? Will the hospital accommodate any of your special dietary needs? Can you speak to the hospital dietitian if you have any questions about dietary needs?

If you have visitors when you are in the hospital, do not let them eat the food on your tray without letting the nurse know. The nurse may be keeping records of what you eat and drink. Similarly, if you are visiting someone in the hospital, do not give them food or drinks that you bring in without first asking the nurse. The food may interfere with medication or the patient may not be allowed any food or may be limited to certain types of food.

Q82: Will you be in a private room or will you have a roommate? Does the room have privacy curtains that surround the bed and are they in working order?

Private rooms usually cost extra. If you have an infectious disease you will be in a private room. If you are able to walk around while you are in the hospital you may want to bring a robe.

Q83: Where are the emergency buttons located in the patient rooms?

Q84: Are there private bathrooms in each patient room? Does the shower or bathtub have safety bars so you can steady yourself while you are in the shower? Are there anti-slip surfaces on the bathtub or shower floor and on the bathroom floor? You are likely to be on pain medication and this may affect your balance.

Q85: Do the patient rooms or the bathrooms have mirrors?

Depending on what you are having done, it may be a good idea to avoid mirrors.

Q86: Are there security guards on the hospital grounds?

If you are being stalked by someone and you do not want them to know you are in the hospital, tell the hospital admissions clerk that you need to be registered under a pseudonym. If the admissions clerk is unable to help you, ask to speak to a social worker at the hospital. Demand that no one is to be told that you are registered at the hospital unless you want them to know. The social worker can help ensure your safety and this can include arranging for a protective restraining order to help protect you from anyone who may try to harm you during your stay in the hospital.

Q87: If the surgery is being done to a child and requires the child to stay overnight in the hospital, does the hospital have a security tracking system?

Some hospitals and nursing homes now have systems that can prevent patients who are wearing a wristwatch-type of monitor from going through certain doorways. The monitor triggers a sensor that locks the door when the person wearing the monitor approaches the door. The monitor can both protect a child from wandering through the halls of the hospital and prevent the child from being kidnapped from the hospital.

Q88: How do you exit the hospital in case of an emergency?

Q89: Where do you park while you stay in the hospital and is there a charge for parking?

Q90: What are the visiting hours at the hospital and where do your guests park?

• THE NURSING STAFF

Q91: Are the staff nurses who will be present during and after the surgery and other personnel trained in emergency services, such as cardiopulmonary resuscitation?

This question may sound out of place but there have been lawsuits based around patients not receiving the most basic forms of emergency treatment when it was needed while they were undergoing medical care.

Q92: What level of training does the nurse who will be present during the operation have and where did the nurse get their training? What educational degree does the nurse carry?

The more help the doctor receives while he is operating on you, the more attention he can give you. A registered nurse has more training than a practical nurse.

The nurse should have gone to a legitimate school. You should not trust yourself with a nurse who received their degree from some third-rate career training center or correspondence school.

Q93: If the registered nurse (RN) is certified through the American Nurses Credentialing Center, what year were they certified?

A certification is valid for five years. After five years the nurse will have to be recertified to show they have continued to maintain an up-to-date knowledge of the profession.

Q94: Does your state have a Board of Nursing, and if not, what health authority regulates the nurses in your state?

Does this authority release information on disciplinary actions taken against specific nurses?

Q95: Does your state require nurses to be licensed and to take continuing education courses?

Q96: Is the nurse who is caring for you legally working in the country?

Q97: How long has the nurse worked at the hospital or with the doctor?

A temporary nurse who is filling in for the regular nurse may not be familiar with the layout of the hospital or where the emergency supplies are stored.

Be careful what the nurse writes on the record. The doctor may base his decision on inaccurate information that was written on your record by other people.

• THE SURGICAL TEAM

Q98: Is the entire surgery performed by the doctor or is part of it to be performed by a surgeon who is in training or another person?

To have a less expensive operation you can go to a medical school and have a student operate on you with a physician's supervision. That is an option and is your decision to make. If you want only the full-fledged doctor whom you hired to perform the operation, include this in the consent form.

Q99: Will there be any students, medical equipment company representatives or other people present during the operation who are there simply to observe the procedure?

Q100: Will a registered, licensed, board-certified anesthesiologist or a registered nurse certified anesthetist be present during the operation?

Again, the more well educated help the doctor has in the operating room, the more attention he can give you. An anesthesiologist or nurse anesthetist can become very valuable if there is a complication during the operation.

> **You want the person administering the anesthesia to have a thorough knowledge of the complexity of anesthesia.**
> - If you choose a physician-anesthesiologist, find out if they are board certified by checking with the American Board of Anesthesiologists. The phone number is in the Research Resources section of this book under the heading of Anesthesiology.
> - If you choose a nurse-anesthetist, find out if they are a registered nurse and a member of the American Association of Nurse Anesthetists. The phone number is in the Research Resources section of this book under the headings of Nurses and Anesthesiology.

• PRICE, PAYMENT AND INSURANCE

Q101: Is the price you are quoted all inclusive or are you going to have to pay separately for the doctor, the anesthesiologist, the operating room, and the post-surgical care such as physical therapy?

Ask the doctor's office manager if you can get a discount on the price you are paying for the surgery.

Q102: Are the follow-up appointments included in the price?

Q103: What is the total cost of having the surgery? How will it affect your financial status?

This includes the doctor's fee, the operating room, the anesthesiologist, the medicines, any money spent because of the surgery and the amount of money being lost by time spent off from work.

Q104: Does the doctor accept your insurance? Is your insurance going to pay for any of this and exactly how much?

Some doctors have become rich by supplying false information to insurance companies. Some doctors will make their patients think they are doing them a favor by getting the insurance to cover part or all of an operation by supplying the insurance company with inaccurate information. Sometimes this act is legitimately sympathetic and helps the patient out of a struggle. Other times the doctor may be doing it out of greed. The doctor gets the money while the patient receives an operation they do not need and is further inconvenienced by the recovery and possible complications. Where is the favor in that?

Q105: Do you need to supply the doctor's office with the insurance forms?

Q106: Will the surgery interfere with any future health insurance coverage?

Q107: If you are financing the operation on credit, how much will you need to pay per month? How much is it going to cost altogether with the interest charges added in? How many years will you be making payments?

Q108: Does the hospital have a patient services department that will help you sort through insurance forms and medical bills? Call the hospital billing department if you have any questions about your bill. (See the Billing Problems heading of the Research Resources section of this book for the phone number of companies that can help you figure out your medical bills and correct overcharges.)

• SIGNING THE CONSENT FORM

Q109: Can you get a copy of the consent form weeks or days ahead of time so that you can read it carefully and make sure it describes the operation you are, in fact, there to have?

Does the doctor have any apprehension about you making alterations to the consent form to make sure you get what you want?

One way to protect yourself is to cross out anything on the consent form that you do not agree to. Customize it to fit your needs and so it is in your best interest. Make sure the doctor knows the changes you have made and discuss any concerns you or the doctor has about the changes.

Q110: Have you had the name of the doctor who is to perform the surgery written into the consent form?

Q111: Have you written into the consent form that an anesthesiologist or nurse anesthetist is to be present to administer the anesthesia and also is to remain immediately physically available if he/she is needed during the surgery and is to be physically present at the time the surgery is finished until you have recovered from the surgery?

Q112: Have you had it written into the consent form what side of the body the operation is to be performed on?

If you are undergoing surgery that is to only take place on one side, be sure to have this noted in the consent form. Medical mistakes are known as "misadventures" in the medical community. A hospital in Florida that had admitted to mistakes where doctors amputated the wrong foot on one patient and operated on the wrong knee of another implemented the practice of writing "NO" in black felt pen on the side that is not to be operated on.

Q113: Is the doctor asking you to sign a waiver or release that aims to limit the legal action you can take in case the doctor or the medical team is negligent?

Contact a malpractice lawyer and ask for advice before signing anything that seeks to limit your legal abilities.

• WILLS

Q114: Have you made out a will?

You can find information about wills at the library or your local bookstore. There are also lawyers who specialize in this area.

Q115: Do you have a living will and does the doctor know about it?

Q116: Have you signed a "donor card" so your healthy organs can be given to someone else who needs them if you die?

See the heading of Organ Donation and Transplants in the Research Resources section of this book.

• SPECIAL HEALTH CONSIDERATIONS

Q117: Were you honest with the doctor about your health history? Do you have a medical condition requiring specialized treatment?

This is not a time to overlook health problems that could cause or contribute to complications with your surgery and the healing process. People who already have health problems are more likely to have complications. If you have diabetes, asthma, bleeding problems, high blood pressure, heart problems, are currently on medication or have other health concerns, you need to be honest with the doctor and let him know. Smokers also have a higher rate of complications after surgery than non-smokers. Contact your other doctor and ask him if having this operation will cause problems with your health.

• WOMEN'S CONCERNS

Q118: If you are having a breast exam you should make sure a female nurse is in the room at the time the doctor is examining you.

Q119: When is your menstrual period?

Women should avoid elective surgery just before their menstrual period.

Q120: If your are planning on getting pregnant, do any medications you are taking because of this surgery have side effects that can interfere with the development of the fetus?

Contact Healthy Mothers, Healthy Babies Coalition, 409 — 12th Street SW, Washington, DC 20024, Phone (202) 863-2552 or 863-2458.

Q121: If you are nursing a baby, what is the waiting period for the anesthetic to clear your system before you can nurse again? Will any other medications interfere with your child's needs?

Ask the obstetrician or pediatrician about these concerns.

• MEDICATIONS

- Do not take medications that have been prescribed to another person.
- Do not mix medications without first asking your doctor and/or pharmacist if the two medications are safe to take

at the same time. This includes over-the-counter medicines.

- Do not expect your doctor to remember all of the prescriptions he may have written for you. The average doctor writes thousands of prescriptions every year. If you are receiving prescriptions from more than one doctor, this increases your chances of taking a dangerous mix of medications.

    If you use the same pharmacist all the time he may have your prescription history in his computer database and can warn you when you may be "crossing medications."

- Dispose of medications at their expiration date. Some medications lose their potency as they age and others may become toxic. Keep them out of the reach of children.

- If you are pregnant, do not take medications without first clearing it with your doctor. This includes medications you have purchased over-the-counter. Your pharmacist may also be able to tell you what medications may be dangerous to the fetus.

- Do not give medications to children that are meant for adults.

- Find out if you are supposed to take the medication with food or water or if they are supposed to be taken on an empty stomach.

- If you are on a medication that has to be injected, do not use the same needle twice and never use a needle that has been used on another person. Dispose of needles immediately after use in a container that is not accessible to children.

- Keep your medications out of the reach of children and pets.

- Keep your medications stored in a dry place. The bathroom is not a good place for medicines because the steam from the bath or shower can spoil them.

- Keep your medications away from heat

- Some medications must be refrigerated. Read the label.

- Do not put more than one kind of pill in the same bottle.

- Do not take medication in the dark.

Q122: Do you have a history of addiction to alcohol or drugs? Have you undergone treatment for drug or alcohol addiction?

Do not be shy in letting the doctor know that you have been addicted to substances. He should then be careful with what type and amount of medication he prescribes, the strengths of the medication. Be careful to let the doctor know that you are letting him know delicate information. If he writes about your drug or alcohol addictions in your medical record, this information may be made available to people whom you do not want to be informed.

Q123: Are there any foods or medications you should avoid in the weeks or days before and after the operation?

Q124: What medications will you be taking before and after the surgery?
Purchase any medications before having the surgery and bring them with you when you have your operation. Your insurance company may only reimburse you for the price of the generic version of any drugs that you are prescribed. Check with your insurance handbook or call your insurance company to find out if there is such a requirement.

Q125: How often do you have to take the medications?
If you are prescribed a drug that is to be taken four times a day, taking four pills all at the same time in the morning is not an option and may be dangerous. Find out if you are to take the medications on a timely basis. For instance, will you have to wake up in the middle of the night to take the medication?

Q126: What are the side effects of the medications?
Have you been taking any medication in the last few months that will interfere with the medication? Inform the doctor of any over-the-counter or prescription medications you have taken within the past few months.
What happens if you do have side effects?
Be aware that some of the positive information you may find about a medication may be information published by the manufacturer or another party who will make money if people choose to use the product. Information from those sources may be misleading. (A book titled *Worst Pills/Best Pills* is available through Public Citizen's Health Research Group. For ordering information see the Publications heading in the Research Resources section of this book.)

Q127: How long will you have to continue to take the medication after the surgery?

Q128: What happens if you run out of medication and you need more? If the doctor is going out of town and you will not be able to speak with him directly, does he have an arrangement with another doctor who will fill any additional medication prescriptions for you?

• TESTS

Q129: Has the doctor performed all the necessary tests to confirm his diagnosis?

Do you know if the doctor has looked at the test results? Did you take the test results with you when you had your second opinion?

Q130: How much do the tests cost? The testing lab may require payment before a test is performed or they may bill to you or your insurance company.

Q131: What tests will be done before you undergo the operation? Where and how are they done?

Q132: Does the doctor own or is he a part owner of the testing equipment or facility where the tests are done?

Q133: Do they plan on taking x-rays of you? What does the doctor expect to find on the x-ray? Are there x-rays of the same body part that another doctor or medical facility has already taken of you that can be sent to the doctor so you can avoid repeat exposure to the radiation that x-rays give off?

Are the personnel who operate the x-ray equipment formally trained about radiation safety and hazards through an approved course given that teaches how to correctly operate x-ray equipment? Have the personnel attended continuing education courses to keep updated on radiographic techniques and new developments?

Every time you are given an x-ray you are exposed to radiation. Some of this electromagnetic radiation remains in the tissues of your body. This can lead to future health problems. X-rays should only be given when they are essential.

Most states do not monitor the personnel who take x-rays and many states do not conduct radiation safety inspections of x-ray equipment and do not know if something is out of place unless a patient makes a complaint with the proper authorities.

When undergoing an x-ray make sure
- The person operating the machinery is properly trained
- You are wearing a protective apron
- If you are undergoing x-rays of the teeth, make sure the technician is using a disposable/sterilization film holder to lower your risk of contracting hepatitis
- The radiology technician who is giving you the x-ray is wearing a radiation monitoring film badge that records their exposure to radiation

Q134: Does the test involve injection of a dye such as iodine? Are you allergic to any of the substances contained in the injection?

Q135: Will experiments be done on any of the tissue that is removed from your body? What is the purpose of these experiments? Is your tissue being used by other people in a way that will bring them financial gain?

Get pathology reports on any tests done on tissue removed from your body.

Q136: How long does it take for the test results to come back?

Do not let the doctor forget to inform you of the test results. If you are not scheduled for an appointment when the test results are expected back, call to find out what the test results are. Get a copy of the results for your personal records.

• FOOD INTAKE

Q137: When is the last time that you can eat before the surgery?

Usually there will be a limit on food and liquid intake for several hours and as much as a day or two before the surgery. This will prevent some complications with anesthesia and the possibility of vomiting during surgery. If the surgeon tells you not to eat, do not eat or you may create problems for yourself. If you vomit during surgery some of the vomit can be breathed into your lungs and this may cause pneumonia.

During surgery the nurse may wet your mouth by putting a wet paper towel in your mouth. This prevents you from getting too dry. When this is done during nasal, sinus, or oral surgery it can make it easier to swallow the blood that will be gathering in your throat. As the blood coagulates, it can irritate the throat and give the feeling of a sore and dry throat and make you cough. Sometimes people who undergo nose jobs vomit up this blood during or after the operation.

Q138: When can you eat after the operation?

Facial surgery patients may be told to avoid foods that require chewing so the muscle movement does not interfere with healing. If the person has had any facial bone damage caused by the surgery and those bones have been set into place, the chewing motion may interfere with the healing of the bone.

There may be other limitations on what you can and cannot eat. Ask the doctor.

• THE SURGICAL PROCEDURES

Q139: What is the name of the procedure you are looking into?

Doctors do not all use the same terms when describing operations and do not all use the same techniques.

Q140: What will you be wearing during the operation?

You may be in your street clothes during the operation or you may have to change into a gown. Whatever you wear, it should be loose fitting and not anything that you will have to pull over your head. Avoid tight clothing, nylons, shoes that need to be tied, or any clothing that is difficult to remove in case a complication arises during surgery.

Q141: What position will you be in during the operation? Will there be any restraints put on you during the surgery to keep your arms, legs, torso, or head immobile?

Some operations require that the patient be tied down to prevent any type of movement that could interfere with the operation.

If you have a physical injury such as a back problem that would require limitations on the position you are in during the surgery, arrangements can be made for your comfort and safety.

Q142: Are any of the procedures experimental or considered to be in an experimental stage?

If it is a new technique, where did the doctor learn it? Who did the original research? Who came out with the technique? Where can you learn more about it?

Q143: Would it be safer to undergo the surgery in stages?

For instance, if you are to undergo eye surgery, would it be better to have one eye operated on and let it fully heal before undergoing surgery on the other eye?

Q144: How long does the operation take?

Q145: What are the steps of the operation from beginning to end?

Q146: Will there be needles or tubes placed in your arms or other areas (between the toes, in the thigh, in the neck, on the tops of the hands, or other areas)? Will you be fed intravenously? Will there be a portacath implanted (this device provides an opening where the nurse can easily draw blood and administer medication)? Will these be placed while you are awake? How long will they remain in place? What kind of pain is involved?

Q147: Do the intravenous pumps have free-flow safety clamps to safeguard against overdoses of medications and IV liquids?

Make it an absolute requirement that any IV used on you be equipped with a free-flow protection device. It can save your health and may save your life.

Q148: Will you have a breathing tube at any time during or after surgery?

When a patient has a tube that goes into the mouth and down the windpipe so a machine can breathe for the patient, it is called being "intubated" or "tubed." The other end of the pipe is connected to a respirator that pumps out oxygen. The tube is called an "ET," or endotracheal tube. The oxygen can also be pumped into the tube manually with a balloon-type device that a nurse squeezes.

The patient is not able to talk during the time the tube is in place. For this reason, you may need to have a pen and writing pad to be able to communicate with others.

Q149: Will any part of your body be shaved? Why, when and by whom? Are you sensitive to razors, or do you easily develop skin rashes? Have you experienced sensitivity to shaving creams? Do you have coarse, curly, thick-stranded hair that twists back into the skin when it is shaved and that causes pimpling or infected hair follicles? These may cause or contribute to infection.

Q150: Will you be under local or general anesthesia?

What is the name of the anesthetic? What are the side effects?

When you wake up from general anesthesia, do not be surprised if the first thing you remember is a nurse standing over you telling you to cough. This coughing will help wake you up and stimulate your lungs and cardiovascular system. You may also be asked to, with the nurse's help, get up and walk around.

Q151: How will the anesthetic be applied? Where are the needles inserted?

Q152: Will there be music playing during the operation? If not, could you bring your own headset and listen to music of your choice?

   The music may help the doctor relax and for you it can drown out any sounds you will hear during the operation. A study by University of Buffalo behavioral researcher Karen Allen, published in the September 21, 1994, issue of the *Journal of the American Medical Association* reported that doctors' stress levels dropped when they played music during surgery.

Q153: What kind of sterility procedures are taken in the operating room? Are the tools heat treated or sterilized with liquids? Who prepares the tools?

   Improperly cleaned tools are one of the leading causes of post-operative infections. Post-operative infections are one of the leading causes of post-operative death. Infections that are acquired in the medical facility where a patient received treatment are called "nosocomial infections."

Q154: Will you be given antibiotic orally or intravenously before the surgery?

Q155: Where and how will the incisions be made?

   Are there different techniques of doing the incisions for the operation you are getting? Will a laser or a scalpel be used to make the incisions? Will there be efforts taken to create the most minimal scar possible?

   If the doctor says the scars will be invisible you should question what he means by this. Scarring after any incision can be expected. They may not end up being very noticeable after a few years and may fade a lot, but more than likely they will always be noticeable upon close inspection. There are certain operations where the incision is made in an area not commonly seen (inside the nose for instance if you are having a nose job). Other incisions can be made where there are naturally occurring folds in the skin (in the folds of the eyelids for instance if you are undergoing eyelid surgery). Some of the most noticeable scars created by cosmetic surgery can occur after a tummy tuck, which leaves a smile scar from hip to hip. Of course a patient should not be concerned about the vanity issue of scars if the operation is something that will overwhelmingly improve the health of the patient.

Q156: Does the operation entail the cutting of any muscles that will no longer be functioning?

During facial cosmetic surgery some cosmetic surgeons, if they think a patient's face is too animated, and without telling the patient beforehand, will cut muscles in the patient's face during surgery. This is sometimes done during nasal surgery when the muscles in the upper lip are cut away from the nasal spine (the bone at the bottom of the septum between the nostrils and above the upper jaw). Some doctors, though they do not inform the patient beforehand, do it every time they do nasal surgery because that is what the doctor was taught to do. This may leave the nose unnaturally stiff. It also changes the shape of the upper lip line and affects the way the upper lip moves. Some doctors will, as stipulated in plastic surgery manuals, alter other muscles in the face, so the face does not move as much, to prevent wrinkles from forming (so they claim). Altering any of the muscles in the face can leave the face unnaturally stiff and with uneven animation or animation that is not in sync with the rest of the person's expressions.

Q157: Is there a chance the surgery will rupture or damage another organ or nerves that control an organ or function of the body?

Q158: Will there be any flesh, muscle, cartilage or bone removed during the operation?

Know what parts of you are going to be altered during the operation so there are no surprises later. One of the rudest surprises that can happen after surgery is when a patient finds the doctor did more and took away more than the patient ever expected. Later the patient finds out that the doctor's definition of a slight change was very different from their own. Once something is cut off the body, it cannot be put back.

Q159: What kind of bleeding occurs during the operation? Is there any chance that you will need to receive blood?

If the surgery causes a large loss of blood, and the chance that you will need extra blood, you may elect to donate your own blood. This can be done starting weeks before the surgery. Even if the blood you have stored is not used, it is better that you have it on hand if there is a chance that it may be needed. This will reduce your risk of contracting a blood-related disease or receiving the wrong type of blood. (See the Blood heading in the Research Resources section of this book.)

Q160: What kind of suture material is used? Are the stitches permanent, dissolvable, or will you have to come in to have them removed? Will there be any staples used instead of sutures on any of the incisions?

There are various thicknesses of suture material (surgical thread). The closer to the number 100 the suture material is, the thinner it is.

Q161: Will there be any drains inserted at the site of the surgical wound? How long will the drains be left in place?

Sometimes drains are used that remain for a few days. This is done so that any excess blood can be eliminated, thus preventing infection.

Sometimes blood clots will form inside the body where it has been operated on. These clots may need to be surgically removed. Blood clots can also travel to other parts of the body. If they settle in the lungs they can halt breathing.

Q162: What kind of bandages are used?

Some bandages are made out of cotton whereas others are a cotton-synthetic blend. Some people are allergic to synthetic materials. This may interfere with healing.

Q163: Will the operation interfere with your sex life, in what way, and for how long? Is there a risk of sexually responsive nerves being cut or damaged during surgery? How close are the incisions to these nerves? (If you are planning on undergoing nasal surgery, read about the VNO in the Nose Job heading in The Deeds section of this book.)

• PAIN

Q164: Is there pain associated with this surgery and what kind of discomfort will you experience during and after the surgery and for how long?

Some pain or discomfort is expected after all surgery because it involves cutting into the body. One patient may feel little pain while another patient who underwent the same operation can experience a lot of pain. The amount of pain after surgery depends on how the operation is done, the patient's pain tolerance, the patient's state of mind and other factors.

If you feel the pain medication that you are prescribed is too strong, ask the doctor if there is another type of drug that is not as strong or if there is a weaker dose available of the same drug, or if cutting the individual pills in half with a knife would be reasonable. Becoming addicted to pain medication is one risk of taking pain medication.

• THE SURGICAL WOUND

Q165: What kind of swelling, bruising and bleeding should you expect to have?

When seeing your bruised and swollen body or face you may wonder what you did to yourself. It can sometimes look as if you have been in a horrible accident and can incite or contribute to post-surgical depression.

Many patients are surprised by the amount of swelling and bruising that occurs in the days after their surgery. You want to be prepared for the vision of yourself being bruised and swollen. The doctor may have photos that he can show you of other patients at the peak of their swelling and bruising period after they have gone through the same or similar surgery.

Any uneven or excessive swelling or pain, or pain that comes on suddenly, may be a sign of complications. You should inform the doctor if these occur.

Q166: Are you supposed to apply ice packs to the wound to control swelling?

This may require that you purchase plenty of plastic zipper bags to put the ice in. Frozen peas, corn or small ice cubes may be better to use on facial wounds than large ice cubes because they are lighter — but have a variety of ice packs ready. Placing a thin cloth over the skin so the ice bag does not sit directly on the skin will prevent the skin from getting too cold and will also absorb any dripping water that should not get on the wound.

• POST-SURGICAL CARE

Q167: How will the bandages be applied and are you supposed to change the bandages when they become dirty, or is the doctor or his staff supposed to do that?

If you are going to have to change your bandages, you will have to know what supplies to purchase. Purchase everything days before you undergo the surgery so that you or someone caring for you will not have to run around buying it when you should be in bed recovering.

Q168: How are you to keep the area of the incisions clean?

You may need to clean the incision areas gently with a sterile cotton swab or gauze dipped in hydrogen peroxide. Ask the doctor what he recommends and purchase these materials before the surgery.

You may be limited in the way you can shower, bathe and wash your hair for days or weeks after surgery.

If you had surgery on your scalp, the use of hair sprays, gels, creams and lotions will also be limited before and after surgery until the stitches have been removed. Ask your doctor when it will be safe for you to start using hair products.

Q169: Who is going to take care of you and be with you for the first 1 to 10 days after the surgery?

Because you may be on medication that can distort your judgment or you may be overwhelmed by the surgery, it is important to have someone around you for the initial healing period. This should be someone who can make a responsible and safe decision as to what medical attention you need.

If you are going to need a visiting nurse, physical therapist or other person to come to your home to treat and assist you after the surgery, the discharge planner or social worker at the hospital, your insurance company or your doctor may arrange for this or supply you with the phone number of an agency that supplies the services you will need.

Q170: Will you need any special equipment (wheelchair, hospital bed, oxygen, crutches, cane, etc.) for your recovery at home?

Where can you get this equipment? Can it be rented or do you have to purchase it?

Q171: Is the doctor available for you to call if you have questions during your recovery? Who will answer the phone when you call if there is an emergency after office hours? Does the doctor carry a pager? Is the doctor going to be in town during the first two weeks after your surgery?

If the doctor is going out of town within two weeks after your surgery you will want to know about it. In case there is a problem of some sort, you want to have access to a doctor who can give you the attention you need. The doctor may have an arrangement with one or more doctors who take over for him when the doctor goes out of town. Other doctors may use a "locum tenens" doctor who is basically a doctor who is hired from a temp agency that supplies medical professionals to fill in for workers who are on vacation or who are sick or when there is a need for more workers.

Q172: Will there be a day or more when you will be confined to your bed before or after the operation?

Q173: What kind of activities should be avoided in the days, weeks and months following the operation?

Q174: If you are having a facial operation, will wearing glasses interfere with any of the healing processes?
Some surgeries of the face and ears require that the person avoid wearing glasses during the healing process. There is an eyeglass cradle available that attaches to the forehead and elevates the glasses off the face. This is not helpful after ear-pinning surgery because the glasses would still sit on the ears. Check with the doctor to see what the limitations will be if you wear eyeglasses.

Q175: Will the operation prevent you from being able to wear makeup for any period of time?
You may be told to clean the area well the night before the surgery and again on the morning of the surgery. No creams, lotions, oils, perfumes, powders or makeup should be applied to the area that will be operated on. Makeup will probably need to be avoided for a few days after the stitches are removed. If you perm, die, tint or bleach your hair, it is a good idea to do this no later than a few days before surgery if the surgery is being performed on the face or head. Hair coloring and perms may also need to be avoided for several weeks after the surgery.

Q176: How long will it be at longest before you can get back to work?

Q177: How many days will you need to remain off from work?
Everyone heals differently. One person getting the same operation as you may or may not have the same amount of swelling, bruising, soreness and bleeding. Adequate rest and nutrition are important for healing.

Q178: What is the chance that you will experience post-surgical depression or surgically induced post-traumatic stress syndrome?

Have former patients of the doctor gone through a depression after undergoing surgery similar to yours?

Does the doctor recommend that you consult with a therapist before the surgery?

People who are sick recover better if they are exposed to people who care about them and pay attention to them. If you are undergoing breast cancer surgery, statistics show that you will recover better if you attend a breast cancer support group. If you have a life-altering disease or other health problem, the doctor, his office or the hospitals' patient relations office may be able to put you in contact with a support group that deals with your condition.

Painkillers are "downers" and can contribute to post-surgical depression. Limit your use of painkillers to the amount that is necessary to relieve pain. The residue from the pain medication will remain in the body's tissues and can contribute to lingering post-surgical depression.

The same caution should be taken with sleeping pills. If you do not need them, do not take them. If you are staying overnight in the hospital, be cautious of a nurse who wants you to take a sleeping pill when you do not need one. The doctor may have prescribed sleeping pills for you if you need them, but this does not mean that you must absolutely take them. The nurse may want everyone on sleeping pills so she does not get bothered.

Be aware of your demands on the nurse who is caring for you. Nurses who work in hospitals are constantly on their feet and this is very tiring. When they work in a large hospital, they can easily walk several miles during one day at work.

Q179: What will the schedule of follow-up visits be after the operation?

Q180: Who will drive you to your follow-up appointments if you cannot drive yourself?

Q181: If there is a problem with the surgery or if you do not like the results, what will the arrangement be if a second operation is needed or requested?

If the doctor did something to you that you do not like or that he is not satisfied with, he may offer you a free operation to correct it after you have gone through a healing period of what could be months or years. A safe waiting period before undergoing a second operation is usually 6 to 24 months, during which the operation site can heal, revascularize and relax. Your specific needs might dictate that you need surgery sooner. Having a second operation too soon on the same location may cause complications including vascularization problems (restricted blood supply) and increased risk of infection.

Letting a surgeon operate on you after he has botched one operation is probably not a wise thing to do. Get a second opinion from an unrelated doctor and investigate your options.

• YOUR MEDICAL FILE

Q182: Have you obtained a copy of the doctor's file on you?

The patient medical records in a doctor's office belong to that doctor. Some doctors sell information from patient records to pharmaceutical companies and medical equipment manufacturers. Other times the records are sold for medical research purposes. Patient names and other identifying information may have been removed from the records before they were sold. Some doctors may have a paper that you sign that explains that his records on you will not be released to anyone other than you unless the doctor's office has your permission. This is a good for you and a doctor who does this is saying that he understands your need for privacy.

It is your legal right to have a copy of your medical record. A doctor's office may request that you pay a small fee for copying your records. A small charge is understandable, but if they want a dollar or more per page, question them on this. They may be trying to discourage you from getting copies. If you want copies of x-rays or medical tests, you should request a copy at the time these are done. If the doctor's office refuses to give you a copy of your record, contact one of the patients' rights groups listed in the Research Resources section of this book under the heading of Patients' and Consumers' Rights.

9 • STRATEGIC PLANNING

Preparing Yourself for Surgery

If you decide to undergo any type of elective surgery, the chances of a successful result are greatly improved if you understand the procedures and the risks, get a second opinion, know the professional history of the operating team, have the surgery in operating facilities that are well equipped and prepare yourself for an adequate recovery period.

The following are suggested ways of preparing for surgery. Following the steps that apply to your situation can increase your confidence that the surgery will be successful, reduce last-minute stress and may speed your recovery.

A. Write down the names of all of the people you are dealing with at the doctor's office and the names of the staff who are going to be in the operating room.

Know what each person's job is and if they are qualified to do their jobs. Remember that you are hiring them, and they are making money from you. You have a right to know what you are paying for and you have the right to refuse treatment from any health professional.

B. Try to schedule your surgery to take place early in the week.

You are likely to receive better treatment if you undergo surgery in the first three days of the week. If you are in the hospital over the weekend you may be cared for by a part-time or temporary nurse who may not be familiar with the hospital, the doctor or the care you need.

C. In the days before the surgery you may need to give blood, and possibly tissue and urine samples for lab testing. Get a copy of the lab results when they come back. Have the doctor explain the test results. Sometimes a doctor forgets to look at the test results.

If the lab report indicates a serious health concern, get a second doctor's opinion. If no emergency exists, assure that surgery is necessary by having another lab go over the test results, or order more test results from a separate test facility before undergoing invasive treatments.

D. When you have your exam and your blood pressure is taken, find out what it is and keep a record of this for yourself. It will consist of a lower number, the diastolic pressure that occurs between the heartbeats, and a higher number, the systolic pressure that occurs when the heart beats.

Depending on your health condition, you may want to purchase your own blood pressure cuff at a medical supply store.

E. Request that you be given your own copy of any "before" photos that are taken. Also request copies of any photos or videos that are taken during the surgery.

Consider taking your own diary of photos before surgery, during the recovery and after healing has taken place.

F. Take care of as many things as possible days before the surgery both at work and at home so you will not be rushing around at the last moment. You do not want to be so rushed that you forget anything that could interfere with the outcome of your surgery.

Make a list of the things you need to do. Prioritize the list and review it throughout the days before the surgery.

Arrange for your paycheck to be mailed to you or directly deposited.

Arrange for someone to take care of your pets and have enough food for the pets to make it through your recovery.

G. Get any prescriptions days ahead of the surgery. Bring the medications with you when you get the operation in case you need them.

Make sure the doctor knows what other prescriptions and over-the-counter medications you are taking. Make a list of them. This list should include every type of medication you are taking including eye drops, cold remedies, birth control pills and pain killers such as aspirin or Tylenol.

Read the information about the medication that is supplied by the manufacturer.

Know what you cannot eat with the medications, when you are supposed to take them and what the side effects are for each medication.

Know what the pills look like, what they are supposed to accomplish and how much to take.

Avoid taking medication in the dark. One of the most common mistakes made in hospitals has to do with patients being given the wrong medication or an improper amount of the right medication. If someone else is giving you the pills, make sure they are giving you the right ones.

It may be helpful to create a checklist calendar for taking medications according to the proper time intervals so you know you have taken them and do not take double doses. This is especially helpful if you are taking a medication that can distort your judgment, or if you are in and out of sleep.

Make note of any changes in your mood, mental capabilities, vision, and any physical changes you experience after taking a medication. Physical changes may include a rash on the skin, nausea, breathing difficulties, dizziness or rapid heart beat. Tell your doctor if you experience these types of side effects.

Some people experience side effects with antibiotics. If you experience nausea or other sickness from the antibiotics or other drugs, do not just stop taking the medications. Notify your doctor of the problem. There may be different types of medication you can take or there may be ways to avoid the side effects, or you may no longer need the medication.

H. Get a thermometer and take your temperature two or three times a day while you are recovering (Normal body temperature stays around 98.6° Fahrenheit). Keep a chart and note any changes. Contact the doctor if there is any unexpected change. A fever is not necessarily a bad thing as it is part of the body's healing process, but let the doctor know if it gets out of hand. Fever may be a sign of an infection and underlying problems.

Other changes and symptoms to be concerned about that you should report to your doctor include
- If you have injured the surgical wound, especially if it starts to bleed or if you have damaged the sutures
- Your incision burns, especially if mucus is present on the wound or the area around the incision turns red
- Prolonged rapid heartbeat
- You fainted

- Heavy sweating, trembling, dizziness, nausea, or breathing difficulties
- Inability to eat food, and especially if this is accompanied by forceful vomiting
- Sensitivity to sound or sensitivity to light
- A continuous headache
- Unmanageable pain and especially pain that comes on suddenly
     How would you describe the pain?
     - Does it radiate to other areas?
     - Does it throb as your heart beats?
     - Does it only happen when you make a certain movement or is it always present?
     - Is it a dull or a sharp pain?
- Pain when urinating or defecating or inability to urinate or defecate. Be careful not to use too much force when going to the bathroom because the pressure can break open sutures and cause incisions to bleed
- Bloody stool or urine
- Unexpected swelling or bruising beyond what the doctor told you to expect
- Inability to focus your eyes or blurred or double vision
- Loss of function such as speech or inability to move a limb
- Your condition does not improve the way the doctor said it would even though you have done everything he has told you to do

Complications such as infection or bleeding can be a serious threat to your health. They should be given prompt attention.

Many lawsuits have been brought against doctors who did not respond to situations where patients' health was at risk, and many patients have died after complications were ignored. If you are experiencing complications and are concerned that the doctor dismisses your concerns too quickly or does not seem to know how to manage your pain or may not be giving you the attention you need (he seems to be overwhelmed with his workload or for some other reason), it may be time to find the medical attention you need by contacting another doctor or by checking into the local emergency room.

I. Have a few clean hats handy that you can wear if you are having a surgery that prevents you from washing your hair. Baseball caps partially hide the face and provide some protection to anyone receiving a facial operation. If the surgery is going to make the upper head swell, the hats will need to be larger to accommodate any swelling. Do not wear a hat that rubs against an incision or surgical wound. Scarves and bandannas may also be helpful.

J. Pay attention to your nutrition. Your body is going to need nutrients so it can heal itself, and there are certain foods that contain healing properties. Health food stores usually carry books on nutrition. (One such book is The *Food Pharmacy Guide to Good Eating*, by Jean Carper; Bantam Books, 1991.)

K. Spend some time days before the surgery to make meals and freeze them in individual meal-size containers that can be heated in a microwave. If you are having a surgery that requires that you do not chew for a certain amount of days or weeks, you may be restricted to soups and liquid foods. Get a juicer or blender to make fresh vegetable or fruit juice. Fresh juices are also full of the nutrients your body can use to heal itself.

L. Depending on your operation, some activity may help you recover faster and some walking and light exercise may help circulation and prevent blood clots, pneumonia and constipation. Ask the doctor what activities would be appropriate for you in your post-surgical condition.

M. Stock up on books, videos, stationery and stamps, hobbies, puzzles and pillows and put your phone next to your bed. Get access to a tape player or CD player so you can listen to soothing music while you rest.

N. Remember that one of the key complications that can arise after surgery is infection. Infection is caused by impurities getting into your system. To limit your exposure to germs, thoroughly clean all the rooms in your home where you will be spending your recovery time. Use hot water (unless otherwise indicated by the manufacturer of the product) to wash bed linen, towels and any clothing you will be using during your recovery. If you are spending a lot of time in bed during your recovery you may want to change your bed linen — or have someone change them for you — every day.

O. Prepare your bathroom so things can be reached easily in case your movements are limited after the surgery. Remove anything on the floor that may cause you to trip or slip. Find out whether you will need to place a stool or chair in the bathtub in case you cannot bend over, sit or stand (a plastic chair or stool that will not float in the tub may be useful; you may be able to rent one from a medical equipment and supplies store). Apply slip guards to your bathtub or shower (these can be bought at most hardware stores). Washcloths can come in handy if you have an operation that prevents you from taking a full bath or shower.

P.   Ice packs can relieve some of the bruising and swelling. (Check with the doctor to see if you will benefit from applying ice packs). If you are to use ice packs on the area of the operation, make sure you have enough ice or a source for it that will last for as many days as you need it, at all hours of the day. Make at least a dozen individual ice packs using plastic zipper bags. Some people who undergo facial surgery use frozen peas or corn in place of ice. Adding a little water to the ice bags at the time you use them will help them conform to the shape of the body part you are laying it on. Wrapping the bag in a thin cloth, as in a handkerchief or bandanna, will absorb any water drops and prevent the area from becoming too cold. Paper binder clamps are helpful for clipping the bag in place. You will also need someone with you to get the ice for you so you do not have to keep getting up.

Q.   A daily massage during your recovery on areas that have not been operated on, even if it is limited to the hands, feet or scalp can keep you from getting too uncomfortable when spending a lot of time in bed, can help prevent stiffness, can aid body circulation, can relieve tension and can help prevent bed sores.

R.   Let the doctor's office know how and where you can be contacted the day and night before the surgery. The doctor, the anesthesiologist or the doctor's staff may need to contact you.

S.   Do not bring jewelry with you when you get operated on. You are going to be unconscious in a room full of strangers — and this is not the time to try to look attractive. Leave jewelry at home or in your safety deposit box.

If you are staying in a hospital it may be beneficial to wear an inexpensive watch if you are not able to see a clock from your bed. A digital watch that glows or has a light switch so you can see it in the dark may be helpful. If you are sharing a room, be aware that some people are not able to sleep if they hear a ticking clock. A digital watch will avoid this problem.

Do bring your glasses or contacts, dentures and hearing aids if you use any of these. You will be asked to remove them before surgery but may need them once you recover from the anesthesia.

T. With a relative or friend present, have one last conversation with the doctor before the operation to clear up any concerns you have. You can always delay or back out of an operation and leave.

If the anesthesiologist or anesthetist fails to show up, refuse to have the operation.

U. Do not enter the operating room and do not let the anesthesiologist or anyone else stick needles in your arm until you are sure everything is clearly understood by you and the doctor. There should be no discussion of changes to the planned alterations of your body once you are in the operating room. If the doctor starts talking about doing things differently or doing more things to you than you had already agreed to, that is your cue to leave.

Once the anesthesia makes its way through the needle and into your arm, it is too late to change your mind, and the outcome of the surgery is something you will have to live with for the rest of your life. Any freedom you give the doctor to do what he wants can be an invitation for a big surprise when the bandages are removed. You do not want to find out after the operation that there was a misunderstanding.

V. You may feel more secure and also feel comforted if you have arranged for someone you trust to wait in the waiting room while you undergo surgery. Let the doctor and the nurse know your friend or relative is waiting.

W. Get a copy of the operation report. It may be referred to as the "doctor's operative summary" or "op report." This is the typed version of what was done to you during the surgery. Also, get a copy of the pathologist's report (if there is one) that would show the results of any tests performed on tissues removed from your body. Keep copies of these for your own records.

Some doctors who put false information down on insurance forms also will put false information into the operation report. This can affect your insurance eligibility in the future.

10 • THE DEEDS

Some of the Most Common Cosmetic Operations, Their Prices and Risks

The surgery prices quoted in the following pages are approximate and are based on the prices charged by doctors throughout the United States at the time this book was being written. Because doctors set their own prices, the price of the procedure can vary depending on the price the doctor charges, the surgical team needed, the complexity and location of the operation, and the going rate in the area where you live. The doctor who charges the highest price is not necessarily the best. Patients should also not trust their face to the lowest bidder. The doctor who charges the least may also be cutting corners, and this may sacrifice a certain level of the safety and quality.

Whatever procedure a patient is going through, they should not expect the results to be perfectly symmetrical. In a liposuction procedure, the same amount of fat may not be removed on each side and each side may not heal evenly. Eyelid surgery may leave one eyelid slightly or dramatically different than the other. If a doctor is doing a total reconstruction job on the nose, the patient should not be surprised if the nose is off center.

Not all of the procedures or risks are listed here.

The Face

Aging of the body is not a disease but is a natural occurrence. The older you get the more your body will change. More than anywhere else on the body, your face will show your age. Changes in the fat and muscles beneath the skin, decreasing bone mass, skin moisture and elasticity along with gravity are the natural causes of changes to the skin that no one can avoid. Repeated weight gains, sleeping face down, overexposure to the sun, bad nutrition, drinking alcoholic beverages and smoking also contribute to wrinkles — these can be avoided.

There are many procedures that can be done to alter the appearance of the face. Face-lifts can tighten sagging skin but do little to improve skin texture or reduce fine lines. Chemical peels and dermabrasion are done to remove fine lines, dull skin and discolorations. Some patients elect to have injections of fat, collagen, silicone, Avetine (a powder used in operating rooms to stop bleeding which some cosmetic surgeons are mixing with the patients' blood and injecting into wrinkles) or Botox (a purified form of the deadly toxin that causes botulism which, when injected into the face, temporarily prevents muscle movement by paralyzing them. This can affect the muscles that control the eyes and leave the face lopsided if one muscle is more affected than another) injected into facial wrinkles to soften their appearance.

Before you let a doctor rearrange your face you should find out what the surgeon plans to do to your face and how the alterations will affect the appearance, movement and aging of your face. Any surgical procedure done to alter the appearance of your face can result in a desired appearance, may result in something that you do not like or may leave you deformed. What the doctor believes to be a good result may not be what you want.

• Retin-A

One of the many products being sold as a wrinkle remover is Retin-A (retinoic acid), a vitamin A derivative, which is Federal Drug Administration approved as an anti-acne medication. Since the late '80s, Retin-A has been promoted as a miracle anti-aging cream. It may prevent acne by making skin secretions more watery. Retin-A irritates the skin, which causes swelling, thus temporarily making some wrinkles disappear. It is believed to diminish liver spots and splotchy skin by peeling off the outer layer of skin and increasing collagen production. Retin-A can be effective in decreasing fine wrinkles but should not be held as a wonder potion, as some marketing campaigns have claimed it to be. It has to be used at least once a day for months before any results are seen. Retin-A can cause redness and photosensitizing, thus the patient becomes more sensitive to the sun. Moisturizers and sunscreen should be applied when using Retin-A to avoid sunburn and dermatitis-type reactions. If you plan on using this product, read the printed matter that is supplied by the manufacturer.

• Chemical Peels

Also called "chemabrasion" and "chemical exfoliation"
> Price variances depend on the extent of the peel.
> Glycolic acid peel treatments $100 to 700
> Trichloroacetic acid (TCA) peel $400 to 2,000
> Phenol peel $1,000 to 6,000

Chemical peels are done to do away with the dull outer layer of skin, fine wrinkles and surface scarring, but nothing more. Fine lines can be removed partially or altogether, depending on the extent of the wrinkles, by way of chemical peeling. Frown lines between the eyebrows, and smile wrinkles on the cheeks and chin may also be reduced by chemical peeling. Some people who are considering a face-lift may be satisfied with the results of a chemical peel. Others who undergo a face-lift may elect to undergo a chemical peel several weeks after their face-lift.

Peels can be helpful in removing age spots (superficial keratoses). Age spots can also be removed by having a dermatologist freeze them with liquid nitrogen or surgically scrape them away.

Peels range from the mild peels, or masks, that a person can do at home to treatments done in salons to the more radical treatments that only doctors should apply. Over-the-counter peels (cosmeceuticals) that use alpha hydroxy acids (AHAs) are one of the fastest selling products to hit the makeup counters in years. These fruit acid peels, which are derived from such things as apples, olives and sugar cane, work by loosening the dead cells from the surface of the skin. They speed up the natural process of the skin where old cells fall away and are constantly replaced by new cells from the deeper layers of skin. This exposes the underlying layer of skin that is smoother and moister and may have fewer fine wrinkles.

Chemical peels may not do enough or may do too much. Damage to the eyelids, eyesight, tear ducts or nasal passages can result. The raw skin that is exposed is sensitive and if the peel is left on too long, or the acid is too strong, the skin can be burned. Permanent scarring similar to any bad burn can be the result. As the popularity of chemical peels increases, there is also an increase in the number of dermatologists treating people who have been burned in the chemical peeling process.

Peels do not work well on all skin types. Black, brown, or olive skin should not be chemically peeled. Anyone who is highly freckled or would not want to lose their freckles should not have the procedure done. The line where the skin peel stopped can be very obvious on people who have freckles. A chemical peel can also make the skin of a white person more white.

Anyone who has used Accutane (isotretinoin — a drug prescribed to treat cystic acne) within the previous year should not undergo a peel.

Some doctors use a Teflon-coated scalpel before doing a glycolic acid peel to perform what is called a "derma planing" procedure. They say this removes some of the outer epidermis layer by gently scraping dead cells (it also shaves away the vellus hairs — the fine, often lightly-colored hairs that are found on the skin throughout the surface of the body and head). This derma planing procedure may increase the chance of scarring when the patient is receiving a stronger peel. Some doctors question the value of this derma planing procedure and wonder if it benefits the patient or just the doctor's bank account. They suggest that one of the many facial scrubs that can be purchased at any drug store may do a better job and cost a whole lot less.

Before an acid peel, the skin is washed thoroughly with an antibacterial soap and disinfected with alcohol. Glycolic acid, alcohol, iodine or acetone may be used to degrease the skin and cleanse the pores. One of the following procedures is then performed.

Glycolic peel

Glycolic acid, a derivative of sugar cane, is the most mild chemical used in peels done by doctors and is sometimes done in two to six sessions once a week for as many weeks. A mild form of the acid is what exists in the peels that can be bought over the counter. Each week the strength of the acid is slightly increased. The acid is left on for two to five minutes and then thoroughly rinsed off. A soothing lotion is then applied to the skin. The immediate result may resemble a mild sunburn and it may cause swelling and blisters on sensitive kin. The peel may also ignite pimpling and irritate the skin. Mild scarring may appear on people who scar easily. The pigmentation of the skin may become lighter or uneven — especially on darker complected skin types. Makeup should be avoided for several hours after the peel is done. Rinsing the face thoroughly with cool water a few times within the first several hours after the peel can relieve the burn-like sensation some patients experience.

Trichloroacetic peel

Trichloroacetic acid (TCA) peels are done in sections and may cause some pain. This type of peel is often done by a dermatologist. It is more aggressive than a glycolic acid peel, but less intense than phenol peels.

After a trichloroacetic peel the skin turns red as the upper layer of skin dries out and becomes tight before it eventually peels similar to a sunburn. Healing of the skin usually takes one to two weeks. Exposure to the sun should be avoided for six to eight weeks. An increased sensitivity to the sun is to be expected. The peel may lighten pigmentation. People who scar easily should avoid this peel — especially if they tend to develop keloid scars.

Phenol peel

Phenol (carbolic acid) is a caustic burning chemical and is the most radical, aggressive and risky of the chemical peels. The chemical causes a mild, controlled burn that dissolves the outer layer of skin. A mild peel is used around the eyes and a stronger peel solution is used on the other areas of the face. If it is done wrong it can burn holes in the skin.

Similar to other peels, pigmentation of the skin can be affected by a phenol peel. Anemia can interfere with healing. Pregnant and nursing women should not undergo a phenol peel. Some of the chemical travels into the blood system and the patient needs to have a healthy heart, liver and kidneys to eliminate the chemical from the body. The recovery time varies with each individual's healing abilities. Depending on the type and extent of the peel and the patient's healing abilities, it can take anywhere from one to four weeks for healing to take place.

A phenol peel is considered to be surgery of the skin, and is sometimes referred to as "chemosurgery." The patient undergoing this type of peel needs to be under either local or general anesthesia. An anesthesiologist or nurse anesthetist should be present when a phenol peel is given. There have been people who, because of too much acid being absorbed through their skin, have died from this kind of chemical peel.

Anyone undergoing a phenol peel should be prepared for the pain, swelling and scabbing. The swelling may take several days to subside as the face turns red and peels like a very bad sunburn. Doctor approved medications can be used to reduce any pain. Men who have this done will not be able to shave for several days. The newly exposed skin is pink and should be much smoother and softer than the layers of skin that were removed. The treated skin should become less and less pink over the following several months as it continues to heal. Makeup can be used to lessen the pinkish color of the face during this healing period. Check with the doctor to find out when it will be safe to apply cosmetics. The skin may be sensitive to some cosmetics for a number of weeks or months after a peel. Skin that has had a phenol peel will be sensitive to the sun for several weeks.

• Dermabrasion
Full face $1,000 to 4,500
Partial area $400 to 2,500

The dermabrasion procedure involves literally sanding away the top layer of skin with a skin surgery tool called a "dermabrader." This may be done to smooth scars so they are even with the surrounding skin. Like a chemical peel, dermabrasion may also be done with the goal of removing fine lines on the skin by removing the outer layer of skin so that the underlying layer of fresher, younger-looking skin will be exposed. As with the facial peel, this should be considered surgery and should only be done by a doctor such as a dermatologist.

Depending on the extent of the dermabrasion to be done, freezing spray or a topical or local anesthetic may be used to numb the area being dermabraided. Because of the damage done to the skin, swelling occurs for the first three to seven days. During this time the skin will get red and a fluid appears that then turns into a crust. Scabs may also form. Medication may be prescribed to relieve pain. The skin may become itchy as it heals. Scratching should be avoided. Redness can take months to heal and fade. Sunblock should be used to protect the healing skin.

Unlike chemical peeling, there is a lower risk of pigmentation change with the dermabrasion procedure but scars may occur.

• Fat Transfer Injections

Also known as "autologous fat transplants" and "microliporeinjection"

Price depends on what is done. If it is done at the time of liposuction, it may be included in the price of that procedure.

Fat transferring is sometimes referred to as "fat sculpting." It is most commonly done to reduce facial lines, but is also done to enlarge lips and breasts, fill out the skin on hands and fingers, enlarge the penis and for other techniques. Some form of fat transplantation has been experimented with since the late 19th century. The current popularity of fat transferring is the result of it being a byproduct of liposuction as doctors who do liposuction can make extra money doing fat transferring using the extracted fat.

Because the patient's own fat is used, chances are slim that the patient will have a reaction to it. The fat is removed from an area such as the belly or thighs using the liposuction procedure, then placed in tubes and mechanically spun to clarify it and separate it from the blood. The clarified fat is then injected into the part of the body that is to be filled out or enlarged. A syringe with a large-sized needle is used so the fat is damaged as little as possible.

Depending on the extent of the surgery, the operation can take anywhere from 30 minutes to more than two hours as an outpatient procedure using local anesthesia. A few stitches may be required at the donor site. Some swelling, redness and bruising should be expected. Icy water in a zipper sandwich bag applied to the site of the procedure may help relieve any pain and swelling.

The process may be done by a cosmetic surgeon or dermatologist, but many of these doctors will not do fat injections. Some doctors claim that the fat that is transferred stays permanently. Others say that any fat transfer technique should be thought of as temporary because the blood supply that serviced the fat being transferred is not included in the transfer. There is little or no vasculature infusion and the body absorbs the fat cells as they die off. The desired result is lost within weeks or months. The fat may also create an odd appearance by fading unevenly.

Some people who have had the procedure done on their face have been left with bumps that do not smooth out. Further surgery is not always successful in revising these scars. Calcium deposits that form in the breasts after fat transferring may cause future problems with cancer detection, increase the need for lumpectomies, and may increase the chance of tumor growth.

• Collagen Injections
Also known as "collagen implants" or "collagen-replacement therapy"
$50 to 70 test dose
$300 to 1,500 per session

Collagen is a fibrous connective tissue protein that is found throughout the bodies of humans and animals. The collagen used in cosmetic surgery is a purified version derived from cows or pigs and is injected into scars, wrinkles and lips to fill them out. Zyderm collagen is used on light wrinkles and zyplast collagen is used on deeper grooves.

The process of injecting collagen for cosmetic reasons is done in a doctor's office after the injection site has been numbed with a shot of painkiller. Because collagen is partly water, the injections are slightly overdone to make up for the water loss that will take place. Any bleeding is usually limited to dots of blood that appear where the needle was injected. There may be some swelling in the area where the collagen was injected, but this usually disappears within a few days. Healing takes anywhere from three to ten days. Men may need to avoid shaving for a few days on the site where the injection took place.

Collagen that has been injected into a person's skin is not permanent. Depending on the patient's reaction to collagen, it can last anywhere from a few weeks to a year. To maintain the results it is necessary to get repeat injections. The more it is done the greater the risk of creating unwanted scar tissue.

Injections of collagen should not be used around the eyes because the thin skin of the eyelids has a greater tendency to show any lumps or scars that may develop from the use of collagen.

No less than a month before anyone plans on having collagen injections, they should have a skin test done. This is where a small bit of collagen is injected into two separate areas of the person's skin (on the back of the neck, the scalp or the arm, for example) to see what their reaction will be to the collagen.

There may still be allergic reactions to collagen, even after a negative skin test. These reactions to collagen include swelling, firmness or tightness, itching, prolonged redness or rashes around the injection site.

Some doctors now offer a procedure where collagen is extracted from the patient's own body. Human collagen is believed to be less susceptible to side effects, such as transmission of viruses or bacteria.

Anyone undergoing collagen injections should keep a record of the name of the company that manufactured the collagen and the inventory number of the batch of collagen being used on them. As with all medical products that are placed inside the body, a person should obtain the literature published by the manufacturer of the product that details possible complications. The phone number of Collagen Corporation is listed in the Research Resources section of this book under the heading of Materials Used in Plastic, Reconstructive and Cosmetic Surgery.

• Silicone Injections

This is illegal and should never be done.

Dermatologists and cosmetic surgeons have injected patients with industrial-grade liquid silicone to fill in wrinkles and acne scars, to build up cheek bones and to enlarge lips. One doctor has claimed to have injected silicone in tens of thousands of people over the last few decades. People who perform underground sex-change operations have used liquid silicone to inject into the breasts of men in order to enlarge the breasts.

The manufacturers of liquid silicone and the US Food and Drug Administration have warned doctors not to use liquid silicone in the body. Liquid silicone injections have never been scientifically evaluated for effectiveness and safety and have never been approved by the FDA. The FDA has cautioned that people who have these injections are exposing themselves to unknown and potentially harmful risks.

Companies that make silicone have said they do not supply the medical community with this substance for use within the human body. There have been reports that doctors purchase the liquid silicone at auto supply stores.

Liquid silicone can freely travel through the body. If it settles in the internal organs it may result in or contribute to ailments such as arthritis, immune disorders, rashes, hardening of the tissues and breathing problems. The silicone can wrap around nerves and marbleize within the skin and surrounding tissues, causing the skin to twist as scar tissue forms and sometimes calcify around the silicone. The silicone may block the blood flow to areas of the skin, which may cause infection and death of a portion of the skin (necrosis). This may necessitate a skin graft and may leave a burn-like scar that cannot be reduced.

• Nasal-Labial Fold Threading or Lift
$800 to 2,500

The indents that run from where the nostrils join the face down to the corners of the lips are called the nasal-labial folds. These folds accommodate the movement of the face by folding inward when a person smiles. They are a natural part of every person's face. With age, the folds may become more pronounced. Plastic surgeons have developed several techniques to reduce the depth of the folds, all of which may cause unwanted scarring, cause infection and have an uneven outcome.

One technique is to take muscle and tissue from another part of the body and thread it into the folds by way of incisions made at the corners of the mouth and at the top of the folds near the nostril or just inside the nostril. A blood supply may grow into the transplanted tissue and result in a permanent change. Some doctors will partially liquefy the tissue and inject it using a large-sized needle. This may not last because a blood supply may not be established in the tissue.

Another technique is done by making an incision at the top and bottom of each fold and running a thread of Gore-tex (a white leather-like Teflon material that has many surgical uses) through the folds to fill them in.

Another technique uses surgical threads made out of a natural glycerin protein. This suture material is the same that is used to sew up interior organs during major surgery. Within several months the threads dissolve into the body. Some doctors say that the body replaces this with its own natural collagen.

Collagen and can also be used to fill in nasal-labial folds by injecting it into the skin.

• Laser Surgery
Price varies depending on what is being done.

Some face-lifts and other operations are now being done with lasers in place of scalpels to make the incisions. Laser light, produced by a carbon dioxide laser, becomes a cutting tool as the tissue is vaporized in a fine line at the point of contact. The incisions made by a laser are smaller and therefore thought to be safer than incisions that are made with a scalpel. Some doctors say that incisions made with a laser also bleed less and heal faster than incisions made with a scalpel. Because laser incisions may result in less bleeding, there may be less bruising than with the conventional scalpel incision.

Laser skin resurfacing

Lasers are also used for skin resurfacing. This is done, using an Ultrapulse 5000, Surgilase laser, or other brand of laser machinery, on any area of the face and body and may be useful in softening or eliminating fine lines, sun damage, discolorations, scarring and birthmarks. The carbon dioxide laser emits short pulses of laser light that can be focused on the outer layer of skin (a pulse laser should be used for treating facial wrinkles). The pulsating laser light rays create a feeling similar to snapping a rubber band against the skin. Depending on the size of the area being treated with the laser, the doctor may use a numbing cream or the patient may need an intravenous sedative anesthesia. Some scabbing and bruising may result from treating the skin with a laser. Pain medication may also be needed during recovery.

Lasers can permanently damage the eyes, cause blotchy skin on darker complected people, and leave scars.

• Face-lift

Also known as "rhytidectomy"
$2,500 to 10,000 +
Face-lift with forehead-lift
$6,000 to 12,000 +
Forehead-lift
$2,000 to 5,500
Eyebrow or midforehead brow-lift
$1,900 to 6,000 +
Face-lift with eye-lift
$7,500 +

The temples, cheeks, jowls and neck are tightened in a face-lift operation. A face-lift tightens the skin of the face but does not change its texture as chemical peels and dermabrasion do. The face-lift operation usually takes between two and four hours and is often done on an outpatient basis but overnight hospital stays are not uncommon.

Face-lift incisions are made starting inside the hairline by the temples above the ears and brought down past the front of the ears, below the earlobes and back behind the ears into the hair. The skin is lifted away from the temple, sideburn area and jowl area and separated from underlying fat and muscle. The skin is pulled back and excess skin is cut off. Some doctors also tighten sagging muscles and tendons. Sometimes fat is removed from the jowls and neck by way of liposuction. Solid silicone implants may be added onto the chin and cheekbones if the patient desires. Techniques to tighten the chin, forehead and eyelids are sometimes performed during the same surgery to give a total lift to the face — although this may create too much of a change for some people.

The bandages that are placed on the head and the sideburn area cover all but the ear canal, face and the back of the head. These bandages are removed two three days after surgery. There are no bandages placed on the stitches around the eyes if eye-lifts were performed. If drainage tubes were inserted on the neck, these are removed by the doctor two to three days after the surgery. Stitches may be removed in stages, with the stitches by the ears being removed seven to ten days after surgery and all other stitches removed by the end of the second week.

Some results of the face-lift should immediately be apparent upon the removal of the bandages. As the face continues to heal during the following weeks and months, the final results of the surgery become apparent. Swelling and bruising may take two to four weeks to subside. Any kind of action that rubs or pulls on the skin of a freshly lifted face should be avoided for a month or more. Cleaning should be done gently for the first few weeks. Men will need to avoid shaving for five to fourteen days after a face-lift.

The scars caused by the face-lift incisions are usually not very noticeable because they are done in areas where they are partially hidden by the hair and in the natural bends of the skin. When incisions are made in the scalp, a portion of the hair-bearing skin is removed. This may result in a larger forehead because the hairline will be further back. Hairless patches on the scalp and scars behind the ears may be noticeable where incisions were made. The incisions that are made by the edge of the ears normally are not very noticeable because they are in the natural skin crease where the sideburn area joins the ear. All of the scars may fade to where they are barely noticeable.

The incisions by the ears for a face-lift are different for a man than they are for a woman. There are doctors who, when making the incision near the ear actually go behind the ear triangle and into the ear so that the scar will be less noticeable. But the incision on a man should be made outside of the ear or else the hair-growing skin of the sideburns will be moved over the ear triangle, and the man will have a problem trying to shave that hair away. Because part of the skin between the ear and the sideburns is cut away during a face-lift, a man may end up with narrower sideburns, sideburns that are closer to the ears, or sideburns that are at a different angle.

Some face-lifts are done so well and look so natural and subtle that most people would not be able to tell that the person had anything done. Other times the person can end up with a face that looks immobile and plastic. The surgery may change the movement of the face so that it moves unnaturally. If the skin is not draped on the face properly, or if the skin does not heal well, the patient can be left with wavy skin. There is also the extreme of being left with a face that has the appearance of being obviously altered and a surgery that disfigured the face or left it partially paralyzed. Paralysis of a part of the face can occur after a face-lift because the nerves that control facial movement can be damaged when the incisions are made. This paralysis may be permanent or reversible.

• Forehead Lift

The midforehead brow-lift is done to remove skin above the eyebrows and to elevate the muscles above the eyes. This is done through incisions made in the naturally occurring lines of the forehead or through an incision made in the scalp a half an inch or so beyond the hairline and then lifting both the eyebrows and forehead. It is sometimes done at the same time as a face-lift.

Forehead lifts sometimes result in permanent paralysis of the forehead muscles. A forehead lift can leave the person permanently unable to move their eyebrows or with a permanently stunned type of expression.

• Eyelids

Known as "blepharoplasty"
Done on all four eyelids $3,000 to 7,000
Done on two eyelids $2,000 to 4,000

Eyelid surgery, or "blepharoplasty," can remove excess fat deposits above or beneath the eyes that cause baggy eyelids, remove wrinkles from the eyelids to give them a younger appearance, remove excess droopy skin on the upper eyelids to improve vision, fix a lazy eyelid; or create a fold in the upper eyelid to make an Asian person look more Western.

Bags under the eyes are caused by weakening of the ligaments with age and drooping of the fatty deposits composed mostly of water that surround and protect the eyes. Some people have droopy bags that appear on their lower eyelids at a very young age. The bags can be removed either by making an incision in the natural crease directly under the lower eyelid lashes — far enough away so the lashes are not damaged — and cutting the fatty pouches out, or by the transconjunctival blepharoplasty technique which is done by making an incision in the inner lining (the conjunctiva) of the lower eyelid. This procedure removes fat that causes puffiness on the lower lids but does not tighten the skin.

One New York doctor uses a tiny, heated needle to eliminate puffiness around the eyes. The procedure is done through a small incision of about 1/4 inch. The needle is inserted and vaporizes the fat in seconds. Because there is no cutting of the tissues other than the small incision there is less damage done with this technique than by using a scalpel. There is less bruising and blood loss, scarring, swelling and sutures. If the person also has baggy skin it can be cut away after the fat has been vaporized.

To do the upper eyelids, incisions are made in the naturally occurring folds of the upper lids. Fatty deposits can be removed and a sliver of skin can be removed to reduce the bagginess of the eyelids.

Droopy upper eyelids can, in some instances, interfere with vision. This is the reason that the operation to correct this is covered by some insurance plans. A person who is seeking to have insurance cover the surgery will need to visit an ophthalmologist, who will determine that vision impairment is caused by sagging eyelids.

Swelling of the eyelids during the healing period after eyelid surgery may be lopsided and one eye may heal slower than the other. Large sunglasses can be worn out in public during the healing period to hide the stitches and bruising. Stitches are removed in about seven to ten days.

The scars that result may be visible when the eyes are closed or the eyelid is pulled. As the scars continue to fade, they may end up as a fine pale line that is barely noticeable. When the surgery is performed on a woman, she can easily cover the scars with makeup. Some women say that it is easier to apply makeup after this surgery because it brings back the natural folds of the upper eyelids.

The eyes may feel too tight for months after blepharoplasty. If you wear contact lenses you may not be able to wear them for about a month after surgery.

With the removal of any tissue, there is always the chance of removing too much — or at least more than the patient would want. It is particularly important to be cautious about any surgery done on a moving part such as the eyelids. Symmetry is important in eyelid surgery, but the results should not be expected to be perfectly symmetrical. If too much fat is removed, the person may be left with a sunken-in or gaunt appearance around their eyes. The incision on the lower lid comes close to the (pretarsal orbicularis) muscle that shapes the lower eyelid. If this muscle is damaged it can change the shape and expression of the eyes.

One of the most common problems with eyelid surgery is when too much of the skin is removed and the patient is left with eyelids that will not close all the way. This may leave the person with a stunned expression. There also may be a problem with too much white showing on the bottom of the eye, which can give the patient a basset hound appearance.

Because the eyes are coated with a thin tear layer every time you blink, anything that would interfere with being able to close the eyes all the way could result in constant dry eyes. Unclosable eyelids can cause drying of the cornea and a burning sensation. It may be a temporary problem that will fade over months or years as the eyelids age and stretch, or it may be permanent. The patient may also be left with blurry vision, which is usually temporary. Although rare, there have been cases of blindness being caused by injuries received or complications from eyelid surgery.

• Oriental to Western Eye Blepharoplasty
To add skin folds to upper eyelids
$2,000 to 4,500 +

Western eye blepharoplasty reshapes the epicantic fold in the upper eyelids. It is the most popular facial cosmetic surgery procedure performed in the Orient. The "Western Eye" technique is also becoming increasingly popular among Asians in large cities in other parts of the world.

The operation is done by creating a fold in the upper eyelids that is not naturally on the eyelids of many Asian people. This is to give the person more of a "Western" or American image. Some claim it is a career tool and say that having the procedure done has helped them advance in the job market and provides a better chance of getting jobs with firms that do international business. Others criticize and deplore the procedure saying it is a form of ethnic cleansing and that people should not be embarrassed by their nationality. Still others wonder what these people will do if they become parents. Will they be embarrassed by the naturally formed eyelids of their children and expect them to undergo the same procedure?

During the surgery the patient is sedated and given local anesthetic but is kept awake so they can open their eyes when the doctor needs to check symmetry during surgery. An incision is made in each of the upper eyelids. Skin, muscle, and sometimes fatty tissue is cut away. Temporary or permanent stitches may be sewn into the underlying muscle to hold them in place as they heal and temporary stitches are placed in the skin. Some doctors stitch the skin to the levator muscle inside the eyelid.

• Lip Reduction
$1,000 to 4,500

Lip reduction is sometimes done on people who have an abnormally large "protuberant" lower lip. This is another procedure which has been criticized by certain groups as removing ethnic qualities and, when done on people of African ancestry, is performed to make them appear Caucasian.

Like any operation that involves cutting away flesh, too much can be removed, the results may cause unevenness and unwanted scar tissue and may damage nerves.

If you are planning on undergoing this surgery, be especially cautious when choosing any doctor before undergoing surgery on a prominent area such as the lips. Take precautions to make sure the result is something you will be happy with. Using a computer imaging system or doing a plaster cast of the face and altering it first may help you determine what you want when planning and preparing for this operation.

• Cheek Implants
Also called "malar augmentation"
   $1,500 to 3,500

   Cheek implants are made of solid silicone and are positioned
onto the cheek bones through incisions made inside the mouth
above the upper gums. The procedure is done under local
anesthetic. Sometimes, as in chin implants, a piece of Gore-tex is
glued to the back of the cheek implant so it stays in place as
tissue grows into the Gore-tex.
   The implant may cause an infection, may be knocked out of
place and may be larger or smaller or not the shape that the
patient desired. Nerve damage may result from the incisions. If
any problem arises, the implants can be removed. The person will
be left with scars inside the mouth and any nerve damage may
heal by itself, be surgically reversible or may be permanent.

• Neck-lift
   $2,000 to 5,000

   This is often done at the same time as a face-lift. Some
people elect to have only their neck lifted.
   This procedure involves making incisions by the ears and
under the chin. Sometimes it is done together with liposuction of
the neck, jowls, and chin area. In some cases the liposuction
procedure done alone through three small incisions by the
earlobes and under the chin can give the desired result.
   After a neck-lift some doctors leave drain tubes in the neck
that remain for one to three days to drain any excess fluid that
accumulates under the skin. This is a preventive measure that
aids in the healing process and may prevent complications that
can arise from swelling and any excess blood accumulation
(hematoma).
   As with any procedure that involves cutting away at flesh
and soft tissue, there can be too much removed, resulting in a chin
that is too tight or is uneven.

• Chin Jobs
• Chin tuck
Also called "submental lipectomy"
   $1,800 to 2,500
• Chin liposuction

Also called "submental liposuction"
• Chin enlargement
Also known as "chin augmentation" or "mentoplasty"
Done with a silicone implant
$1,000 to 2,000
• Chin repositioning
Also known as "sliding geneoplasty"
Done by moving a piece of the bone
$1,000 to 3,500
• Chin bone shaving reduction surgery
Also called "chin osteotomy"
$1,000 to 3,500

Skin folds that droop over the front part of the upper neck are called a "double chin." This sag is a result of a combination of sagging neck skin, fat and/or muscle. The operation done to change these sagging tissues is called a "submental lipectomy," or a chin tuck, which is the removal of fat and usually a small flap of skin, eliminating the double chin. It is often preferable to leave some looseness in the skin of the neck to match the rest of the face and to prevent it from looking unnatural. A full neck-lift may bring about the desired result.

Chin enlargement, or "augmentation mentoplasty," is done by inserting a solid silicone form on the front of the chin bone to give a person a more pronounced chin. The implant is inserted through an incision inside the lower lip or just under the chin. Excess fat and skin can also be removed during mentoplasty to help eliminate a sagging or double chin.

Chin augmentation is sometimes done at the same time as a nose job. Because a small chin can make the nose look larger than it actually is, some people decide to undergo chin augmentation first before deciding on a nose job. After the chin has healed, the nose may look smaller than it had before the chin enlargement. If the chin enlargement was done with an implant, it is a less permanent solution and the implant can be removed if the patient does not like the appearance it gives them.

In another technique done to augment the chin, the lower part of the chin bone can be sawed off and moved forward. This is done through an incision that is made in the gum below the front teeth. This procedure is called a "sliding geneoplasty" and can be done instead of getting a chin implant. In this technique the bone is secured with screws and the teeth are wired shut for weeks while the jaw bone heals. Because the actual bone is moved, there is no risk of it being knocked out of place as with an implant. There is also a lower risk of infection. This surgery may help lift a droopy neck because the muscles are connected to the part of the bone that is moved forward.

During chin shaving surgery to reduce a chin that the person thinks sticks out too far, the incisions are the same as with a chin enlargement surgery. The bone is then sawed or shaved with a surgical instrument to the desired shape, and the incision is closed.

• Facial Implants

There are risks with placing any unnatural material in the body. These implants are made from silicone rubber, and some people claim that silicone in any form can cause ailments when it is placed inside the body. The implants are sometimes backed with a sheet of Gore-Tex so it will adhere to the surrounding tissues and stay in place. Some doctors say this may cause deterioration of the bone. The change that results from a facial implant may be noticeable immediately. The implant usually stabilizes in the following months as the tissues heal around it. There can be problems with the implants being larger or smaller than the patient desired. There may also be problems with the position of the implant and the scar that forms around it. These may cause the patient to desire more surgery — which will create more scar tissue. Implants can be knocked out of place if the face is bumped. Because the surgery involves creating a pocket to position the implant, there is a chance of facial nerve damage.

• Liposuction of the Face

Sometimes a pocket of fat will cause one area of the face or neck to bulge. These may occur after a person has gained and then lost a large amount of weight. They also occur in people who have never had a weight problem. These pockets of fat may be removed with liposuction or by surgically removing the fat pads with a scalpel.

Facial liposuction is done by inserting a small suction (canulla) tube through an incision just under the chin or in the crease of skin by the bottom of the ear in front of the earlobe and vacuuming the fat out. The procedure is sometimes done in combination with a face-lift, chin tuck or with solid silicone implants placed on the cheek or chin bones.

The expected injuries caused by the surgery include numbness, swelling and bruising that may last anywhere from a few days to several weeks. An elastic neck wrap is worn for several days to weld the skin back in place. This elastic wrap may continue to be worn at night for several weeks to help complete the healing process. The surgery site should be protected from any bumps, rubbing and big movements for four weeks.

As with other liposuction there can be problems with asymmetry if uneven amounts of fat are removed from each side of the face. Too much fat removal can result in hollow, sagging skin, and this may affect the way the skin ages. Complications can result in the death of a portion of skin, although this is rare. Some fluid accumulation may occur, which may require surgical drainage. The skin may also look wavy or spotted. Liposuction of the neck can cause the skin of the neck to reposition back further behind the ears. This may require the male patient to have to shave further back on the neck. Numbness or loss of sensation to the skin is usually temporary.

• Cosmetic Dentistry

In the past doctors yanked out crowded teeth and used braces to align the remaining teeth. This sometimes resulted in a small circle of teeth that did not sufficiently fill out the lip areas, leaving the person with a Mona Lisa-type smirk.

Orthodontia and jaw surgery or "orthognathic" surgery is not commonly thought of as cosmetic surgery but with the advancements in surgical procedures and the dramatic change that can be made in the lower half of the face by making changes to the teeth, jaw surgery is being sought out more and more as a cosmetic procedure.

There are several procedures that can change the appearance of the teeth. These include straightening, whitening, bonding, veneers, teeth-colored fillings, and using fake teeth made out of composite material or porcelain to replace teeth that have decayed, been damaged, have fallen out, or are not shaped the way the patient desires. These procedures may be done by a maxillofacial or oral surgeon, dentist or orthodontist. Sometimes all of these doctors are involved in the treatment of one patient.

All man-made materials added to the teeth may require future maintenance as they may shrink, chip, crack, stain (caused by coffee, tea, eating berries or smoking), or fall off. They may also create crevices where bacteria can grow, and this may contribute to future oral health problems. If a tooth is filed down too much it can become hypersensitive and a man-made material (plastic or ceramic veneer) will need to be bonded to the tooth.

For the person who has teeth that are not aligned — an overbite, underbite or crossbite — the person should consult with an oral surgeon or orthodontist. Braces may be the solution to improving the bite alignment, or an operation where the jawbones are cut and rearranged may bring the desired appearance. If the jaw bones are cut the patient will have their teeth wired shut for weeks or months as the bones heal. The patient may still have to wear braces and/or wear a removable retainer for months or years to complete the procedure.

Teeth whitening or bleaching is done by lightening the tooth enamel and underlying dentin by using a bleaching gel (containing carbamide peroxide) that is applied using a thin, flexible, custom-fitted plastic form when done at home or, in a dentist's office, by application of a chemical solution that is activated by a special light. Most patients who choose the home bleaching kit wear the appliance at night. Some find the application causes temporary irritation to the gums and throat and sensitivity to the teeth and root canal work. The home bleaching process is done in cooperation with a dentist who supplies the materials and checks up on the patient to follow the results and watch for any unforeseen problems. Recently there have been home bleaching kits sold over the counter and through mail order. Anyone using these kits should understand what these kits can and cannot do. People who have bleached their teeth too much or have had bleaching procedures performed too many times have ended up with dull, chalky teeth. A person who thinks they are saving money by using one of these over-the-counter bleaching kits should consider the amount of damage they may end up inflicting on their teeth when they do not have the supervision of a dentist.

Some people choose to have the silver fillings that dentists have placed in their teeth replaced with ceramic fillings for cosmetic reasons because the ceramics are similar to the color of teeth. Others are having the silver amalgam fillings replaced with gold or ceramics because the silver filling material contains mercury, which some reports claim may cause birth defects, miscarriages or other problems. Mercury is toxic in high doses and some people are sensitive to small amounts. The dentists, hygienists and dental assistants are under the highest risk of overexposure, and some tests have shown a higher rate of miscarriages among women who work with amalgams. The American Dental Association has said that there is no cause for concern and no need for people to have the silver fillings removed. It may be wise to listen to both sides of the argument before undergoing procedures to have your silver fillings replaced with ceramic fillings.

Anyone interested in cosmetic dentistry should investigate the available options and the materials that can be used and get an opinion from more than one dentist or orthodontist. The quickest procedure might not be the best choice to obtain a cosmetic dentistry goal.

For information on any cosmetic dental procedure, contact the American Academy of Cosmetic Dentistry or the American Association of Orthodontists. They are listed in the Research Resources section of this book under the heading of Jaw, Dental, and Oral Problems.

• Nose Jobs
Also known as "rhinoplasty," "nose reshaping," "nasal sculpting" and "nose reduction"
$2,500 to 8,000 +
• Septoplasty
This is done to correct a septum that is off center (the center structure of the nose between the nostrils that sits between the two sides of the nasal cavity)
$1,000 to 3,500 +
• Septorhiniplasty
This is a septoplasty done at the same time as a nose job
$2,800 to 8,000 +
• Nose enlargement
Also called "nasal augmentation" or "augmentation of the nasal dorsum" and creating a "French bridge"
$2,500 to 7,500 +
Any of the above done along with chin augmentation
add $500 to 1,000

The structure and function of the nose
The nose can give a person a sense of cultural identity. Some people think of a large nose as aristocratic. People are often very sensitive about their nose. Making remarks about a person's nose has always been an cheap and easy way to insult someone. There have been wars, especially between North and South Korea,

where cutting off the noses of captured solders was used as a form of punishment.

The noses of babies are normally very small and upturned. As a child grows their nose becomes longer and often more defined. By the time a person is in their late teens the nose has done most of its growing, but it is natural for the nose to continue to grow and change shape throughout life.

The nose is made up of an outer layer of skin that covers a structure that is made of bone and cartilage. The joint of the nose, which is about one-third of the way down the bridge of the nose where the bone and cartilage meet, provides for movement and flexibility of the nose. The interior cavity is made up of mucous membranes that cover the bony and cartilaginous skeleton. This membrane moistens the air you breathe, keeps the inside of the nose lubricated and warms the air on its way to the lungs.

The nose is very sensitive and responds to emotions of anger, fright, pleasure and pain. The turbinates inside the nose filter the air and often enlarge when air intake increases. It is normal for the nose to run when you exercise because the moisture the nose puts out increases when your breathing rate increases. Various airborne substances, pollutants and foods can also trigger a nasal reaction. It is normal for one side of the nose to close off as the erectile, reactive tissues of the nose respond to weather changes, smells, and various airborne elements including pollen.

The nose provides a way for a person to smell. Unusual smells are stored in the brain's memory so that a person can recall a smell they smelled years and even decades in the past. Smells can bring back good memories and trigger subsequent pleasurable responses or, in the instance of a fire, chemical or offensive smell, can alert someone to an existing danger and bring a physical response.

When an odor molecule comes in contact with the membrane inside the nose, a surface receptive protein on the cells then triggers a G protein (known as the G protein because it binds to a molecule called guanosine triphosphate — the two scientists who discovered this G protein won a Nobel Prize in medicine) that activates a biological communication switchboard within cells that lead to the area of the brain that recognizes smell.

The vomeronasal organ

Anyone considering nasal surgery should consider the damage that it causes to the vomeronasal organ.

The presence of the vomeronasal organ in animals has been known for some time. It was also known to exist in human fetuses and at birth, but until recently scientists had thought it was non-functioning in the adult human. They are just now starting to understand how it works.

Research done at the Monell Chemical Senses Center in Philadelphia, the University of Kentucky, the Rocky Mountain Taste and Smell Center at the University of Colorado and by researchers at the University of Utah has shown the vomeronasal organ does function in adult humans. It is a tiny structure in the human nose and is located within the mucous membrane inside each nostril on both sides of the septum. The difference between the vomeronasal organ and the olfactory system, which senses smells, is that the vomeronasal organ senses odorless molecules called "pheromones."

Pheromones are chemicals that humans emit through the skin that travel through the air. They access the vomeronasal organ through small slits within the opening of the nose. The information from the vomeronasal nerves travels through a neural pathway to the accessory olfactory bulb into the hypothalamus, which is at the center of the brain and controls basic drives and emotions. These messages have a strong influence on feelings and behavior. One behavior that is influenced by pheromones is sexual attraction. Pheromones that affect women are emitted by men and vice versa.

Erox Corporation of Fremont, California, was founded by Dr. David Berliner, a former researcher with the University of Utah. The company has developed a perfume called Realm that contains pheromones and that comes in two versions: one for men and one for women. The fragrance for men contains female pheromones and the women's perfume contains male pheromones. One other company puts out a fragrance called Athena Phermone 10:13. It contains an additive for women that was developed by Winnefred Cutler, a former researcher with the University of Pennsylvania who conducted research studies on pheromones at Monell Chemical Senses Center in Philadelphia.

Research scientists who examined tissue obtained from nasal surgery patients found the vomeronasal organ in every one of the samples. Other research has shown that the sex life of animals declines if their vomeronasal organ is removed. Because surgery damages or removes the vomeronasal organ, this has raised researchers' concerns about the effects of nasal operations on the patient's ability to detect and react to pheromones, and the extent this in turn impairs sexuality.

Altering the nose

Where anyone got the idea that a smaller nose is better than a larger one is anybody's guess, but cosmetic surgeons have made a killing on the amount of money spent by people wanting to change their noses.

More than any other cosmetic procedure, undergoing a nose job can be agonizing because the nose is so central to the face and can interfere with the basic function of breathing.

People refer to cosmetic surgery on their nose as getting their nose "fixed." If there was nothing wrong with it in the first place, how could it be fixed? "Changed" is more of a correct word. Having a crooked nose is not like having crooked teeth. Crooked teeth can cause tooth decay, chewing difficulties, speech problems and jaw alignment problems. A crooked nose does not affect a person's health, but it can add character to the face and give the person a distinctive, or at least an interesting appearance.

Surgical changes of the nose can easily be justified for someone who has rhinophyma, which causes a red, lumpy and swollen nose and results in scarring and the kind of disfigurement experienced by entertainer W.C. Fields. But most nose surgeries that are performed today are on people who subject themselves to the somewhat barbaric surgery performed by cosmetic surgeons who inject a patient with anesthesia, tie their arms down, immobilize their head and cut, saw and chisel away at the patients nose. This usually results in a nose that is narrow, straight profiled and upturned, as if that is the way all noses should be.

Rhinoplasty is the name of the operation that changes the appearance of the outside of the nose. Rhinoplasty gained its first bit of fame after World War II and became popular by the 50s when the actress Marilyn Monroe had her nose slightly narrowed. In the 60s and 70s, women in large cities flocked to cosmetic surgeons to have their noses made smaller. Many noses that were altered in the 60s and 70s had an artificially cute overdone look as too much bone and cartilage was removed by the doctors who operated on them. Many of these noses were made so narrow that it caused breathing problems. The damage the surgeries inflicted caused permanent difficulties with swelling, as well as muscle, nerve and tear duct damage.

Even today it is estimated that 10% or more of people who have cosmetic surgery performed on their nose go in for additional surgery because of unsatisfactory results. This is not an accurate figure as far as the number of people who are unsatisfied because it is based on the actual number of people who actually go in to get revisions and not on the amount of patients who desire or need revisions. With more than 10% of the people being so unsatisfied that they go in for one or more operations to try for a better result, one can see why it is important to make the right decision the first time.

> *I had a boyfriend who went and had a nose job. I don't know why he did it. He didn't even tell me. It didn't look right. All the sudden half his nose was gone. He had all these ethnic features, and big hands and then all the sudden this little nose. It didn't look natural anymore. It wasn't in harmony with the rest of his face. It didn't match. It was strange looking at him after that. It affected our relationship. All I saw was this nose that had been operated on. He said he liked it but I know he didn't, but what could he do? He was stuck with it and it didn't match. The harmony was gone.*
> — an L.A. woman

Many doctors do the same cuts to every nose as if they are running an assembly line. These are the doctors who are known as "hacks." They end up giving the same nose to everyone regardless of the patient's facial structure, size of the other facial features, skull size or ethnic background. If you are going in for a nose job you should be aware of the doctor's individual taste. If you like your nose big, then you should be sure that you do not end up on the operating table of a doctor who likes to make all noses small. Similarly, if you favor noses that are long and aristocratic do not go to a doctor who seems to think that everyone should have a button nose.

If you are one of those people looking at other people trying to decide what kind of nose you want, it would be a good thing if you were looking at people with your same ethnic background and facial structure. What often makes a nose job so obvious is that the nose is made to look like a nose that does not fit the rest of the face or even made so small that the person appears to have been in an accident.

Within reason there are various things that can be done to alter the appearance of the nose. A hump can be removed, the nose can be shortened, widened or narrowed, and the tip can be altered. A nose can almost always be made smaller, but cannot always be made larger or wider. Some people, rather than let the doctor fully remove the hump from their nose, choose to keep a hump but have it made slightly less prominent. Others go into surgery with the goal of changing only one thing about their nose such as the width or the length.

If you are going to let the doctor make alterations to the cartilages that form of the tip of your nose you are taking a risk. This is where many mistakes are made. More than any other area of the nose, tip cartilages that have been cut can give the nose an odd and unnatural appearance and show the signs that the nose has been surgically altered. Once they have been ruined it is very hard to try to make them appear normal. Each operation costs thousands of dollars and the surgeries need to be spaced far enough apart — usually several months to more than a year — to give the nose adequate time to heal and relax. Multiple operations on a nose can make it become firm. There are some very good medical books in large university libraries that show photos of people who have had very messy nose operations where the tip cartilages have been ruined. There are also some doctors who spend the better part of their time in the operating room redoing bad nose jobs.

Basically, the best things you can do before you make a decision with what you want done to your nose is to find out what can be done, what you would like done, and ask a lot of questions of the doctors you interview — and altering the consent form to place restrictions on what the doctor can do to you.

Some people who undergo nasal surgery to make their nose smaller later go in to have the nose made larger — some even aim to get the original appearance of the nose back. Thousands of people with noses made smaller earlier in their lives have gone under the knife to make their noses larger and especially to build up a profile that was made "too cute" in an earlier nose surgery. Some doctors call adding a peak to the bridge of a nose to increase its profile "a French bridge." The thought behind this is that the nose of the '90s is sturdier and less perky — a strong nose shows strong character. One New York doctor has appeared in the media claiming that he has performed hundreds of these nose enlargements — and that probably comes to a total of hundreds of thousands of dollars for his bank account.

Adding onto the nose can be a very agonizing operation to go through. There are various materials that can be used to build up the bridge and columella of the nose. The natural sources obtained from your own body include septal cartilage, ear cartilage, skull bone, rib cartilage, hip bone and fascia (a connective tissue that binds body structures together). If artificial materials are used, there is less surgical trauma because it saves the time of harvesting tissue from another part of the body. Artificial materials are coral and silicone rubber. Other doctors also use bovine (cow) cartilage that has been prepared for use in the human body.

It is very hard to recreate the appearance of a nose as it was previous to surgery. Any doctor who makes it sound easy is being unrealistic, and you should question his motives for agreeing to perform the operation on you.

If the nose is being restructured, the cartilage and bone that make up the structure of the nose is actually being broken and/or cut into pieces, some pieces are taken out and disposed of and the remaining pieces of the nose are pieced together.

The size of a nose can be reduced by doing things to the structure of it, but there will be the same amount of skin draped over a smaller structure. The tent of skin covering the nose will have less support and the skin will fall differently around the nose, eye and cheek areas, and may make the crease in the eyelids change. All of this will result in a nose and central face that has different angles, and this will cause light to be reflected off the face in a different way, thus the appearance of the person's face may be dramatically different. It can increase the depth of wrinkles between the eyebrows. Scar tissue can change the contours of the nose and prevents it from moving in its natural way. Male nose jobs can end up looking too delicate, narrow, straight, smooth and feminine or unnaturally upturned. Making the nose smaller can make the ears and other features look bigger and disproportionate to the nose.

Some of these procedures done to alter the appearance of the nose can cause more problems than they are meant to solve, especially if it involves altering the nasal bone. If the nose is narrowed it may cause breathing problems and the sides may be set so far in that they collapse into the nasal cavity. The septum may be damaged. Changes in the weather, exercise and increased heartbeat can sometimes cause pain in a nose that has been operated on. Some people continue to have problems with swelling many years after their surgery along with nasal headaches and facial pain that may be permanent or may come and go. The menstrual cycle can also affect a nose that has been operated on.

Repairing nasal damage

If you have significantly broken your nose, you should be able to tell just by looking at it. Having had your nose broken does not necessarily mean that you need an operation. If you are concerned about getting the damage repaired through an operation you should take into consideration the amount of damage the operation is going to cause. One may outweigh the other. If there is not a noticeable difference and the damage is not interfering with breathing, you should probably rule against undergoing nasal surgery. The operation can cause more damage than the simple break would cause. The outcome of the surgery may cause more long-term problems than the slight bit of original damage would have ever caused.

An operation where the sharp edges from a damaged bridge of the nose are shaved can take as little as 10 minutes. Because the bones are not broken when there is only shaving performed there is less injury and the healing time is shortened considerably and the person can get back to their normal activities much sooner. There is less risk of pain and infection and other complications, and a shorter recovery period.

Improving breathing

Structural formations within the nose that can cause breathing problems include a deviated septum (the center of the nose is off center), enlarged adenoids (enlarged mass of lymphoid tissue at the back of the pharynx), large or displaced turbinates inside the nasal cavity, tumors or polyps.

Allergies and nose jobs

Proceed with caution when seeking to improve breathing airways. There are some nasal problems that improve by themselves with time — months or years. The trauma of surgery may aggravate the condition. Swelling of the nasal mucous membranes may be a seasonal reaction to humidity and airborne particles like pollen, smoke or smog. Changes in the body or outside temperature may also affect the mucous membranes. A condition called "vasomotor rhinitis" causes a stuffy and runny nose when a person is exposed to sudden bright light, changes in humidity and temperature, and exposure to strong odors. It is best to treat these problems with medications, nasal mists, Chinese herbs, allergy treatments or by avoiding foods that cause allergic responses in the nasal area rather than undergoing a surgical procedure which may magnify the problem or may be altogether unnecessary. Nasal surgery will not improve asthma or reactions to pollen or mold. Narrowing the nose by way of a nose job can make any nasal congestion worse and cause breathing problems that did not previously exist.

Septoplasty

If there is any cartilage or bone of the central structure of the inside of the nose (the septum) that is interfering with breathing, it can be altered in the operation called a "septoplasty." When this operation is done together with a nose job to change the appearance of the nose it is called a "septorhinoplasty."

No changes to the outside of the nose need to be made to improve breathing. Nearly 80% of all people have deviated septums. So, simply having a deviated septum is not reason enough to have surgery. Though it is one of the more commonly used reasons to have surgery to try to get insurance to cover part or all of the cost of a nose job, having a deviated septum does not automatically mean you have a breathing problem or even have to consider taking the risks of surgery.

Complications that can result from septoplasty include having a hole in the septum and damage to the senses of smell and taste as well as damage to the vomeronasal organ.

Nose surgery

Most nasal surgery is done while the patient is aware of what is going on in the room but anesthetized enough so they do not feel any pain and cannot move. The patient wears a surgical gown and a surgical hat. They lay flat on their back and their arms are immobilized by tying them down. The patient receives an intravenous anesthetic and Novocain is injected at the base of the nose. The patients eyes are closed and they may feel as if they are sleeping or may fall asleep.

Incisions are made just inside the nostrils and sometimes across the skin between the nostrils (columella). If the columella was cut the entire structure of the nose can be exposed by lifting the skin up off of the nose structure. After this is done there will be a slight scar on the columella that will normally fade to the point where it is not very noticeable. By working through these incisions the doctor can alter the bone and cartilage that make up the structure of the nose. The appearance, size and breathing capability of the nose can be changed.

The patient may hear conversations between the surgical team and may hear the suction tube that is used to remove blood and mucous from the nasal area during surgery. If the bone of the nose is to be altered the patient will hear the hammering and chiseling sounds as the doctor breaks and cuts the nasal bone into pieces. All this time there will be some blood that will trickle into the throat and this is normally swallowed. The patient can receive moisture by having the nurse hold a wet towel in the mouth. Depending on the amount and type of anesthesia that the patient is given they may be able to converse a little with the doctor.

Recovery

Expected injury from nasal surgery can include extreme bruising, red blotches on the whites of the eyes which can take several weeks to heal, and swelling of the entire frontal half of the head and neck. During the healing period after nose surgery you will have to keep ice on your face around the clock off and on every few minutes for at least the first three to six days. Most of the swelling will disappear within three weeks of the surgery but do not be surprised if the nose is still noticeably swollen after four to six weeks — especially if you allowed the doctor to alter the bone. It can take three or four months for swelling to go down and one to two years to loosen, especially if the bone was altered. It can take from one to three years before the final form of the nose is established. Some people continue to treat this swelling for several months after surgery by placing ice on their nose at night.

Immediately after surgery the nose may feel tight and have a throbbing sensation. Bleeding may continue for the first several hours after surgery. This requires having a role of gauze taped under your nose like a mustache. This gauze will have to be replaced several times during the first day after the surgery as it gets soaked with the blood that leaks from the incisions inside the nose. You may need to continue wearing this gauze mustache for two to three days. Any large amounts of bleeding should be reported to the doctor immediately.

Blood-tinged mucus will have to be gently hocked up or swallowed. The nose might be packed with cotton bands, which makes it necessary to breathe through the mouth. This can result in dry mouth, chapped lips and a sore throat. If you get sick during the days that the nose is packed and have to vomit, it can be quite uncomfortable. The mouth should be kept wide open when sneezing, vomiting or coughing to prevent pressure on the face and nose. Do not blow the nose for two to three weeks after nose surgery. The doctor can use an instrument to suction mucus and blood clots out of the nose during your visits with him in the days following surgery.

The swelling caused by nasal surgery can be quite severe to the point that you will not be able to open your eyes or comfortably close your upper lip — one reason it may be uncomfortable to close your lips is because you may not be able to breath out of your nose because it will be swollen and packed. The bruising and swelling will usually get worse on the second or third day after surgery. If the bone of the nose was altered the bruising will become very dark and the swelling will be intense. If the bone has been worked on you should also not do any hard chewing that can move the facial muscles.

The bruising can get quite severe to the point where your upper and lower eyelids and upper cheeks may turn deep purple. The bruising will spread to lower parts of your face as it fades away over the first couple weeks and may fall all the way down to the bottom of the neck or upper chest before completely disappearing. The eyelids may become deep purple and stay that way for weeks as they casually fade. The whites of the eyes might turn blood red which can take over a month to clear up.

During the first week or two after nasal surgery you may notice a particular smell. It is the smell of the scabs inside the nose and will last as long as they remain in there. The scabs should not be picked at as this can cause additional bleeding, infection, unwanted scarring, lead to complications that may require additional surgery and generally delay healing. Large scabs inside of the nostrils can partially or wholly block breathing and may remain for one to two weeks before they fall out.

Blood tinged drainage from the nose can go on for one to two weeks and even longer depending on the extent of the surgery and your body's own healing process. You should sleep sitting up for the first four to seven days so the drainage from the nose does not choke you in your sleep and so the blood pressure in the head will be kept to a minimum.

The inner rim of the nostrils may be cleaned with a cotton swab dipped in hydrogen peroxide. Antibiotic ointments such as Neosporin, Polysporin or Bacitracin may be helpful in keeping the inside of the nose moist and reduce bacteria growth around the dissolvable sutures, thus helping the healing process. These antibacterial ointments can also be applied with a cotton swab. Ask the doctor before using any ointment on any surgical wound.

You may be told to avoid the shower or even the bathtub for the first few days after surgery. The steam from the bath or shower may cause bleeding. You may need someone to wash your hair, or tilting your head backwards under the shower while keeping the water off the face and holding a towel on the face may be an option — just be sure to keep your balance. A damp wash cloth can be used to clean the face.

Glasses should not be worn on the nose for a month or more if the bones of the nose were broken during the operation.

Ongoing risks from nasal surgery

Infection is not common after nasal surgery because of the rich blood supply to the nasal area. Bandages, splints and packing placed in the nose after the surgery and that is too tight can contribute to infections and in the worst case can cause toxic shock syndrome (a potentially fatal infection of toxins produced by bacteria). If a fever occurs you should notify your doctor.

Altering the bone during surgery may cause injury to the lacrimal (tearing) apparatus and this may cause dry eyes. Altering the bone may also cause inflammation of the membrane of connective tissue (periosteum, a skin-like tissue that covers bones) that surrounds all bones except at the joints. Sometimes these problems are due to swelling from the surgery and improve as the nose heals. Facial pain may occur as the weather changes and facial pain similar to headaches may be temporary or permanent.

A Los Angles woman who had a nose job had to be rushed from a family picnic a month after her surgery after her nose started bleeding profusely with no obvious reason. She was given blood to replace the blood she lost.

Ongoing problems with bleeding after nose surgery may be temporary or permanent and may have to do with the way the membrane inside the nose healed. If the size of the breathing passages was altered during surgery, the sounds of breathing through the nose will also be different. Swelling problems of a nose that has been operated on can interfere with breathing and voice resonance and may last for months or may be permanent.

Breathing difficulties caused by a nose that was narrowed too much may be permanent or reversible through a second surgery. Problems with dryness inside the nose may be temporary or permanent.

If muscles were damaged or cut the nose may not move as much as it used to. If the bridge was reduced during the surgery, a portion of the nasal bone was removed, which is where a muscle is connected that goes up into the forehead. Once this muscle is cut, the lower forehead between the eyes may appear slightly different and may not move the same after surgery. The cut muscle may also occasionally spasm or twitch.

The cuts to the bone and cartilage may be felt through the skin. They also may be noticeable under certain lighting conditions.

The incisions inside the nostrils may change the curve of the nostrils and leave little indents on the skin of the outside of the nose.

Complications of nasal surgery that may affect the skin are the occurrence of spider veins, dimpling where underlying bone and cartilage were altered and crossed nerves on the flesh where touching one part of the nose results in feeling it on another part of the nose. Numbness of the nose often occurs after surgery but normally fades as time goes by but may be permanent.

• Hair Transplants
Various procedures called "Anteroplasty," "Galeoplasty, " hair plugs," "plug grafting," "strip grafting," "pedicle flap," and "scalp reduction"
$500 to 35,000+ depending on procedure

From razor blades to electrolysis, the hair removal industry is a two billion dollar a year industry. Nearly thirty million dollars is now being spent each year on hair removal creams and lotions. Hair replacement is also a billion dollar industry as techniques to surgically restore hair are becoming more accessible and popular.

Both men and women can have thinning hair. Hair loss may be the result of bad diet, stress, disease, heredity, hormones, burns or other conditions. Everyone loses some hair every day as the body randomly sheds and replaces hair. In the natural aging process, genetic patterns trigger certain hair follicles to slow down (androgenetic alopecia) and eventually stop producing terminal hair (the thick strands of hair as opposed to vellus hair which is very fine and often very light in color and is found throughout the surface of the skin). Most people, including women, will lose some hair, especially along the hairline. This is normal and is not a "deformity."

In what is called "male pattern baldness," the hairline recedes and the top (vertix) of the head eventually becomes bald as the male hormone, which is normally present in both men and women, affects the hair follicles. On most people, the hair on the sides and back of the head continue to grow for a lifetime.

Some people are not bothered by their hair loss. A bald head is thought by some to make a man look aristocratic, dignified, wise and even sexy. Other people cannot accept their hair loss and have decided it is unappealing.

In the past, the most common ways to cover bald spots were by using some very fancy hair styling that usually did not hold up in a strong wind or by using various shapes and sizes of wigs. There have always been lotions and potions marketed as cures for baldness, and some people have made a lot of money by selling these miracle cures. In 400 BC, the Greek physician, Hippocrates, known as the Father of Medicine, applied opium, spices and pigeon poop to try and reverse hair loss (don't try this at home). In the 1840s, there were pills sold in America that were guaranteed to cure cholera, jaundice and baldness. In recent years, while some people have resorted to purchasing specially made spray paints for the scalp, the more promising, but also more expensive choice has been to purchase high quality custom-made partial wigs that are woven into the person's natural hair and worn for weeks without being removed. These can be maintained with monthly salon visits where the weave is adjusted.

The most involved and expensive way to replace hair is found in the offices of cosmetic and dermatologic surgeons who will surgically transplant hair from the sides and back of the head to bald areas. One way of doing this is by cutting small pieces, or "plugs," of hair-bearing scalp from the sides and back of the head and grafting these into the skin on the bald areas. Another way is to cut away at bald spots and replace that area with a piece of hair-bearing scalp that has been surgically stretched in what is called "scalp reduction surgery."

One hair transplant technique is called "micrografting" or "minigrafting." This is where the plugs of hair that are taken from the back or sides of the head are cut into smaller pieces containing only two or three hair follicles. These micrografts are then put into tiny incisions in the bald area of the scalp.

Minigrafting results in the most foolproof final appearance and avoids the "doll head scalp" appearance that is the result when micrografting is not used and rows of hair plugs give the scalp a plantation look. Some people say that because the hairs are not all at the same angle it can look scruffy and be hard to manage.

There is some scabbing that occurs after the transplants. These should be left alone to fall off on their own. Antibiotic ointments or prescription pills can be used to prevent infection and irritation of the transplants. Any unexpected bleeding should be reported to the doctor. Because of the length of time it takes to transplant the fine hair grafts and the necessity to space them far enough apart to give each graft adequate blood flow, it may take several sessions with the doctor to adequately fill in the balding areas — though some doctors now do hundreds of minigrafts in one session. Sessions may be spaced weeks or months apart and may take a year or more to complete. The transplanted hair follicles lose the hairs contained in the grafts after about a month. Weeks or months later new hair grows out of the grafts and then continue to grow in a normal manner.

In the process called "scalp reduction," the galea layer of the scalp on the crown of the skull is surgically undermined. This frees the scalp so that it can be stretched over areas where bald scalp has been cut away in a star shape.

Another method of hair replacement is done by using scalp flaps. This is done by surgically cutting sections of the scalp and, while keeping the section partially attached to the scalp to keep a blood flow, rotating it to another position on the head where a bald area has been cut away. This gives immediate results but can leave an unnaturally defined hairline. Scarring may be covered with the hair but may be visible when the person is caught in the wind or rain.

The most radical technique for filling in bald spots is done by surgically placing small balloons (tissue expanders) beneath the hair-bearing scalp on the sides of the head. The balloons are then filled with saline (a saltwater solution) and remain there for months. During this time the person has to live with the large bump on the scalp caused by the underlying balloon. Saline is injected into the balloon through a "port" that also sits beneath the skin. The completely filled balloon can create a bump on the head nearly the size of a typical soda can. When the skin is sufficiently stretched, the stretched-out hair-bearing scalp is pulled onto the area where the bald skin was cut away.

The type of anesthetic used during any hair transplant depends on what procedure is being done. If the patient is awake during the surgery, some doctors provide a selection of videos the patient can watch during the surgery.

The more complicated the surgery is, the greater the risk of complications including bleeding, unwanted scarring, infection, death of skin (necrosis), nerve damage, poor blood flow (vascularity) to the tissue after healing, bald patches along incision sites and loss of hair on the transplanted scalp.

The challenge with surgical procedures to transplant hair is getting the hair replacement area to look natural. Not all people are good candidates for hair transplants. If a person chooses to undergo a hair transplant, they should, as with any planned surgery, do research and take great care in choosing a doctor. The outcome cannot be guaranteed and the naturalness in the final appearance is a gamble. With all hair transplant techniques the final result will never result in the fullness of the prebalding state. If there were scalp reductions done or any other technique that caused scars, the scars may eventually show as the hair continues to thin as the person ages.

Other ways to treat thinning hair

Rogaine — a solution containing minoxidil (a blood pressure drug) can be obtained through a prescription. It is applied to the scalp twice a day and has been proven to increase the size of some hair follicles — but it is not a permanent solution for people who are concerned about hair loss.

Some people claim that the use of biotin dietary supplements can improve both fingernail quality and hair thickness. It is sold in healthfood stores.

• Ear Pinning
Also called "otoplasty"
$2,100 to 4,800

Otoplasty is performed through incisions behind the ears and alters the structure of the back of the ears to change their contour and place them closer to the head. This surgery is often performed on children as young as kindergarten age to avoid any teasing the child may experience from other children.

Bandages are worn for several days after the surgery to hold the ears in place. The sutures are then removed. The ears should be protected for several weeks to allow them to heal. Eyeglasses that are worn too soon after surgery may pull the ears out or irritate the incisions.

• Port Wine Stain Removal

Port wine stains are pink, red or purple patches that contain a dense system of blood vessels beneath the surface of the skin. They often appear on the face or neck and are commonly referred to as "birth marks." They may darken with age and develop a lumpy texture with small bumps or nodules made up of blood vessels that can bleed excessively if they are cut.

Though some people do not mind having a port wine stain and it sometimes becomes part of their identity, others do not like the attention the stains give them and seek ways to have them removed.

The most common and successful way to fade port wine stains is by using a laser that emits microsecond-long pulses of yellow light that destroy the blood vessels. These treatments are done in short sessions and may need to be spread over a number of months or years. Because there is some pain involved, the patient is often given an anesthetic. The younger the patient is the easier it may be to treat the port wine stain.

• Permanent Makeup

Also known as "dermapigmentation"
$150 to 1,500 per area

Permanent makeup is applied by injecting pigmentation into the bottom layer of the skin that is called the "dermis." In other words it is a tattoo. This is usually done to give permanent coloring in place of eyebrow liner, eye shadow, eyeliner, lipstick, lipliner and blush. It also can be used to restore color to an area of skin that has lost its color such as an injury to the lips.

The technique of applying permanent makeup is not taught in medical schools. Some states limit who can do it. It is done by some cosmetic surgeons but is most commonly done by dermatologists or in a salon by an aesthetician or a person with no formal training. Even when the person has had training it may have consisted only of a two-day class or simply by watching a videotape. No special license is needed to purchase the equipment, and a person who has the equipment can be in business as soon as they find a paying customer.

Tattooing involves poking color into the skin with a needle and this causes pain. When it is done by a doctor, an injectable anesthetic can be used or a topical anesthetic may be applied. There may be some bleeding, swelling and bruising. After the scabs have healed some touching-up may need to be done.

Some of the advertising for permanent makeup salons and the people who apply the "makeup" claim that the dyes are gamma-irradiated and FDA approved and are not the dyes that are used in a common tattoo parlor. The FDA was contacted by the author of this book and they said they have not approved any dyes for tattooing the skin. Some of the dyes used for tattooing purposes have been approved for other uses but they have not been reviewed by the FDA for tattooing purposes.

As is the case with other tattooing, some people have later regretted having had permanent makeup applied. The results may be uneven — sometimes very uneven. The color that was used may not look the same as the skin ages. The color can also fade unevenly. Damage to the eyes can occur when this tattooing is done around the eyelid area. The colors that are used contain various metals and chemicals that can cause an allergic reaction. Some people experience ongoing pain and swelling on and around the tattooed area. Laser light and skin peels may sometimes remove some of the dye from the skin, but these procedures include other risks and are expensive.

The Body

• Breast Reconstruction
$6,000 to 30,000 +

Some women choose to have their breasts reconstructed after damage caused by cancer, accident or after a breast has been destroyed by leaking silicone-filled breast implants.

Breast reconstruction uses the woman's fat, muscle, blood vessels and skin taken from the abdomen, hips, back, thighs or buttock, which is then rotated to the chest while keeping it connected to its original blood supply. If the woman wants a nipple, that is created in a second surgery done at a later date — usually months later.

Breast reconstruction is complicated and is major surgery. Therefore, any women seeking this surgery should interview a number of doctors who have performed the surgery before undergoing this procedure.

Breast reconstruction takes several hours and carries unique risks, including blood transfusions during surgery and loss of blood flow in the flap. Patients need to plan for a lengthy recovery and must consider all the risks and possible complications including the need for additional surgeries. The donor site will have scarring. Not all women are candidates for breast reconstruction.

(For more information contact the breast cancer support groups that are listed in the Research Resources section of this book under the heading of Breast Cancer.)

• Breast Lift or Reduction
Also called "mastopexy"
   $3,000 to 6,000
• Breast reduction
Also called "mammoplasty"
   $3,000 to 7,500

Breasts that have changed shape because of age or lactation can be reshaped by way of a breast lift surgery.

Overly large breasts (gigantomastia) may cause or contribute to back pain, cause sore shoulders and restrict movement. Because of this, insurance may cover a breast reduction surgery.

Reducing large breasts may improve posture, make it easier to buy clothing and get people to look at the face rather than the chest. It may also prevent people from assuming that a woman is sexually preoccupied simply because she has large breasts.

Just because a woman has large breasts *and* back problems does not mean the back problems are being caused by the weight of the breasts. Back problems may be the result of weak stomach muscles, bad posture, past injuries that were never treated properly, damaged spinal disks or vertebrae, slipped or ruptured disks, tumors putting pressure on the spinal cord, inherited abnormalities, arthritis, ulcers, kidney or hip problems, diseases of the colon or prostate or menstrual pain.

If the breasts are very large, the operation can be done in two stages scheduled over a year apart. This may be done to save the nerves connecting the nipple and to preserve the lactating capabilities. Rather than risk losing nipple sensation and the ability to breastfeed by cutting the nipple off and replacing it at the end of the operation after the breasts have been reduced, the nipple can stay attached to the underlying tissue as the breasts are reduced a little. Then if the woman wants her breasts made smaller, another operation can be done a year or more later.

Both breast reduction and breast lift surgery require that the nipple be repositioned higher. If this is not done properly the nipple may die because of poor circulation or infection. There is also a risk of change in sensation and coloring of the nipple.

Depending on the extent of the reduction, the surgery may take from two to seven hours to perform. It is usually done on an outpatient basis but may require a hospital stay. Excess skin is removed during breast reduction and lift surgeries. Liposuction may be performed to shape the area around the breasts. When this is done the doctor should take care to preserve the contours of the cleavage

One complication of the surgery is that the breasts may swell too much, tearing the skin around the stitches and resulting in scarring. The final result may be breasts that are uneven, pointy, cross-eyed, or lopsided. There can be loss of sensation to the breasts. There will be scars where the incisions were made and these scars may be very obvious or may fade considerably.

After breast surgery, the patient needs to avoid sleeping on her sides or stomach for several weeks. Lifting or any action that could strain the chest area will also need to be avoided.

• Breast Enlargement with Implants
Also called "augmentation mammoplasty" or "breast augmentation"
$ 2,100 to 5,000

> . . . the American Board of Otolaryngology has stated on their own stationery that with regard to breast augmentation mammoplasty that the board does not believe that this is within the purview of the specialty of otolaryngology head and neck surgery. Yet when an otolaryngologist undertakes to increase a woman's breasts and they are doing it and that is the concern that we have that he is acting in direct opposition to their own board.
> — Dr. Norman Cole, past president, American Society of Aesthetic Plastic Surgery; treasurer, American Society of Plastic and Reconstructive Surgery, testifying at Congressional subcommittee hearings on plastic surgery industry, 1989

Making the Decision to Have Reconstruction with Silicone Gel Breast Implants

Although breasts reconstructed with implants are not the same as natural breasts and are sometimes troublesome, many women have reported they are happy with their appearance, size, and feel or texture.

Learning why some women choose reconstruction with implants and why others do not may help you decide whether this surgery is for you. The reasons are varied and highly personal:

- To replace an external prosthesis
- To avoid being constantly reminded of their cancer
- To allow for a more comfortable active lifestyle
- To avoid embarrassment in public dressing areas
- To help create a look that makes them feel more comfortable with or without clothes

A few reasons why some women decide against reconstruction with implants :

- They want to avoid more surgery
- They feel the risks outweigh the benefits
- They are happy with their external prosthesis
- They are concerned over the unknowns about breast implants

Special Medical Considerations

Before making your decision to have implants, you should discuss with your doctor the following important medical matters and how they might affect your decision:

- Whether only the initial surgery will be required or if additional corrective surgeries might be needed on your reconstructed or other breast
- The possibility of rupture of your implant(s), signs to watch for, and what is involved if your implant(s) ruptures
- Gel bleed (the sweating of microscopic amounts of silicone through the implant envelope) and how it might affect you
- Capsular contracture (the tightening of scar tissue that forms around implants) and how it might affect you
- What is currently known about an association of autoimmune disease with silicone gel breast implants
- The effect of past or future radiation (x-ray) therapy treatments for breast cancer

- *Your personal or family history of immune-related disorders, such as scleroderma and lupus*
- *The effect of medicines, especially any taken for chemotherapy*
- *Previous problems with breast implants you may have had*
- *The movement of your implant when you lie down or raise your arm*
- *Discomfort when lying on your stomach*
- *Your breasts' response to heat, cold, touch, and sexual activity*
- *Effect on breastfeeding*
- *The chance that you may be able to feel the edges of the implant*
- *The appearance of your cleavage*
- *Matching both breasts*

You should know that your breasts may not match after surgery for a number of reasons, such as:
- *Capsular contracture*
- *Your implant(s) may shift*
- *Side effects resulting from the use of cortisone around the implants(s)*
- *The use of different-sized implant(s)*
- *The difference in the healing processes between the two breasts*
- *Changes in the thickness of your chest skin after mastectomy*
- *Tissue changes resulting from radiation treatments*
- *Other medical reasons*

Your Expectations

Your expectations about your reconstruction may be influenced by the way you feel about the results of your mastectomy and the way you think it affects your life. Although the final outcome of the reconstruction surgery is not entirely predictable, your expectations of the final result should be realistic. So, with this in mind, it's important for you and your doctor to discuss the breast size and shape you want, the range of surgical possibilities and outcomes for you, and to take into account the special medical considerations.

To help you get an idea of what results may be possible, look at "before" and "after" pictures of patients who have had this surgery. Your doctor may have some to show you.

Keep in mind, however, that there is no way to assure that your results will compare with those of any other woman.

Your results will depend on many factors — your overall health, your chest structure and body shape, how your body heals, the effects of any other breast surgery you may have had, the skill of your plastic surgeon, and the type of reconstruction procedure you have. Usually it takes more than one operation to get the results you want, especially if you want your nipple rebuilt.

Scarring is a natural outcome of surgery, but your doctor will try to keep scars as subtle as possible. He can explain the location, size, and appearance of the scars you can expect to have. For most women, they will fade over time to thin lines, although the darker your skin, the more prominent they are likely to be. To avoid a new scar, your doctor may be able to insert your implant through the mastectomy scar (if there is enough skin).

The pocket where the implant is placed may be located behind (submuscular) or in front of (submammary) the chest muscle. Ask about the pros and cons of each technique. Sometimes a tissue expander is surgically put in place to stretch the skin. This can take months, and when the skin is stretched enough, it is replaced with the implant.

Keep in mind that an implant is artificial and the body reacts to it. Like anything else, implants age over time and may need to be replaced. Therefore, you should not expect your implant to last indefinitely, even though it may last for many years.

Insurance Coverage

Most insurance companies cover the costs of breast reconstruction after mastectomy. Before surgery, be sure to ask your insurance agent whether

- *Your policy covers the cost of the implant surgery, the implant, the anesthesia, and other related costs.*
- *The policy covers treatments for medical problems that may be caused by either the implant or the reconstruction.*
- *The policy covers the cost of removing (explanting) the implant.*

— from FDA breast implant information packet, October 1993

There are four ways of installing breast implants
- Through the nipple (peri-areolar approach)
- Through the arm pit (auxiliary approach)

- Under the breast (inframammory approach)
- Through the belly button (navel or transumbilical approach)

In the belly button technique the implant is installed by way of the navel then filled with saline. This sometimes still requires an incision under the fold of the breast or on the nipple to do the final adjustment to the implant.

A breast that has been implanted can remain tender for weeks and up to several months before they settle and relax and show the final results of the surgery

One of the problems with breast implants is positioning them. Placing the implants improperly can cause the breasts to look saggy, too perky, lopsided or too high. There was a woman in Los Angeles whose doctor placed her implants so high they touched her collarbones. Some women who have had their breast implants below the muscle complain that the implant moves around whenever they move their arms.

Anyone with breast implants should be aware of any changes in texture and shape of the breast, which may be signs of a ruptured implant.

Depending on your source of information, the complication rate from breast implants can run anywhere from as little as 2% to over 70%. Some believe that all women who have implants will eventually have problems with the implants.

Antibodies attack foreign substances, such as bacteria and germs. For years it was thought that silicone was inert, that the body was incapable of forming silicone antibodies. Medical scientists are now saying that the body may form antibodies against silicone in any form.

Before you make the decision to get breast implants, educate yourself about the options, future implant materials that may become available and the known risks. Contact the breast cancer support groups and the breast implant groups listed in the Research Resources section of this book.

• Male Breast Reduction

Done to reduce overly large male breasts or "gynecomastia"
   $ 2,000 to 5,000

Some men develop unusually feminine breasts. This is a condition known as "gynecomastia." Some medications, such as

Digitalis and Tagamet, can induce this condition. It may also be caused by hormones, tumors or a high body fat content. If a man is at his ideal weight and still has large breasts, these can be surgically altered to remove any excess tissue. Liposuction may provide the desired result.

Any unusual growth in the breast should be looked at by a doctor. A breast exam should take place before any type of breast surgery.

Risks of this surgery (other than the obvious breastfeeding complications) are the same as with a female breast reduction.

• Tummy Tuck
Also called "abdominoplasty"
$ 3,500 to 7,500 +

This operation is done through a long smile-shaped incision at the bottom of the tummy between the hip bones. An incision is also made around the belly button and the skin is lifted up away from the abdomen. The muscles in the abdomen are tightened. Fatty deposits can be removed and excess skin is cut away. Because the skin is pulled downward, a new hole has to be cut for the belly button. The incision is closed and the skin is sewn around the belly button. Drainage tubes may be inserted and left in place for a day or more.

As with all surgeries there can be problems with healing, infection, and hemorrhaging. If too much fat is removed the skin may not heal properly and parts of the skin may die (necrosis).

Tummy tucks can be painful because the torso moves with every breath. It is major surgery and should always be done in a hospital and include a stay in the hospital of two to four nights. Usual recovery time is from three to six weeks. A scar is left around the inside rim of the belly button and between the hip bones. As time goes by the scars may fade considerably. The long scar at the bottom of the tummy is usually low enough to be covered by a reasonable bathing suit.

Other than the stretch marks that are on the skin that is removed during the procedure, stretch marks cannot be removed by undergoing a tummy tuck.

• Liposuction
First area $1,500 to 3,500
Each additional area $250 to 600

- Liposuction of the neck, chin or face
  $2,000 to 5,000
  With chin or cheek implants add $500 to 1,500

> *Consider the most popular procedure, liposuction, the surgical removal of fat by a machine not unlike a vacuum cleaner. A cosmetic surgeon can buy $4,000 worth of equipment on Monday morning, do two procedures on Monday afternoon, and then make money all day Tuesday.*
> — Congressman Ron Wyden, during Congressional subcommittee hearings on plastic surgery industry, 1989

> *The doctor I had was board certified and highly recommended.*
> *It was never told to me that there was a chance of infection, and it was never conveyed to me that I could hemorrhage . . . three weeks after the operation the front of my right leg caved in. There was an area of six inches long and six inches wide which I could place my hand into which I could feel muscles and bones in my leg. The doctor told me to rub my leg. Every time I went back to him it was the same story. He told me to keep rubbing my leg. He told me to have my husband rub it too, wink, wink — "just think of all those great rub downs."*
> *I could not bend my leg, I could not put my leg over the other leg. The pain was too much.*
> *. . . I went looking for a doctor who could fix my leg. On this particular doctor's walls he had a cartoon that said, "Treat yourself to a tummy tuck on your VISA card and a buttock lift on your MASTER CARD."*
> *For the little bit of fat, I ended up with a nightmare. Because when I awoke, I have not been the same person.*
> — Angela Brown, telling a Congressional subcommittee about her botched liposuction surgery, 1989

Liposuction was pioneered by a French abortionist in the 1970s. Reportedly over 100,000 Americans had liposuction in 1992. It is a procedure that has became popular and provides a cash harvest to doctors who can learn the procedure at a weekend seminar.

Liposuction can be done on the body to reduce sagging knees and ankles and to reduce breasts in men who have large breasts or as part of a breast reduction surgery performed on women who have overly large breasts. It is often done to reduce a double chin and baggy jowls during face-lift operations. Most commonly it is used to reduce love-handles on the lower back, stomach bulges and fat in the butt and thighs.

Liposuction is done with a suction "cannula" tube that is inserted through an incision usually about 1/8 to 1/2 inch long that is made in natural skin folds when available. Some of the incision areas to perform liposuction on the body include the inside rim of the belly button and the crease of the buttocks and the side of the hips. The cannula tube is connected to a vacuum device and is inserted into the skin where it is moved back and forth around the fatty areas to loosen and suction out the unwanted fat cells. A small cannula is believed to be safer and provide better results than a large one.

To prevent as much blood loss during surgery as liposuction patients experienced just a few years ago, doctors now add sterile saline solution along with Epinephrine (adrenaline) to the local anesthetic used to numb the surgical site. This reduces the amount of blood lost during the procedure and may provide for a better result.

Liposuction should only be used as a way to adjust the contours of the body and face. Liposuction is not meant, nor should it be used, to reduce weight or to correct obesity. It also will not cut down on the body's cholesterol level. Liposuction should not be used as an excuse to avoid eating or exercising properly. It can remove fat from surfaces under the skin but cannot remove fat from areas surrounding the interior organs where too much fat can cause serious health problems. Only diet and exercise can cut down on the amount of fat in the inner body.

Some doctors say that once the number of fat cells in a certain area have been surgically reduced by liposuction they do not return, while other doctors say that some areas of the body will create more fat cells when a person gains weight. If the patient then gains weight, the areas where the fat cells were removed can remain thin while other areas will gain the weight. This can result in an unusual wallowing appearance around the uneven areas of the liposuctioned location. Liposuction may occasionally worsen the appearance of cellulite.

Besides the doctor's skills and the technique used to perform the procedure, the outcome of liposuction depends on the resiliency of skin and how well it contracts and reshapes to the new contours. Any excess weight should be lost months before liposuction so the body and face and the skin covering them have time to adjust to the weight loss. This will help determine what contouring can be done, what the patient wants done, can give the patient a more realistic expectation of what can be done and may contribute to a more satisfactory result.

The surgery site is usually wrapped after the surgery to bind the skin back in place — this can include wearing a compression girdle. The garment collapses the tunnels so that they heal together. Recovery may take a few months as the swelling and bruising subside.

Nerves may be damaged during liposuction, resulting in temporary or permanent numbness. There have been patients who have had their muscles ripped and intestines and other vital organs torn open and partially suctioned out by the vacuum of the canulla tube used in liposuction.

When fat is removed electrolytes are removed also. Severe complications can result from excess fat removal and can send a patient into shock similar to that of people who have suffered a bad burn. Too much blood or fluid loss during liposuction can send a person into shock and may result in death. The wife of one doctor in Oklahoma died from too much blood loss while she was undergoing liposuction performed by her husband. One teenager died while undergoing liposuction when the doctor gave him an overdose of anesthesia.

The thousands of dollars spent to undergo liposuction might be better spent on a week or more at a health resort. Many of the health spa vacations cost less than undergoing liposuction surgery. The week spent at the spa is equal to the week that may be spent recovering from liposuction. Because the guest is taught healthful eating and proper exercise, the whole person is revitalized rather than just the part that had been suctioned of fat.

• Butt-lift (lipodystrophy)
$4,000 to 8,500+

During this procedure, incisions are made in the fold of skin at the top of the legs. Long, wide wedge-shaped strips of skin and fat, extending from the butt crease to the sides of the hips are cut off and the incisions are closed.

For best results the patient should lose excess weight and remain at an ideal weight for three to six months before undergoing this procedure.

To avoid damaging the incisions and the healing of the skin, the patient must avoid sitting for two or more weeks.

• Varicose Vein Removal

Also called "sclerotherapy"
- Spider vein removal/hyfrecation
- Varicose vein surgery/stripping
  $ 300 to 4,500+

The evaluation and treatment of vein disease is called phlebology. Bulging veins known as varicose veins can be caused by heredity or by hormonal changes during pregnancy. They happen when blood gathers where vein structures have broken down. They can cause discomfort, pain, burning and itching sensations and can lead to phlebitis or ulcerations. Various procedures can be done to soften the appearance of or eliminate varicose veins. Removing the veins may be beneficial in relieving the discomfort that is caused by them.

The varicose vein removing procedures include sclerotherapy, phlebectomy, hyfrecation, treatments with lasers and electrical clotting. With every technique to remove varicose veins there are recurrences seen. Some people find the recurrence rate of varicose veins to be acceptable and go in every few years for more treatments. (Pregnant or nursing women should not have these procedures performed on them.)

Sclerotherapy is a technique that has been widely used. It uses injections of either a saline or a chemical solution. The injections cause inflammation within the veins which causes them to collapse. The compressed vein walls grow together and the vein is closed. There is little or no pain caused by the procedures because the needles that are used are very small. There may be some muscle cramps during the procedure that usually last only a few minutes. Because saline is saltwater and is a naturally occurring body fluid there is little chance of an allergic reaction. There may be some bruising that will heal within a week. Some discoloration within the veins can occur and this normally fades in the following weeks and months.

The treatment is not always successful and more than one treatment may be needed to obtain the desired result. Because it may relieve pain, it is covered by some insurance plans. With some sclerotherapy, compression stockings need to be worn for two to three weeks for large veins and a few days for spider vein treatments. Regular activities are not interrupted by the healing, although heavy exercise should be put off for two or three days. Exercise may aid in the healing and prevention of future varicose veins.

Some of the doctors who criticize the procedure cite studies that show that sclerotherapy can cause more varicose veins and discoloration and a high rate of dissatisfaction. The chemical that is used may aggravate the immune system. The chemicals can also cause an allergic reaction, which has resulted in patient death.

Sometimes the removal of veins can make more veins appear. The end result may be scar tissue that creates white streaks on the legs. This is one procedure that can be performed on a small area to determine the chance of successful results.

Ambulatory phlebectomy is a vein elimination technique that may be longer lasting and less expensive than sclerotherapy. This procedure involves making small incisions in the leg and teasing the vein out with a hook. It may take weeks to heal. More veins may appear over the next several years but they may not be as extreme as the veins that were removed.

Hyfrecation can also be done with electrical clotting of the vein for the very tiniest veins. With hyfrecation no bandages need to be worn afterward.

Many of the people who are performing these procedures in some of the hard-sell vein clinics that have large ad campaigns are not vascular surgeons. Some doctors who work in these clinics have been ordering thousands of dollars worth of diagnostic tests.

• Scar Revision

How a scar affects the person can depend on the location of the scar and what caused it. Some people wear their scars proudly and show them off as if they are some type of award of courage. A scar that gives a model or actor character can make that person more in demand. The person with a scar may look more rugged, threatening or appealing as the scar brings attention to the surrounding features, as a beauty mark would.

Scars may also be reminders of tragic incidents such as an accident or crime and may be physically as well as psychologically deforming. Facial and neck scars can be particularly damaging to the person's image and erode the person's self-esteem because they can attract the rude comments of insensitive people. A person with dramatic facial scars can become a recluse and avoid activities that would expose the scar to people they knew before they had the scar. In this type of situation, a successful scar revision surgery can resurrect the person's esteem. Eventually some or all of the mental duress caused by a scar can fade as the person gets used to the scar. Sometimes a scar may also represent a struggle that made the person stronger.

Scars are made of collagen, a protein found throughout the body. During the healing of a wound the wounded area produces more collagen than normal. The blood vessels also increase in size as they bring nourishment to the wounded area. Some of the collagen usually breaks down as the wound heals and the blood vessels decrease in size. This is what causes the scar to fade, loosen and sometimes shrink.

The final outcome of a scar can take more than a year. In young people a scar may fade to the point where it is nearly undetectable by adulthood. Certain areas of the body are more likely to produce wider, thicker scars. Common areas for this to happen are on areas where the skin is pulled and stretched by common movements of the body.

The intensity of a scar depends on the location of the wound and the person's ability to heal. Some people form light scars while others form thicker scars. People with dark skin are more prone to form keloid scars. These are the kind of scars that are thick, raised, sometimes shiny, and in some people can continue to grow as the site produces more collagen and fails to break it down.

There are various ways to alter a scar so it becomes less noticeable. Scars need to heal and mature, usually for a year or more, before any surgery is performed on them. Not all scars are candidates for scar revision, and in some cases the procedures done to fade the scars can cause them to become more noticeable.

Steroid treatments to a scar can retard the collagen buildup. Some scars can also be surgically altered to remove the most dramatic areas. Surgery to remove a scar can be as simple as cutting away at the scar and sewing the skin back together in a way that it heals with as fine a line as possible. Sanding a scar with a dermabrader tool (a surgical process called "dermabrasion") can be effective in toning down a scar and bringing it to the level of the surrounding skin. There is a limit to the amount of dermabrasion that can be done.

Sometimes temporary surgically implanted skin-stretching balloons (tissue expanders) are placed beneath the unscarred skin near the scar. The balloons are then filled with a saline solution (salt water) over weeks and months. When the skin has been adequately stretched the balloons are taken out, and the scarred skin can be cut off and the stretched unscarred skin can be pulled over the area of the amputated scar.

Though there will always be some scarring caused by the incision to perform scar reduction procedures, the outcome can be successful in giving the area a more normal appearance.

• Tattoo Removal

People have probably been getting tattoos since the earliest of times. Tattoos have became popular in the last century with servicemen who get tattoos of the name of the ship they served on, names of the battles they fought and, the always popular, muscle movement tattoos that feature dancing girls.

In the last ten years there has been a surge in the popularity of tattoos as tattooing has become a mini industry with several magazines solely dedicated to "skin art." Tattoo parlors have popped up in every city. Some tattoo parlors in small resort towns specialize in giving people "skin photos" so tourists can remember special vacation moments. People who have gained fame through their music, acting, modeling or self-promotion display their tattoos in magazines and on TV talk shows. Some of them test the TV censors by confessing to strategically placed tattoos or by rearranging their clothes to show talk show hosts and audiences their newest tattoo.

Some couples have gone in for his-and-hers matching tattoos as a way of showing their dedication to each other. Some clubs and criminal gangs require their members to get a specific tattoo. Other people have had company logos tattooed on their bodies. There are people who have gotten tattoos on every possible square inch of available flesh of their body and face. Some crime victims have been able to identify their assailants by the criminal's unique tattoos. In one case that centered around a tattoo, a parent was charged with child abuse after having given his child a homemade tattoo.

Whatever a person's reason had been for getting a tattoo, many have gone on to regret the decision — especially when the tattoo is a symbol of a past romance gone sour or of people with whom they no longer associate.

Past techniques of tattoo removal involved dermabrasion, burning or surgery. These techniques caused scarring. Tattoos are now removed by dermatologists who use laser light and fruit acid treatments on tattoos that have been numbed with anesthesia.

The length of time required to remove a tattoo depends on the size of the tattoo; the amount, type and color of ink used; and the depth of the tattoo in the skin. The ink then fades in the following weeks and months as the skin naturally rids itself of the impurity. There will probably always be signs of the tattoo on the skin.

• Penis Lengthening/Enlarging
About $3,500 to 6,000

One of the new "breakthrough" procedures being touted in advertising that has been popping up in newspapers in the last couple of years is that of penis enlargement. The surgery is most commonly performed by either a urologist or a cosmetic surgeon. The procedures are done by transferring fat from one part of the body (via liposuction), usually the abdomen, into the penis to give it thickness (girth) and by cutting two suspensory ligaments that attach the penis to the pubic bone. The ligament-cutting procedure is done to extend an internal portion of the root of the penis further away from the body.

In the fat transfer procedure, as with all fat transfer procedures, the blood supply that fed the fat is not included in the transfer and some or all of the fat will fade away over time. This may result in gaps and unevenness. Doctors warn that fat transferred into the breasts to enlarge them can leave behind lumpy calcium deposits that may hide tumors or trigger their growth. The same may be true for fat transferred into the penis, though penile cancer is very rare. The operation may also cause infection and scarring. These scars may cause the penis to be twisted or curled.

The ligament-cutting procedure is attributed to a Doctor Long Daochou of Wuhan, China, where he is chief of the plastic surgery department at the First Affiliated Hospital of the Hubu Medical College. Doctor Long Daochou claims he developed this penis lengthening technique after experimenting on corpses. This procedure usually results in a gain of less than an inch, and this is mostly seen only during the flaccid state, with little gain in an erection. Some doctors warn that this can damage the nerves and blood vessels that service the penis and this may result in impotence or less feeling in the penis and could interfere with the ability to ejaculate. The suspensory ligaments that are cut also are the ones that center and steady the penis when it is erect. The erect penis might then be at a lower angle and off center after these ligaments have been cut. If there is any length gained in the erect state, the hair-bearing skin at the base of the lengthened penis will be pulled out during an erection and will cover part of the shaft.

Both of the procedures are done on an outpatient basis. Sex is out of the question for at least a month.

For the man who has a penis that is so large it should carry its own birth certificate, there is no operation to reduce the size of it.

• Sex-Change Operations

Among the people who undergo plastic surgery are those who have their sex organs surgically altered from male to appear female or female to appear male. Some refer to the process as "gender reassignment surgery."

Most transsexuals are men who have become women. The female-to-male operation is less common and more complicated to perform. The process of changing a man to appear as a woman includes hormone therapy, electrolysis to remove facial and body hair and sometimes a nose job or other cosmetic surgery to make the male face more feminine. The procedure to give a female the appearance of a male includes hormone therapy, removal of the breasts, removal of the uterus, and the surgical construction of a penis, which is a very complicated surgery with a price range of anywhere from $30,000 to $100,000.

The number of Americans who have had sex-change operations is estimated to be from three to six thousand and 30,000 worldwide according to the International Foundation for Gender Education in Waltham, Massachusetts. There are only a small number of doctors in the world who have any real experience at performing sex-change surgery. One doctor in Trinidad, Colorado, claims to have performed 3,000 male-to-female surgeries and 250 female-to-male surgeries.

Anyone considering a sex change should do research, investigate all of the ramifications and understand that relatives, especially parents, and sometimes the patient, may go through a grieving process as they lose the person they knew. Know that all gender-specific physical characteristics cannot be changed, especially the size and shape of the shoulders, arms, hands, feet and other physical structures related to sexual identification. There may be limited or no sexual feeling at all on the surgically redesigned organ. This can include the breast area if surgery is done there. Some doctors claim that over 80% of their sex-change patients have some sexual sensation on their redesigned sex organs. The redesigned sex organ will not appear exactly like a natural organ, especially if it has been a surgery to create a penis. The more natural-appearing surgically created sex organs are those of the female.

Among the precautions that can be taken before a person undergoes a sex-change operation is extensive psychotherapy. The patient also may be required to live as the new sex in clothing and by name for about a year before any surgery takes place. This means dressing like the new person he or she will be and taking on the new name legally and professionally. Some surgeons will take other precautions before the major change. These additional precautions may include performing the less dramatic parts of the sex change such as electrolysis on the man to remove facial hair or a nose job to make it more feminine. Other surgeries that may be done before the main surgery takes place can include having breast implants or other cosmetic surgery to give the person a more feminine or masculine appearance. Men being surgically changed to appear female sometimes elect to have some of the cartilage shaved from the Adam's apple to create a more feminine-looking neck. These can all be done months or years beforehand so that the patient can go through a gradual change and have time to decide if it is in fact what they want to do before the main surgery is performed where the genitals are altered.

Just as in other types of surgery, there have been botched sex-change operations and surgery performed on people who were unprepared. Even after all of those preventative measures, there are some people who later, after having all of the surgeries completed, realize they had made the wrong decision for themselves. Some of these patients have gone on to form support groups to help them cope with their situation.

11 • RESEARCH RESOURCES

Educating Yourself

If you are considering any elective surgery procedure, doing your own research can answer a lot of questions. Being well-informed can also play a part in your recovery, as studies show that well-informed patients recover faster. Any good doctor would not feel attacked by a patient who has made the effort to inform themselves by doing research.

The medical professional you are communicating with may not be aware of all the options out there for you because that person may not have read all of the information there is on your condition. Many procedures and forms of treatment have been developed after a patient inflicted with a condition was relentless in finding a way to improve their health. You may be one of those patients who is paramount in the development of a new form of treatment or operational technique.

If you are planning to undergo elective surgery, you should take responsibility to protect yourself. Investigate the doctor's training and experience. Know what the operation entails, what the risks are, what kind of injury it can cause, the healing process, and what can be done to fix the problems that may arise if the operation does not give the desired result.

Doing your own research and studying medical books found in any good library or bookstore can prepare you to deal with the world of medicine. No matter what your health concern is, there is information somewhere that can help you understand it and find the right help. Some doctors, medical schools and hospitals may let you use their private libraries for your medical research. The National Network of Libraries may be able to help you locate a library that contains the information you need (800) 338-7657.

Library research:
A librarian can help you locate specific information you need in reference books. Most libraries have a variety of

directories, indexes and encyclopedias that cover many
health topics. They also have other resources, such as
- **Directories that include information on associations**
There are thousands of support and specialty
information groups that exist to help people with specific
health needs. Associations provide a valuable network of
resources through publications and services such as
newsletters, conferences, seminars and professional journals.
Many of their publications contain the most recent
developments in medicine.
- **Computers for research**
Some large libraries have a computer database that you
can use to find information about specific subjects. Some
libraries are connected to the Internet.
- **Books**
Many guidebooks, textbooks and manuals on health are
published annually. To find the names of books not in your
local library check *Books In Print*, a directory of books
currently available from publishers.
Medical information in books can become quickly
outdated as advances in some areas of medicine are
happening rapidly.
- **Magazine, professional journal and newspaper articles**
Magazines and newspapers provide information that is
often more current than that found in books and textbooks.
There are a number of indexes available in libraries that can
help you find specific articles in periodicals.

You may not be able to understand all of the technical terms
used in medical books. Medical language is filled with phrases
such as "in vitro fertilization," which is simply the term for test-
tube fertilization. Using complicated terms is one way the
medical community keeps itself ambiguous. Meanwhile, to find
definitions of medical terms, look in a medical dictionary — or
ask your doctor.

Do not judge the simplicity of an operation on the clean line
drawings that are often used in medical texts to show how an
operation is performed. A textbook understanding of a surgical
procedure and actually performing the surgery are two very
different things. Also, remember that medical books often use
photographs of the worst case scenarios. So, if you are diagnosed
with a condition and are looking into a medical book and find
photos of people who have experienced severe reactions to the

same condition you have, do not assume that you will one day appear the same way.

Some doctors think that the patient should only know so much, and some act as if medical information should only be read by people who hold a degree in medicine. Some believe the patient should put their trust in the doctor. That is one way to open the door to future disappointment. If after surgery you discover that the operation was not what you expected, then it is too late to do library research, ask questions, get second and third opinions, assure that you understood every word of the informed consent form, and receive detailed explanations from the doctor of his intentions for you.

When you consider that many people spend thousands of dollars on operations to repair what other doctors have done to them, that other people are stuck with bad results from cosmetic surgery because they cannot afford to have it fixed or it is beyond repair, and that people have been injured, maimed and killed during cosmetic surgery, you should see very clearly that doing your own research before undergoing any of these surgeries is a very wise thing to do.

Do not be surprised if during your research you find out something that the doctor does not know. The human body is a very complex mechanism and not one person knows everything about it. There are also new procedures being developed and new discoveries about the body being found every day by the many people around the world dedicated to the study of the human body.

Medical Health Organizations, Information Resources and Personal Support

I tried to include groups that deal with everything that is mentioned in the book. Some of the organizations listed here are nonprofit and support themselves solely by donations; therefore, they may welcome any kind of financial help you can give them (check with them before sending a donation). Some will require that when you request information, you send them a self-addressed, stamped envelope.
— the author

Phone numbers

Because phone numbers are subject to change, if any of the following phone numbers do not work, simply call information by dialing the area code followed by 555-1212 and ask for the new number of the organization.

Books

There are many books available on most subjects. The books that are listed are some of the books the author has read and that can generally be found in book stores or libraries. More technically detailed books are available in medical libraries.

Organizations

A listing here does not mean a company is completely legitimate. Consumers should take steps to protect themselves and beware of the credibility and safety of any service, business, association or professional mentioned in this research section.

• ABUSE

Books :
- *Come Here: One Man Overcomes the Tragic Aftermath of Childhood Sexual Abuse*, by Richard Berendzen with Laura Palmer; Villard Books, 1993
- *Confronting Abuse*, by Anne L. Horton, B. Kent Harrison and Barry L. Johnson; Deseret Book Company 1993
- *The Courage to Heal: A Guide for Women Survivors of Child Sexual Abuse*, by Ellen Bass and Laura Davis; Harper Collins, 1993
- *Family Violence*, by Mildred Daley Pagelow; Praeger, 1984
- *The Right to Innocence*, by Beverly Engle, M.F.C.C.; St. Martin's Press, New York, 1989
- *The Sexually Abused Male*, by M. Hunter; Macmillan, New York, 1990
- *Silent Sons*, by Robert J. Ackerman; Simon & Schuster, 1993
- *Trauma and Recovery*, by J.L. Herman, Basic Books/Harper Collins, New York, 1992
- *Verbal Abuse: Survivors Speak Out on Relationship and Recovery*, by Patricia Evans, 1994
- *The Verbally Abusive Relationship: How to Recognize It and How to Respond*, by Patricia Evans; Bob Adams, Inc., 1992
- *Victims No Longer: Men Recovering from Incest and Other Sexual Child Abuse*, by Mike Lew; Harper Collins, 1990
- *Wednesday's Children : Adult Survivors of Abuse Speak Out*, by Suzanne Somers; Putnam, 1992
- *Woman-Battering: Victims and Their Experiences*, by Mildred Daley Pagelow; Sage Publishers, 1981
- *You Can't Say That to Me!: Stopping the Pain of Verbal Abuse*, by Suzette Haden Elgin; John Wiley & Sons, 1995

Many people undergo plastic surgery to repair physical damage that was the result of physical abuse and criminal assault. People who have been the subject of other forms of abuse might also seek a physical transformation through surgery to change the part of their physical structure that was the target of abusive criticism or cruel comments.

Abuse and assault are about power and control. It can be done in several ways including sexual, verbal, psychological, physical, spiritual, ritual and financial. The physical and emotional damage caused by abuse makes it one of the most horrible violations a person can experience.

Often a person who has regularly been mistreated in their own home does not recognize the seriousness of the problem and does not know the damage that has been done to them. Many times they lack healthy communication skills and proceed to mistreat others or allow others to mistreat them.

Simply leaving an abusive relationship does not cure a person from it. They take a suitcase of memories that affect their thought patterns, dreams, actions, body language and the way they treat and relate to other people.

People involved in abuse should seek outside help through counseling and/or support groups. The best understanding of abuse may come from people who have had to cope with severe abuse. There are many books written about the different kinds of abuse. Reading books about abuse that were written by people who have been through severe abuse may be very helpful to people who are currently experiencing it or who need to work through their feelings about what happened to them in the past.

A support group is a group of people who share a common concern and who are seeking information, strength and support to cope with an ongoing personal issue. A doctor or other "expert" is usually not present and the groups are run by an organizer who is part of the group. There is usually a small donation requested but people with financial troubles can attend for free and should not feel embarrassed to do so.

Center for Adult Survivors of Sexual Abuse
205 Avenue I, Suite 27, Redondo Beach, California 90277; Phone (310) 379-5929

Child Help USA
6463 Independence Avenue, Woodland Hills, California 91367; Phone toll-free (800) 422-4453

Domestic Abuse Hotline
Phone toll-free (800) 288-3854

Family Violence & Sexual Assault Bulletin
1310 Clinic Drive, Tyler, Texas 75701; Phone (903) 595-6600

Incest Resources Women's Center
46 Pleasant Street, Cambridge, Massachusetts 12139; Phone (617) 492-1818

Incest Survivors Anonymous
P.O. Box 17245, Long Beach, California 90807-7245; Phone (310) 428-5599

Incest Survivors Resource Network, Inc.
P.O. Box 7375, Las Cruces, New Mexico 88006-7375; Phone (505) 521-4260

National Association for Child Abuse and Neglect
Phone (800) 4-A-CHILD

National Center for Elder Abuse
810 First Street, Suite 500, Washington, DC 20002; Phone (202) 682-2470

National Coalition Against Domestic Violence
P.O. Box 18749, Denver, Colorado 80218-0749; Phone (303) 839-1852
— or —
P.O. Box 15127, Washington, DC 20003-0127; Phone (202) 638-6388 or 293-7764 or toll-free (800) 333-SAFE

National Resource Center on Child Sexual Abuse
Phone (800) 543-7006

National Victim Center
Infolink
P.O. Box 17150, Fort Worth, Texas 76102; Phone (817) 877-3355 or toll-free (800) FYI-CALL

Rape Abuse & Incest National Network
Phone (800) 656-HOPE

Survivors of Incest Anonymous (SIA)
P.O. Box 21817, Baltimore, Maryland 21222; Phone (410) 433-2365

• ACCREDITING HEALTHCARE FACILITIES AND SETTING HEALTHCARE STANDARDS

To find out whether a hospital has been certified by Medicare, contact your local Medicare office (a Social Security office can supply you with the phone number). Your state health department can tell you if a hospital has been suspended from participating in Medicare or is on probation. The United States Government Printing Office prints a yearly *Medicare Information Report*. It is available in some libraries or can be purchased through the

United States Government Printing Office
Phone (202) 783-3238

American Association for Accreditation of Ambulatory Plastic Surgery Facilities
1202 Allanson Road, Mundalein, Illinois 60060; Phone (708) 949-6058

The American College of Radiology accredits radiology facilities that, among other things, conduct mammograms.

American College of Radiology
1891 Preston White Drive, Reston, Virginia 22091; Phone (703) 648-8900

American Hospital Association
Order Processing Department
840 North Lake Shore Drive, Chicago, Illinois 60611; Phone (312) 280-6000

American Managed Care and Review Association
1227 — 25th Street, NW, Number 610, Washington, DC 20037; Phone (202) 728-0506

Association for Ambulatory Healthcare
9933 Lawler Avenue, Skokie, Illinois 60077-3702; Phone (708) 676-9610

The *Consumer's Guide to Hospitals* is published by the Center for the Study of Services and contains information compiled by the Healthcare Financing Administration which collects data on hospital mortality rates. The book is available for $12 through the

Center for the Study of Services
Phone (800) 475-7283

Commission on Accreditation of Rehabilitation Facilities
2500 Pantzano Road, Tucson, Arizona 85715; Phone (602) 748-1212

Foundation for Healthcare Evaluation
2901 Metro Drive, Suite 400, Bloomington, Minnesota 55425

For information on hospital mortality rates, contact the

Healthcare Financing Administration
Health Standards and Quality Bureau
2-D-2 Meadows East Building, 6325 Security Boulevard, Baltimore, Maryland 21207; Phone (410) 966-1133

The Joint Commission on Accreditation of Healthcare Organizations offers educational programs for people in the healthcare industry and inspects medical facilities to see if they are in compliance with national standards. The commission is sponsored by the American Medical Association, the American Hospital Association, the American College of Physicians, the American College of Surgeons, and the American Dental Association. The survey consists of more than 2,000 quality standards, including safety of the buildings, infection control, patient services and records, staff training, use of pharmaceuticals and administrative procedures. The survey does not cover specific medical procedures and their outcomes. About 80% of US hospitals are accredited.

The JCAHO will tell you whether a particular hospital is accredited. In October, 1994, the commission agreed to begin to make once-secret report cards issued to 11,000 US hospitals, nursing homes and other health facilities available to the public. This action drew complaints from hospitals about the fairness of the reports and claims of inconsistencies in the inspections conducted by the commission. The detailed performance reports, which are prepared every three years with participating facilities, were previously confidential. The cost of obtaining a report is $30.

Joint Commission on Accreditation of Healthcare Organizations
1 Renaissance Boulevard, Oakbrook Terrace, Illinois 60181; Phone (708) 916-5800 or 5600

To find out if a hospital has been certified by Medicare, contact your local Medicare office (a Social Security office can supply you with the phone number). Your state health department can tell you if a hospital has been suspended from participating in Medicare or is on probation. The United States Government Printing Office prints a yearly Medicare

Information Report. It is available in some libraries or can be purchased through the

United States Government Printing Office
Phone (202) 783-3238

The National Committee for Quality Assurance accredits Health Maintenance Organizations. The Committee keeps report cards on HMOs. The report cards are based on an evaluation system called the HEDIS Indicators. These report cards may be available directly from the HMOs and helpful in evaluating the services a person may receive under a particular HMO plan.

National Committee for Quality Assurance
1350 New York Avenue, NW, Suite 700, Washington, DC 20005

• ALLERGY AND ASTHMA

Books:
- *The Complete Guide to Food Allergy and Intolerance: Prevention, Identification, and Treatment of Common Illnesses and Allergies Caused by Food*, by Dr. Jonathon Brostoff and Linda Gamlin; Crown Publishers, 1989
- *Sinus Survival*, by Dr. Robert S. Ivker; Perigee Books/Putnam Publishing 1992

Allergy Alert Newsletter (published quarterly)
Allergy Foundation of Canada
P.O. Box 1904, Saskatoon, SK, Canada 57K 3S5; Phone (306) 652-1608

The Allergy and Asthma Network publishes the Mothers of Asthmatics Report. The newsletter presents educational, medical and resource information on asthma and allergies.

Allergy and Asthma Network
3554 Chain Bridge Road, Suite 200, Fairfax, Virginia 22030; Phone (703) 385-4403

Allergy Control Products
96 Danbury Road, Ridgefield, Connecticut 06887; Phone toll-free (800) 422-DUST

Allergy Foundation of America
801 Second Avenue, New York, New York 10017; Phone (212) 684-7875

American Association of Certified Allergists
800 East Northwest Highway, Suite 1080, Palatine, Illinois 60067; Phone (708) 359-3919

American College of Allergy and Immunology
85 West Algonquin, Suite 550, Arlington Heights, Illinois 60005; Phone (708) 427-1200 or toll-free (800) 842-7777

Asthma and Allergy Foundation of America
1717 Massachusetts Avenue, NW, Suite 305, Washington, DC 20036; Phone (202) 265-0265 or (800) 624-0044

Asthma Information Center
P.O. Box 790, Springhouse, Pennsylvania 19477-0790; Phone toll-free (800) 727-5400

Canadian Society of Allergy and Clinical Immunology
Victoria General Hospital, P.O. Box 5375, 800 Commissioner's Road East, London, Ontario N6A 4G5; Phone (519) 685-8167

The Food Allergy Network
4744 Holly Avenue, Fairfax, Virginia 22030

4Health (detoxification products)
5485 Conestoga Court, Boulder, Colorado 80301; Phone (800) 525-9696

Gluten Intolerance Group of North America
P.O. Box 23053, Seattle, Washington 98102-03543; Phone (206) 325-6980

ZAND Herbal Formulas
P.O. Box 5312, Santa Monica, California 90409; Phone (310) 822-0500

• ANESTHESIOLOGY

Upon request, the American Association of Nurse Anesthetists will send you pamphlets that will familiarize you with anesthesia and the process of preparing for, administration of and recovery from anesthesia. The name of the pamphlets are: *Anesthesia and Patient Responsibility; Before Anesthesia: Your Active Role Makes a Difference;* and *After Anesthesia: Your Active Role Assists Your Recovery.*

Prior to entering the Master's Degree nurse anesthesia educational program, nurse anesthetists must have at least one year's acute care experience. Additional continuing education is required for recertification every two years.

American Association of Nurse Anesthetists
222 South Prospect Avenue, Park Ridge, Illinois 60068-4001; Phone (708) 692-7050

American Board of Anesthesiology
100 Constitution Plaza, Hartford, Connecticut 06103; Phone (203) 522-9857

American Osteopathic Board of Anesthesiology
17201 East Highway 40, Suite 204, Independence, Missouri 64055; Phone (816) 373-4700

American Society of Anesthesiologists
520 Northwest Highway, Park Ridge, Illinois 60068-2573; Phone (708) 825-5586

American Society of Post Anesthesia Nurses
11512 Allegheny Parkway, Suite C, Richmond, Virginia 23235; Phone (804) 379-5516

American Society of Regional Anesthesia
1910 Byrd Avenue, Suite 100, Richmond, Virginia 23230-1086; Phone (804) 282-0010

Association of University Anesthetists
Department of Anesthesia, University of Washington, Seattle, Washington 98121; Phone (206) 305-3117

The AWARE (Awareness with Anesthesia Research and Education) Foundation was founded by Jeanette Tracy. She had an "explicit awareness" experience during hernia surgery during which she could not move or communicate but could feel all pain and hear what was going on in the operating room. The foundation is working to find a way to monitor when a person becomes aware of pain during surgery.

AWARE Foundation
Phone (800) 65-AWARE (29273)

Canadian Anesthetists' Society
1 Eglinton Avenue East, #209, Toronto, Ontario M4P 3A1; Phone (416) 480-0602

• BILLING PROBLEMS

Book
  • *Getting the Most for Your Medical Dollar*, by Charles Inlander and Karla Morales; People's Medical Society [462 Walnut Street, Allentown, Pennsylvania 18102 Phone (610) 770-1670]

Although some overcharges might be honest mistakes, most hospital bills contain errors and these are usually not in the patients' favor. Often these charges are false, and some charges are for tests and procedures that were ordered and never carried out because they were overlooked or were canceled.

When services are not coded correctly it can cause interference with insurance coverage. When you cannot get clear definitions of the codes and abbreviations on your hospital bill you may want to contact the patient account representative at the hospital billing department, the doctor, or the claims representative of your insurance carrier to find out what it is you are being charged for. Keep a record of who you spoke with, the date and what was said. If all else fails you might want to contact your state's insurance commissioner.

If you send your medical records to one of the private auditing services be sure to request that your records be returned to you unless you possess your own copy. Whenever possible keep the originals for your own files and send copies to the auditing service.

CostReview Services is a company with three medical price review departments. CostReview works with insurance companies, MedResolve works with doctors, and MedReview works with patients.
MedReview will review patient bills generated by hospitals, doctors, clinics and laboratories. A person using MedReview's service sends the company copies of medical records and itemized billing statements and any records relating to each bill. A nurse-auditor will make a report of the discrepancies and work with the patient to straighten out the bill. If a claim for adjustment or reimbursement is appropriate, MedReview will act as your advocate in filing an appeal. The fee for the audit of hospital bills is based on the amount billed by the hospital. All fees, for both hospital and physician reviews, are subject to 8% sales tax.
According to MedReview, there are discrepancies on 98% of hospital bills that are sent to patients.

MedReview
3724 Executive Center Drive, Suite 101, Austin, Texas 78731; Phone (512) 338-9196 or toll-free (800) 397-5359

ProMediClaim is not associated with any insurance agency.

ProMediClaim
113, McHenry Road, Suite 274, Buffalo Grove, Illinois 60089; Phone (708) 634-6212

• BLOOD

Emergency surgery and some medical conditions account for the majority of transfusions. For this, a public blood supply is maintained. Most types of planned surgery patients generally lose so little blood that they do not need blood transfusions. Few plastic surgery procedures require any type of blood donation. If a blood donation is needed, there are questions that should be asked and precautions to take.

A "team approach" with your doctor, the blood collection facility, and you, the patient, is needed to determine what the safest transfusion procedure is that may be taken.

Seven Important Questions to Ask Your Doctor (before undergoing surgery)
1. *Will I need blood for my operation?*
2. *Can I give blood in advance in case I need it?*
3. *Is there enough time before the operation to give the blood I will need?*
4. *Where should I go to give blood for my operation?*
5. *Can my blood be saved during the operation and given back to me if I need it?*
6. *What are the risks in giving or receiving my own blood?*
7. *Will I have to pay extra if I use my own blood?*
   — from the publication *Your Operation — Your Blood,* by the National Heart, Lung, and Blood Institute, a branch of the National Institutes of Health

Some of the more common operations in which enough blood will be lost to require transfusing are orthopedic, cardiac, chest, gynecological, and blood vessel surgery. Under rare circumstances blood transfusion may also be needed during pregnancy and delivery.

The procedure where a person donates blood before getting an operation is called "autologous" blood donation (blood intended for use by someone other than the donor is known as "homologous"). It is based on the fact that donating before surgery, and receiving your own blood during and after surgery, is better and safer than receiving someone else's blood.

Some advantages to donating one's own blood for later use are

- *reduced risk of infectious disease transmission*
- *reduced risk of transfusion reactions related to differences between donor and recipient, such as blood type*
- *more rapid replacement by your body of blood lost during surgery, since the bone marrow where blood cells form has already been activated by the process of donating blood*
- *less demand on the community blood supply*

In autologous donation, a person can often give one unit of blood a week for up to six weeks, depending on the anticipated need. Each unit is just under a pint and is about 10 percent of the total blood supply of an average-sized adult. The last donation is usually made no closer than three days before the scheduled surgery. This allows the body time to replenish the fluid that has been removed. It is possible that iron supplements may be prescribed to build up the number of red blood cells to avoid anemia.

As public interest in blood donations has increased, a number of entrepreneurs have entered the market. These facilities will — at their locations around the country — collect, freeze and store your blood, and then deliver it to you — thawed and ready to use — when and if your physician calls for it.

Costs can be high, and shipping charges may be added. There is no guarantee the blood would be available when needed or that there would be time to thaw and ship it. (Under present FDA regulations, frozen blood may be kept for only 10 years and cannot be shipped between states.) In addition, frozen blood contains only red blood cells. If you need blood platelets or plasma, you may have to turn to the public blood supply. (As liquid blood, the donated units can be kept for up to 42 days, depending on the preservative used.)
  — from *Who Donates Better Blood for You Than You?*; *FDA Consumer Magazine*

You should inform your doctor of your blood type. Receiving the wrong blood type can kill you. Transplanted organs and tissues also need to originate from a person with the same blood type as the receiver.

During surgery the volume of blood in the body must be maintained. A depletion in the volume of blood in the circulatory system can lower blood pressure and threaten the delivery of oxygen and the removal of waste products from the vital organs. A sustained minimal blood flow is called shock, and can lead to infection, irreversible organ damage — including damage to the brain, and death. On the other hand, if blood pressure is too high, blood clots may be dislodged and this can contribute to more bleeding.

When an operation is being performed that causes a large amount of blood loss, autotransfusion devices may be used to collect the patient's own blood shed during surgery and return it back into their body. This is called "blood salvage" or "intraoperative blood collection and reinfusion" and is often done during heart, vascular, and orthopedic surgeries, solid organ transplants and other very complicated operations. The amount of blood recovered during surgery varies with the operative procedure but may amount to 50 percent or more of the blood lost. Blood salvage is not done with patients who have infections (because there is no existing system that can effectively clean the blood), cancer (because of a risk of transferring malignant cells to another location) or other risk factors.

Two ways of salvaging blood and reinfusing it into the body exist. The first is to reinfuse the blood after mixing it with an anticoagulant. The second is to clean the blood with special equipment before reinfusing it. The first method, which is the fastest of the two, processes a unit of salvaged blood in just a few minutes. The process that cleans the blood is believed to be safer than the one where the blood is not cleaned because cleaning the blood can remove tiny bits of tissue and other debris introduced into the blood during the surgical procedure. When blood is salvaged during surgery a specially trained person whose job is to run the machinery that treats the salvaged blood is required to be present with no other responsibilities during the surgery.

Sometimes blood is collected after surgery through the use of drains located at the surgical sites and reinfused without being processed.

Another form of self-donation is called "acute normovolemic hemodilution." This is done by drawing blood from the patient before surgery and immediately infusing the patient with fluids to compensate for the blood that has been removed. The blood is collected into labeled blood bags and mixed with an anticoagulant. It can then be stored at room temperature for up to four hours or refrigerated if more time is needed. After the surgery the patient is reinfused with the blood that was drawn. This preserves red blood cells by preventing them from being lost through bleeding during surgery. The procedure may be performed by the attending anesthesiologist. Some in the medical community question the safety of this procedure.

Some items to consider if you are going to need to receive blood during a surgery and you are going to donate your own blood:
- You may need more blood than the doctor predicts.
- One surgery might not be enough to correct what the surgery is meant to correct.
- You may have complications that could require further surgery.
- The blood you donate may be contaminated after you donated it because of a lab accident or neglect.
- The blood you donate may be mislabeled.
- Some people have contracted blood-related illnesses from donated blood when they received donated blood after autologous donations were used up.
- Depending on the facility where your blood is stored, unused autologous donations may be discarded upon your release from the hospital or may be stored until the blood is expired. Your interests might best be served if the blood is kept until it expires in case you need it. Find out what the policy is at the facility you are dealing with. Extended storage can usually be arranged.

There are currently more types of blood tests than ever before. This has made today's blood supply safer than any time in the past. But blood reinfusion (receiving your own blood) remains the safest option.
- The FDA has said that the chances of an allergic reaction to transfusion is as high as 1 in 25
- The FDA has said that blood that harbors the HIV virus sometimes gets through the testing system — 1 in 61,000 to 1 in 225,000
- Blood with the hepatitis C virus is believed to still be a risk in about 1 in 900 transfusions
- Blood taken from people who are infected with dangerous viruses can test clean because the tests actually screen for antibodies and not for the actual virus and the body can

take weeks or months to start producing antibodies after a person is infected
- Not all viruses have been discovered
- There is no fail-safe screening test for a toxic bacterium called Yersinia which can cause massive blood clots
- Most blood banks are not required to be federally licensed and are not required to report mistakes to the FDA
- The FDA records several thousand blood bank errors every year including mislabeling of blood with the wrong blood type, inaccurate or inadequate blood testing, and improper storage
- Some blood products used in America are imported from other countries where testing procedures may not have been done properly
- The possibility of lawsuits being filed against blood banks is a serious consideration, so when they and medical facilities learn that a patient may have received tainted blood they do not always notify the patients even if they know who the patients are and how to contact them

Other blood facts:
- The process of donating blood stimulates the bone marrow to produce more blood cells
- It takes the body about 24 hours to replace the fluid lost during donation of one unit of blood but up to two months to replenish the supply of red blood cells contained in that unit — taking iron supplements can assist the body in replacing blood cells faster
- Red blood cells survive for about 110 days
- Liquid blood can be stored for 42 days
- Frozen blood can be stored for ten years
- A unit of blood is just under a pint
- The average person carries about 10 units of blood and a healthy person can quickly recover from the loss of 10 percent of their blood volume
- When donating for autologous collection the last donation is usually collected no later than 72 hours before surgery
- Many patients preparing for surgery can give blood as frequently as every 3 days, although once a week is most common when donating for autologous purposes
- Some patients, such as those needing cardiovascular surgery, may risk deterioration of their condition if they delay surgery in order to donate autologous blood. The risk

of contracting a contagious disease through America's donated blood is generally very slim. In cases when the patient is delaying needed surgery while the health condition is deteriorating much more risks are created than any risks presented by receiving blood from another person.

People with healthy blood should donate blood regularly. To find out about donating blood for yourself or for others, contact the Red Cross or a local blood bank at the phone number listed in your phone book or one of the following groups.

American Association of Blood Banks
8101 Glenbrook Road, Bethesda, Maryland 22207; Phone (301) 907-6977 or 215-6480

Council of Community Blood Centers
725 – 15th Street NW, Suite 700, Washington, DC 20005; Phone (202) 393-5725

Department of Health and Human Services
Public Health Service
Food and Drug Administration, Office of Public Affairs, 5600 Fishers Lane, Rockville, Maryland 20857

National Hemophilia Foundation
1101 – 17th Street NW, Washington, DC 20036; Phone (202) 833-0085

The Red Cross
Phone (800) 974-2113

• BREAST CANCER

Books:
* *Breast Cancer*, by Steve Austin and Cathy Hitchcock; Prima Publishing, 1994
* *Breast Cancer, The Complete Guide*, by Yashar Hirshaut and Peter I. Pressman; Bantam Books, 1993
* *Breast Cancer? Let Me Check My Schedule!: Ten Women Meet the Challenge of Fitting Breast Cancer into Their Busy Lives*; Innovative Medical Education Consortium, Inc. [(800) 205-4632], 1994
* *I Can Cope*, by Judi Johnson and Linda Klein; DCI Publishing, 1988
* *Long-Term Tamoxifen Treatment for Breast Cancer*, by V. Craig Jordan, MD; University of Wisconsin Press, Madison, WI 53715, 1995
* *Dr. Susan Love's Breast Book*, by Susan M. Love; Addison-Wesley, 1991
* *Recovering after Breast Surgery: Exercises to Strengthen Your Body and Relieve Pain*, by Diana Stumm; P.T. Hunter House Publishers [(510) 865-5282], 1995
* *Save Yourself from Breast Cancer*, Robert M. Kradjian, MD; Berkeley Publishing Group, phone (212) 951-8913
* *Surviving Cancer*, by Danette G. Kaufman; Acropolis Books, 1989
* *What to Do if You Get Breast Cancer*, by Lydia Komarnicky, and Anne Rosenberg; Little, Brown and Company, [(212) 522-8070], 1994
* *You Don't Have to Suffer: A Complete Guide to Relieving Cancer Pain for Patients and Their Families*, by Susan S. Lang and Richard B. Patt; Oxford University Press [(800) 451-7556], 1995

American women have one of the highest incidences of breast cancer in the world. Although there has been research that shows there are certain risk factors for developing breast cancer, no one really knows what causes breast cancer. All that is known is that the incidence of breast cancer is believed to have doubled in America from 1940 to 1980.

> During the eight years of the Vietnam war, 54,000 Americans died. This year alone, 46,000 women died of breast cancer.
> — The Breast Cancer Research Foundation, 1994

While doing research for this book I compiled the following list of items that various sources of information mentioned may play a part in determining whether a woman does or does not develop breast cancer:
- Taking the pill (though some studies show that the pill reduces the incidence of ovarian and uterine cancers)
- Taking DES (diethylstilbestrol) treatments during pregnancy
- Having a menstrual cycle that started early in life
- Going through menopause late in life
- Having a family history of breast cancer

    In September 1994, it was announced that researchers at the University of Utah identified a breast cancer gene now called BRCA1 that is estimated to be carried by 600,000 American women and may account for 5 percent of breast cancer cases.

    Researchers Mark Skolnick, Lisa Cannon-Albright and David Goldgar were aided by genealogy records kept by Mormon families in Utah who are known for keeping detailed family history charts that go back for centuries. Using records from Mormon families, the Utah Genealogical Data Base was specifically set up to be used for genetic research.

    Some question whether making a test that screens for this gene widely available would result in emotional stress for the women who have it and a false sense of security for those who test negative for the gene when only a small percentage of women with breast cancer have a family history of it.
- Having an induced abortion (increases risks)

    A study done by the Fred Hutchison Cancer Center in Seattle and that was printed in the Journal of the National Cancer Institute found that, among 1,815 women studied, women who had an abortion were 50% more likely to develop breast cancer. If the abortion was before the age 18, the women were 150% more likely to develop breast cancer. The risks were higher if the pregnancy had proceeded beyond eight weeks.

- Having children early in adulthood (lowers risks)
- Breast feeding (lowers risks)
- Regular exercise (lowers risks)

A 1986 study done by Rose E. Frisch of the Harvard School of Public Health and Center for Population studies came to the conclusion that long-term athletic training establishes a lifestyle that somehow lowers the risk of breast cancer and cancers of the reproductive system.

A study done by Leslie Bernstein at the University of Southern California's Norris Comprehensive Cancer Center that was published in the September issue of the *Journal of the National Cancer Institute* concluded that exercising at least four hours a week significantly reduces breast cancer risks. Working out lowers the levels of estradiol (a form of estrogen) and progesterone, both of which can play a part in breast tumor formation, and subsequently diminishes the breast's exposure to hormones.

- Taking lactation suppresser drugs (increases risks)
- The accumulated effect of x-rays done over the years
- Having estrogen therapy after hysterectomy

Estrogen may be beneficial in preventing heart disease and osteoporosis but also may promote breast cancer (for updated information on the subject of hormone replacement therapy, contact A Friend Indeed Publications, Inc., Box 1710, Champlain, New York 12919-1710, Phone (514) 843-5730, Fax (514) 843-5681. Ten issues a year are $30.)

- Consumption of soy protein (lowers risks)
- Having a diet low in nutrition and especially low in fresh fruits and vegetables

Women who eat a mostly vegetarian diet have lower levels of the kind of estrogens associated with breast cancer. According to the University of California in Los Angeles, a diet high in plant content helps to prevent breast cancer because plant fiber slows down the reabsorption of hormones associated with increased risk of breast cancer.

- Having a high-sugar diet

- Having a diet that is high in fat

  A study of women in the country of Greece that was done by epidemiologists at Harvard School of Public Health that was published in the *Journal of the National Cancer Institute* reported that women who had consumed olive oil in their daily diets had a 25% lower risk of breast cancer compared to women who consumed olive oil less frequently. The study's authors cautioned that they do not yet know what substances in olive oil may help to prevent breast cancer. Olive oil does contain vitamins and is a monounsaturated fat.

- Eating foods that contain artificial colors, flavors, preservatives and other artificial additives

- Eating foods that contain growth hormones and other chemicals fed to farm animals

  One such hormone that has received a lot of attention is the milk-production stimulant known as recombinant bovine growth hormone. The hormone induces a marked and sustained increase in levels of the insulin-like growth factor-1 (IGF-1) in cow's milk. Some say that it is likely that IGF-1 promotes transformation of normal breast tissue to breast cancer and that it maintains malignancy of human breast-cancer cells, including their ability to spread to distant organs.

  The FDA has said they have found no unusual problems with cows that have been injected with the bovine growth hormone.

  In a letter written to the FDA, Dr. Samuel Epstein, a professor of occupational and environmental medicine at the University of Illinois School of Public Health, warned that the effects of IGF-1 could include premature growth stimulation in infants, breast enlargement in young children, and breast cancer in adult females. In an article written for the Los Angeles Times, Epstein noted that the Council on Scientific Affairs of the American Medical Association stated: "Further studies will be required to determine whether the ingestion of higher than normal concentrations of bovine insulin-like growth factor is safe for children, adolescents and adults."

  Hormone-treated cows are believed to have a higher incidence of painful udder infections, and this results in pus contaminated milk. The antibiotics used to treat these infections also end up in the milk products that are sold for human consumption.

The FDA has said there are no risks involved with the ingestion of the milk from cows that have been treated with the hormone.

On December 14, 1994, the unresolved human health issues related to Bovine Growth Hormone caused the European Council of Ministers to impose a ban through the year 2000 on the commercial use of the product. (Citizens for Health Report, Volume 3:1, 1995)

(For more information on this subject, contact The Humane Farming Association at [415] 771-CALF or the Pure Food Campaign at [202] 775-1132)

- Exposure to pesticides used on farms, in homes and businesses, and sprayed over cities

  Researchers at the Strang Cancer Prevention Center at Cornell University Medical School found that pesticides appear to raise levels of a harmful form of estrogen. The study was done with the expectation that it would show that pesticides had no effect on estrogen.
- Exposure to tobacco smoke
- Exposure to household chemicals
- Exposure to certain chemicals found in toiletries and hygiene products
- Exposure to industrial chemicals and waste
- Exposure to exhaust fumes and air pollution
- Living in neighborhoods with an abundance of electrical transformers

On October 18, 1993, members of the national Breast Cancer Coalition handed President Bill Clinton a stack of petitions containing 2.6 million signatures of American citizens urging the president to initiate more research to find what may be causing breast cancer.

According to the American Cancer Society, breast cancer is the most common form of cancer in America and is the leading cause of death among women ages 15 to 54 years. Many professionals consider it to be an epidemic as it is now expected to afflict 182,000 American women a year and cause the death of 45,000 of these women. Women who get breast cancer when they are young are more likely to die from it. One in nine American women who live to their full life expectancy are expected to develop some form of breast cancer. Whereas three quarters of all breast cancer cases occur in women over 50, the incidence of breast cancer has risen steadily among women in every age group. Because of medical advances, most women who do get breast cancer will not die from it. Additionally, women with breast cancer who attend support groups have a better chance of surviving the disease.

The National Cancer Institute recommends that all women do monthly breast self-examinations (BSE) to feel for lumps or thickenings, swelling, puckering, skin irritation and pain or tenderness of a nipple (all lumps are not cancerous, but should be checked by a doctor). For women who menstruate, the best time to examine the breasts is two or three days after the menstrual period ends, when the breasts are least likely to be tender or swollen. Women who no longer menstruate should examine their breasts at the same time each month. (As about 1,000 American men are diagnosed with breast cancer each year and an estimated 300 die each year from breast cancer, men too should regularly examine their breasts.) The breast exam should cover the entire chest area from underarm to underarm and from the collarbones to the underside base of the breast.

The NCI also recommends that, starting in their teens, women should have breast exams once every three years performed by a doctor. The breast exam should include the area behind the areola, where many lumps are overlooked.

One way of finding lumps is through mammography. A mammogram is a special x-ray picture of the breast done with minimal amounts of radiation. It is designed to find cancer in its earliest stages — even years before a person can feel a lump or have any other symptoms and sometimes when a lump is still the size of a pinhead. Women should have mammograms performed at facilities that are certified by the FDA (Food and Drug Administration). A facility that is certified by the FDA should have the certificate prominently displayed.

> Quality standards for mammography were required by a law passed by Congress in 1992, and the deadline for certification was October 1, 1994. Facilities lacking such certification are operating illegally. To find an accredited facility call the Cancer Information Service at 1-800-4-CANCER.

During the mammography procedure, the breast is placed between a compression paddle and an x-ray plate and pressure is applied to flatten the breast in order to get a clear x-ray picture.

Some women may feel a little discomfort, but the exam takes only a few minutes. Over the past 20 years, the technique has been greatly improved. During the same visit at which the mammogram is performed, a physical exam of the breast should be performed by the radiologist (not by the technician). (Most mammograms range from $70 to $150 for a routine screening mammogram to $250 for a diagnostic mammogram for women with symptoms. Some health insurance plans cover the cost.)

Breast tissue and cancerous tumors can have the same density. Mammography is more accurate in older women who have gone through menopause because the breasts are less dense and have more fatty tissue. When a lump is found, the use of high-resolution digital ultrasound can help distinguish between cancerous and non-cancerous lumps.

Digital mammography that uses computers to sharpen mammographic images can make it easier to detect tumors of the breast. Magnetic resonance imaging (MRI), a high-powered imaging device, has proven to be helpful in detecting abnormalities within the body and especially in screening for brain and spinal cancer. At a cost of $1000, MRI is more expensive than mammography but has been shown to be more beneficial in detecting breast cancer in younger women because their breast tissue is more dense. Dr. Steven Harms of Baylor University Medical Center designed an MRI technique specifically designed to detect breast cancer and that has detected cancer that did not show up in mammography. Unlike mammograms, MRI does not use radiation, which is believed to be one of the causes of breast cancer.

It has long been the advice of specialists in the area of breast cancer for a woman to have a first mammogram at about 35 years of age, then every other year during the 40s and annually after age 50. Other experts believe that the additional exposure to the radiation used during mammography can lead to breast cancer. The Illinois-based Cancer Prevention Coalition says that some studies show a link between exposure to premenopausal mammography and breast-cancer mortality.

The Food and Drug Administration encourages women with breast implants who are in an age group for which routine mammograms are recommended to be sure to have these examinations at the recommended intervals. Women with implants should always inform the radiologist and technician about the implants beforehand. (Mammograms can rupture implants. Xeromammography and MRI are believed to be safer for women with breast implants.)

The key to surviving breast cancer is early detection. The sooner a problem is found, the greater the chance of successful treatment. And, in many cases, less extensive surgery can be used to treat the disease, often saving the breast. When breast cancer has spread beyond the breasts and the lymph nodes, it usually settles in three places — the lungs, the liver and the bones. The further it has spread, the lower the chances are of survival.

If a lump is found in your breast, ask if needle biopsy techniques (fine needle aspiration or core biopsy) are used in the doctor's office. Needle biopsies are less invasive than surgery. They have been common in Europe and are becoming more popular in America. One of the breast cancer information organizations listed in the following pages may be able to help you find a doctor in your area who is experienced in performing needle biopsies.

Studies have shown that women are more likely to have the proper testing done if they go to an obstetrician/gynecologist who is female because they follow screening guidelines for mammograms and pap smears better than male doctors. A woman should be forewarned that unnecessary mastectomies and hysterectomies are more common than any other type of surgery. (Read the books *Male Practice: How Doctors Manipulate Women*, by Robert S. Mendelsohn, MD; and *No More Hysterectomies*, by Vickie G. Hufnagel & Susan K. Golant.)

Alta Bates Comprehensive Cancer Center
Cancer Risk Counseling Service
Berkeley, California; Phone (510) 204-4286

American Cancer Society
Phone toll-free (800) ACS-2345

The American College of Radiology is the certifying organization for radiologists and conducts a five-step accreditation process for mammography clinics.

American College of Radiology
Mammography Accreditation Program
1891 Preston White Drive, Reston, Virginia 22091; Phone (703) 648-8900

Breast Cancer Fund
1280 Columbus Avenue, Suite 201, San Francisco, California 94133; Phone (800) 487-0492

Breast Cancer Research Foundation
Box 9236, GPO, New York, New York 10087-9236

Breast Lump & Cervical Cancer Information Hotline
Phone toll-free (800) 4-CANCER; In Alaska phone toll-free (800) 638-6070

Cancer Care
Phone (212) 221-3300

Coloplast is the manufacturer of the Intrigue falsies that can be placed in the bra to make up for what mastectomy has taken away.

Coloplast
Atlanta, Georgia; Phone (404) 426-6362 or toll-free (800) 741-0078

Coping Magazine is written for cancer patients and their families. Subscriptions are $18 a year.

Coping Magazine
2019 North Carothers, Franklin, Tennessee 37064; Phone (615) 790-2400

Dana-Farber Cancer Institute
Boston, Massachusetts; Phone (617) 632-2178

The Health Resource will put together an individualized, comprehensive research report on your specific medical problem. Contact them for current prices.

The Health Resource
564 Locust Avenue, Conway, Arkansas 72032; Phone (501) 329-5272

Lombardi Cancer Research Center
Comprehensive Breast Center, Georgetown University, Washington, DC; Phone (202) 687-2104 or 687-2113

Mammatech sells an educational kit that teaches how to properly do breast self-examination. The kit includes a video and a silicone model of a breast.

Mammatech
P.O. Box 15748, Gainsville, Florida 32604; Phone (800) 626-2273

My Image after Breast Cancer
6000 Stevenson Avenue, Suite 203, Alexandria, Virginia 22304; Phone (703) 461-9616

National Alliance of Breast Cancer Organizations
9 East 37th Street, 10th Floor, New York, New York 10016; Phone (212) 719-0154

To obtain information about accredited facilities where mammograms are performed, call the National Cancer Institute. The Institute also provides information on comprehensive cancer centers.

National Cancer Institute
Phone toll-free (800) 4-CANCER

New Hampshire Breast Cancer Coalition
18 Belle Lane, Lee, New Hampshire 03824

North Center Cancer Clinic
Phone (612) 520-5155

Susan G. Komen Foundation (breast cancer information)
5005 LBJ Freeway, Suite 370, Dallas, Texas 75244; Phone toll-free (800) 462-9273

Terri's Post-Surgical Boutique Catalogue sells prostheses, accessories, brassieres, swim wear, lingerie and sleeves for women who have had breasts removed or damaged by accident, cancer or breast implants. Call for a catalogue.

Terri's Post-Surgical Boutique Catalogue
2570 North McCarn Road, Palm Springs, California 92262-2240; Phone (619) 325-2612 or toll-free (800) 925-3676

United Center for Breast Care
333 North Smith Avenue, St. Paul, MN 55102; Phone (612) 220-8300 fax 220-7203

UCLA Breast Center
Phone (800) UCLA-MD-1

A technique that involves injecting a blue dye into a breast tumor to determine if cancer has spread into the lymph glands was developed by surgeons at the John Wayne Cancer Institute. Often the lymph glands, part of the body's immune system, near the breast that is being removed are removed at the same time.

John Wayne Cancer Institute
1328 – 22nd Street, Santa Monica, California 90404; Phone (310) 315-6125

For all cancers, blacks have about a 39% survival rate, compared with 55% for whites. Breast cancer is the leading cause of death of all black women, and they die from breast cancer at higher rates than whites. A study released by Emory University School of Public Health in Atlanta came to the conclusion that the higher breast cancer mortality rates among black women are the result of socioeconomic reasons. Blacks are less likely to have health insurance and this limits access to healthcare.

A donation-supported breast cancer education and support group specifically targeted to women of color was started in Los Angeles and is branching out to other cities. For information contact the

Women of Color Breast Cancer Survivor Support Project
Phone (213) 418-0627 or (310) 532-5128

The donation-supported Y-Me National Organization for Breast Cancer Information and Support has put together a booklet titled "*When the Woman You Love Has Breast Cancer*" that addresses the emotional issues a man may face when his wife has breast cancer. They also publish a pamphlet called *For Single Women with Breast Cancer*. Another one of their publications, *If You've Thought about Breast Cancer*, contains up-to-date information about breast cancer risk, mammography screening, diagnostic techniques, therapies, breast reconstruction and clinical trials on prevention. Call for ordering information.

Y-Me National Organization for Breast Cancer Information and Support
212 W. Van Buren Street, 4th Floor, Chicago, Illinois 60607-3908; Phone (708) 799-8220 or (312) 986-8228; Toll-free (800) 221-2141
Spanish-speaking individuals can call (312) 986-9505

• BREAST IMPLANTS AND SILICONE POISONING

Books:
- *Breast Implants: Everything You Need to Know*, by Nancy Bruning; Hunter House Publishers, [(510) 865-5282], 1995
- *The Silicone Breast Implant Controversy: What Women Need to Know Now*, by Frank B. Vasey and Josh Feldstein; Crossing Press [(800) 777-1048], Freedom California, $20.95
- *Silicone-Gate*, by Henry Jenny [(800) 574-2978]

To find out information on the $3.75 billion breast implant settlement reached in Birmingham, Alabama, on March 23, 1994, phone 1-800-887-6828. Obtain a copy of the court settlement document and study it. Contact the silicone survivor groups and listen to their interpretation of the settlement. Contact the American Trial Lawyer's Association for a referral to a lawyer in your area who is well versed in the breast implant mess.

The Food and Drug Administration and Silicone-Filled Breast Implants

Mentor Corporation (the sole active manufacturer of gel-filled implants at this time) has announced that it will stop manufacturing silicone gel-filled breast implants within the next couple of years. McGhan Medical Corporation intends to resume manufacturing silicone gel-filled implants, but it is uncertain when that will happen.
> — from FDA information packet on breast implants, October 1993

In 1991 the FDA launched an investigation to find out what problems were being caused by leaky breast implants. On April 16, 1992, the FDA announced that it would allow silicone gel-filled breast implants to be available only through clinical studies that would be conducted in three phases: The first, the Urgent Need phase; the second, the Open Availability or Adjunct phase; and last, the Core Studies. The first phase began in the summer of 1992, the second in the fall of 1992. The FDA estimated that it would take 3 to 5 years to conduct each study once they had begun.

The silicone-gel version of testicular implants were also withdrawn from the market. The remaining device is a solid version that contains no silicone gel.

The FDA continues to state that the possible link between gel-filled implants and the various health problems that have been brought to light is uncertain. Depending on the situation, any woman experiencing the symptoms should see a rheumatologist or other type of specialist for further evaluation.

The literature put out by the FDA in 1993 detailed the specific requirements under which implants will be available (for updated material, contact the FDA at the phone number given in this section).

Because of FDA's concerns about the possible risks of silicone gel-filled breast implants, these devices are only available to women who are enrolled in a clinical study sponsored by the implant manufacturer and approved by the FDA. At this time, one manufacturer, Mentor Corporation, has been approved by FDA to conduct a study.

Any woman who needs the implants for breast reconstruction can enroll in the study. This includes those who have had breast cancer surgery or a severe injury to the breast, or who have a medical condition causing a severe breast abnormality. Those who must have an existing implant replaced for medical reasons, such as rupture of the implant, are still eligible. Women who want the implants for breast augmentation (enlargement) cannot be enrolled in these studies.

Later, more strictly controlled studies are planned to investigate the safety of the implants in greater detail. Those studies will enroll a limited number of women who want the implants for breast augmentation, as well as those having them for reconstruction.

The research studies will not address all of the safety issues related to silicone gel-filled implants. The studies are prospective clinical investigations. This means that they are designed to follow new patients after they receive the implants and look for specific benefits or problems. Other types of safety questions will be answered in other studies.

For example, questions about possible long-term effects, such as immune-related disorders or cancer, will be answered by studies of those who already have the implants. Two of these studies, sponsored by implant manufacturers, are underway at New York University and the University of Michigan. The results are projected to be available in 3-5 years. A third study on long-term effects will begin this year [1993] under the sponsorship of the National Cancer Institute, part of the National Institutes of Health (NIH).

Other kinds of safety questions will be answered by laboratory studies conducted by the manufacturers under an FDA-imposed timetable. These include the chemical makeup and effects of silicone material that "bleeds" out of the implant shell, the strength of the implant shell and its resistance to rupture, and the physical and chemical changes that implants may undergo in the body

To enroll in a study, a woman who needs silicone gel-filled implants for breast reconstruction should first contact the doctor who chooses to perform the implant surgery. The *doctor will then make the necessary arrangements with the implant manufacturer.*

Before the woman can be enrolled, her doctor must certify that she qualifies medically for the implant. She will have to sign a special consent form, certifying that she has been told about the risks of the implants, and enroll in a registry so that she can be notified in the future, if necessary, about new information on the implants.

The FDA recognizes that women who have lost a breast because of cancer or trauma, or who have a serious breast malformation, may have a special need for an implant. So we are not setting a limit on the number of these women who may enroll in the studies.
— from FDA information packet on breast implants

In 1993 the FDA reported that no study had been done to determine whether, and it is still not known for certain whether, silicone that bleeds from gel-filled breast implants can find its way into breast milk, or if this were to occur, what effect it could have on the child. Some doctors in America have claimed to have found symptoms of unusual immune disorders in some children of mothers with silicone gel-filled breast implants. This raises the question of whether silicone might be seeping into the women's wombs or mixing with breast milk.

If a gel-filled implant has ruptured, it should be removed. Signs and symptoms of rupture may include pain, tingling, numbness, burning, changes in the breast size or shape, and changes in sensation.

An implant may rupture without causing symptoms, but women should not have routine mammograms (breast x-rays) just to detect these "silent" ruptures. Other methods of detecting implant rupture, such as ultrasound, computed axial tomography (CAT) scans, and magnetic resonance imaging (MRI), are still being studied and are not recommended for routine screening.

The chance for rupture may increase the longer the implant has been in the body. Injury to the breast also increases the chance of rupture.
— from FDA information on breast implants, October 1993

According to the FDA, there is no widely available test to detect silicone in the body. Even if simple techniques to detect silicone were available, they might not be useful in detecting a rupture because small amounts of silicone bleed from even intact implants. Furthermore, because silicone is found in food and many products, including commonly used medicines and cosmetics, the tests may not be able to easily determine whether the silicone came from the implant or another source.

> *The life span of the implants is not known; future studies should help to answer this question. Implants can last from a very short time to many years, depending on the patient and the implant. In any case, breast implants should not be considered "lifetime" devices. Women should be followed by their physician for as long as they have their implants.*
> — from FDA information on breast implants, October 1993

Anyone getting implants or who already has them should keep a record of the name of the implant manufacturer, product name and catalogue number, style, size and lot number (some of this information is found on a sticker that is in the package of the implant). Also keep a journal of the dates of the surgery and dates on which any problems were recognized and the nature of these problems and a record of all visits or phone calls made to the doctor's office, insurance companies, lawyers and any other organization. Keep copies of all letters where you mention your implants and write detailed notes of each conversation and action that took place regarding your implants including dates, names, locations, position of the person spoken to and the address and telephone numbers of the individuals and the organization they work for.

Saline-Filled Breast Implants

Saline implants are more liquid-like, which causes them to bounce more than silicone and some women who have had both types of implants say saline implants ripple and show through the skin more than silicone implants.

Because saline is saltwater, which is a naturally occurring body fluid that is not thought to be harmful, saline-filled implants are now being advertised as safe. Saline-filled implants are believed to be less dangerous than silicone implants, but health risks still exist.

About 40,000 women received saline implants in 1992. On January 5, 1993, as saline-filled implants were beginning to fill the void left after silicone implants were removed from the market, the FDA announced that, in order for them to keep the implants on the market, manufacturers of saline-filled breast implants would be required to submit evidence of their safety and effectiveness. The final FDA decision on saline-filled breast implants is expected to be made in 1998.

The FDA has said that women should carefully read the patient information sheets that accompany the implants and discuss the risks with their doctor before undergoing implant surgery.

> *The FDA has notified the manufacturers of saline implants that they will be required to submit safety and effectiveness information, just as the manufacturers of the gel-filled implants were required to do. The saline-filled implants will be allowed to remain on the market only if the FDA decides that the information submitted by the manufacturers shows that they are safe and effective. The FDA will be calling for this information within the next few months.*
> — from FDA information packet on breast implants, October 1993

The FDA says it does not have enough scientific evidence to determine whether the silicone rubber shell of saline-filled implants can cause immune-related diseases or cancer and has said that these and other risks should not be ruled out. (Also to be investigated for safety are testicular implants that are used for cosmetic purposes to replace testicles lost through cancer, accident, or crime, and inflatable penile implants that are used to treat impotence.) In December 1994, the FDA announced that saline breast implants would be allowed on the market for at least another three years while studies continued to be conducted to determine their safety.

Saline implants have been available since 1969. Their development in 1968 has been attributed to a Doctor Henry Jenny of Palm Springs, California. Dr. Jenny warned against the use of liquid silicone. He claims to have never used anything but saline implants because he always believed the silicone gel was poison to the body. In 1978 he testified before the FDA's new office of medical devices. There he presented his research findings that showed silicone gel implants were a health hazard to anyone who received them. He showed the advisory panel some sticky and leaking implants that he had removed from women's breasts. He believed there was no difference between the risks of this leaking silicone and the silicone that had been used to inject into women's breasts before breast implants were developed. (The FDA has banned the practice of injecting silicone into women's breasts and, because of the dangers of it, in some states it is considered a criminal offense.)

It has been estimated that about 10% of the women who received breast implants before 1992 received saline-filled implants. As saline-filled implants were on the market before the Medical Device Amendment of 1976, which gave the FDA authority over implant devices, saline-filled implants were allowed, under the law, to remain on the market with the understanding that the FDA would later require manufacturers to demonstrate their safety and effectiveness.

Saline-filled implants are believed to rupture easier than silicone implants, and, when they do rupture, they often deflate rapidly. In 1992 the FDA received over 1,000 reports of problems associated with saline-filled breast implants. Because saline-filled breast implants are filled by the surgeon at the time of surgery by way of a tube (called a port), this tube may cause additional problems with the way it sits in the body. It has been the cause of additional surgeries in some women. Mold, bacteria, and fungus can grow within the implants and cause serious infection if the implant leaks. Some saline-filled implants that have been removed are clouded with murky moldy growth floating in the saline.

Getting Mammograms When You Have Breast Implants

Both silicone gel-filled and saline-filled breast implants can interfere with the detection of early breast cancer. Not only do implants make mammography more difficult to perform, they also can hide the abnormalities that mammograms are meant to find. The tissue surrounding the implant can become compressed and dense. Precancerous microcalcifications, which cannot be felt during a breast exam, are especially likely to be hidden by breast implants. Additionally, any abnormalities caused by the breast implants may lead to a false alarm.

If a woman has breast implants, it is important to ask whether personnel at the mammography facility are trained and experienced in special techniques for performing mammography on patients with implants. If these techniques are not used, breast cancer can go undetected. Because mammograms involve compression, the implant can be ruptured by an untrained technician. Facilities that are accredited by the American College of Radiology are more likely to have appropriately trained personnel.

Some doctors question whether the additional views needed to do a mammogram on a woman with breast implants, which increases the amount of radiation the woman would normally be exposed to, also increases the chance of developing breast cancer.

American College of Rheumatology
60 Executive Park South, Suite 150, Atlanta, Georgia 30329; Phone (404) 633-3777

AS-IS provides information about breast implants and breast reconstruction and can refer women to local support groups. They have put together a brochure that explains the various procedures available for rebuilding breasts and includes a list of questions to ponder. They also have other informative material on breast implants that is available for sale. The group publishes a newsletter that is available for $25 and is a non-profit organization that survives on donations.

American Silicone Implant Survivors
1288 Cork Elm Drive, Kirkwood, Missouri 63122; Phone (314) 821-0115

Breast Implant Information Foundation
Marie Walsh, P.O. Box 2907, Laguna Hills, California 92654-2907; Phone (714) 830-2433

Breast Implant Litigation Group
Fax (617) 557-7187

The Food and Drug Administration will send you a package of printed materials about breast implant manufacturers, consumer groups, and physician's groups. Write or call the

Food and Drug Administration
Breast Implant Information Service
Office of Consumer Affairs (HFE – 88), 5600 Fishers Lane, Rockville, Maryland 20857; Phone (303) 443-5006 or
FDA Breast Implant Info Line toll-free (800) 532-4440
To report problems with your breast implants, phone (800) FDA-1088

The Breast Implant Litigation Group of the American Trial Lawyer's Association can refer you to lawyers in your area who are involved with breast implant lawsuits.

Breast Implant Litigation Group of the
American Trial Lawyer's Association
1050 – 31st Street NW, Washington, DC 20007-4499; Phone (800) 424-2725 or 2727

Breast Implant Relations Network of the American Society of
Plastic and Reconstructive Surgeons
Phone (800) 635-0635

Children Afflicted by Toxic Substances was founded by a woman who started the group after she realized her silicone gel-filled breast implants may be affecting the health of her children.

Children Afflicted by Toxic Substances
60 Oser Avenue, Suite 1, Hauppauge, New York 11788; Phone toll-free
(800) CATS-199

The Coalition of Silicone Survivors was started to assist women with
silicone and saline-filled breast implants. The group continuously
researches information on medical testing and safety of implants as well as
implant legal matters. The group publishes a monthly newsletter available
for $25 US funds/$35 foreign US funds. They also publish a list of tests
that are recommended for implant patients and information on how to get
these tests. Tapes of their national conference are available for $75. The
COSS is a not-for-profit, tax-exempt corporation that supports itself with
donations. For an information packet, write or call the

Coalition of Silicone Survivors
P.O. Box 129, Broomfield, Colorado 80038-0129; Phone (303) 469-8242

The Command Trust Network is a nonprofit organization that was
created to assist women who have breast implants. They publish literature
about breast implants. They supply information on implant-related
problems, research, testing, removal, legal referrals, psychological support,
support groups, and information on breast implant studies, government
intervention, and manufacturers.

Command Trust Network
Reconstructive Surgery Division, Sybil Goldrich, 256 South Linden Drive,
Beverly Hills, CA 90212; Phone (310) 556-1738

Command Trust Network
Cosmetic Surgery Division, Kathleen Anneken, RN, P.O. Box 17082,
Covington, Kentucky 41017-0082; Phone (606) 331-0055

**Implant Patients Relations Information Line of the
International Breast Implant Registry**
Phone toll-free (800) 892-9200

The International Implant Registry is a confidential database that keeps
complete current information about people with implanted medical devices.
In the case of a notification of a problem with an implant from an implant
manufacturer or by the FDA, the Registry responds immediately to notify
your physician and surgeon that you have that particular device so that
appropriate action may be taken.

International Implant Registry
2323 Colorado Avenue, Turlock, California 95380; Phone (800) 344-3226

La Leche League International (promotes breastfeeding)
9616 Minneapolis Avenue, P.O. Box 1209, Franklin Park, Illinois 60131-
8209; Phone (708) 455-7730, toll-free (800) LA-LECHE

National Women's Health Network
1325 G Street, NW, Washington, DC 20005; Phone (202) 347-1140

Public Citizen's Health Research Group, which has lobbied to have
silicone gel breast implants removed from the market entirely, has a
newsletter and offers referrals to attorneys who are handling breast
implant litigation. They offer an information packet about breast implants
that they will send you if you send them $6 and a self-addressed 9x12-inch,
stamped envelope. Donations are accepted.

Public Citizen's Health Research Group
2000 P Street, NW, Suite 700, Washington, DC 20036; Phone (202) 833-
3000

Call the Explanted Implant Evaluation Lab before having explant surgery to make arrangements to send your implant to them for testing.

Dr. Saul Puszkin, Professor of Pathology
Department of Pathology, Box 1194
Mount Sinai Medical Center
1 Gustave L. Levy Place, New York, New York 10029-6574; Phone (212) 241-5635

The Silicone Information Network is an information resource center for women who have concerns about their silicone-filled breast implants or silicone-induced health problems. S.I.N. is listed with the national registry of Silicone Support Groups. They have gathered information from across the country about implant research and support groups for women who have problems with their breast implants. It is their intent to bring about awareness of silicone disease by educating and informing the victims, public, medical community and legislators.

Silicone Information Network
P.O. Box 414905, Kansas City, Missouri 64141-4905; Phone (816) 478-4229

To report problems with breast implants, with the guidance of a lawyer, write for the Medical Device and Laboratory Product Problem Reporting Program report sheet from the United States Pharmacopoeia, which is under contract with the Food and Drug Administration to collect and organize the problem reports. The USP sends a copy of each report to the FDA. The FDA may contact you for further information about your report to discuss your observations. You will also be asked whether you want your name to be used on the reports given to the manufacturer of the implant, other parties of the FDA and to those who conduct other public and private studies.

United States Pharmacopoeia (USP)
Attention: Dr. Joseph Valentino, 12601 Twinbrook Parkway, Rockville, Maryland 20852; Phone toll-free (800) 638-6725

The Untold Truth is a book about the history of the medical use of silicone and its effects on the body. The book contains a medical dictionary and a reference section listing health and healing books and organizations. It is available for $19.95 through

The Untold Truth
P.O. Box 26923, Charlotte, North Carolina 28221

The Xerox corporation manufactured a machine that is helpful in getting an image that shows if silicone implants have ruptured. The machine is called a Xeromammography device. It is no longer being manufactured but Xerox has a service agreement with the medical centers that own the machines. To find out more about the machine and the location of one closest to you, contact

Xerox Medical Center – Xeromammography Department
Phone toll-free (800) 558-6669; In California call (818) 303-6634

• BREAST IMPLANT MANUFACTURERS

Baxter Healthcare Corp.
1 Baxter Parkway, Deerfield, Illinois 60015; Phone toll-free (800) 323-4533

Bioplasty has been a manufacturer of breast implants. It is also the manufacturer of Bioplastique, which is not yet approved by the FDA in

America, and is a man-made material that has been used in Europe for years to rebuild noses that have been damaged by accident or through bad cosmetic surgery operations.

Bioplasty
623 Hoover Street NE, Minneapolis, Minnesota 55413; Phone (612) 378-1180, toll-free (800) 328-9105

Cox Uphoff, Inc.
1035 Cindy Lane, Carpenteria, California 93013; Phone toll-free (800) 872-4749

Dow Corning Corporation
P.O. Box 994, Midland, Michigan 48686-0994; Phone toll-free (800) 442-5442

LipoMatix is the company that manufactures the Trilucent breast implants that are filled with a natural fat derived from soybean oil and that were introduced in America in the summer of 1994 after being implanted in the breasts of women in Britain, Italy and Germany. The fat is a form of triglyceride, which is a natural fat in the body. The implants still use a silicone shell which some experts believe is not good for the body. The company is partially owned by the biotechnology company Collagen Corporation of Palo Alto, California. It is the same company that markets the collagen that cosmetic surgeons and dermatologists use to inject into facial wrinkles to plump them out.

The company has been issued the patent to a microchip called "SmartDevice" which is about the size of a grain of rice and that is already being used in the Trilucent breast implants. The SmartDevice microchip is manufactured by a subsidiary of Hughes Aircraft Co., Hughes Identification Devices, and it works like a barcode and contains information about the implant manufacturer and other relevant information. The company plans to market the device to manufacturers of other implant devices such as manmade hip joints and heart valves so that all implant devices can be registered with an international information source. A similar type of device is used to implant into the necks of dogs so animal shelters can scan the dogs with a hand-held scanning gun that reads the information on the chip through the skin.

LipoMatrix
Phone (800) 839-3020

McGhan Medical Corp.
700 Ward Drive, Santa Barbara, California 93111; Phone (805) 683-6761 or toll-free (800) 624-4261 or phone toll-free in California (800) 228-8967 Customer affairs fax (805) 967-5839

Mentor Corporation (the only company that still makes silicone-gel-filled implants)
5425 Hollister Avenue, Santa Barbara, California 93111; Phone (805) 681-6000 or phone toll-free (800) 525-6747 or (800) 525-9151; Fax (805) 967-3013

Porex Technologies
500 Bohannon Road, Fairburn, Georgia 30213; Phone toll-free (800) 241-0195

Surgitek
3037 Mount Pleasant Street, Racine, Wisconsin 53404; Phone toll-free (800) 634-4397 or (800) 367-6723

• CLEFT PALATE, CLEFT LIP, AND COSMETIC BIRTH DEFECT CORRECTION

Congenital deformities of the structure of the mouth and lips can disrupt speech, nutrition and other areas of health. Depending on how dramatic the deformity is, the person can also feel they are being judged on the basis of their disfigurement.

The following organizations can provide information to people or parents of children who have facial deformities. Because not all doctors practice the same surgical techniques to correct such deformities, it may be beneficial to contact more than one of the groups to find out about the various techniques that are available.

The American Cleft Palate – Craniofacial Association is an association of doctors, dentists, speech pathologists, audiologists, psychologists, nurses and others involved with the care of individuals with clefts of the lip and palate and other craniofacial deformities.

American Cleft Palate – Craniofacial Association
1218 Grandview Avenue, Pittsburgh, Pennsylvania 15211; Phone (412) 481-1376

Cavernous hemangiomas are composed of red, spongy tissue containing enlarged blood vessels that grow rapidly and can be radically deforming to skin and surrounding structures. The Belle Foundation was started to educate parents of children with these deformities about safe and effective treatments to remove cavernous hemangiomas and to help raise funds for children needing surgery to remove these growths. Donations are appreciated.

Belle Foundation
P.O. Box 385, Gracie Station, New York, New York 10028-0004

The Children's Craniofacial Association functions as a networking and referral service for healthcare professionals, for government officials and for parents of craniofacially disfigured children. The association publishes materials and produces instructional films and videos.

Children's Craniofacial Association
10210 North Central Expressway, Suite 230, Lockbox 37, Dallas, Texas 75231; Phone (214) 368-3590

Children's Hospital of Los Angeles
Plastic Surgery Department; Phone (213) 660-2450

Interplast is a group that sends volunteer medical teams to developing countries to perform cost-free reconstructive surgery on people who are suffering from various deformities caused by accidents and birth defects.

Interplast
2458 Embarradera Way, Palo Alto, California 94303; Phone (415) 424-0123

Let's Face It Newsletter (for people with facial disfigurement)
P.O. Box 711, Concord, Massachusetts 01742; Phone (508) 371-3186

The National Foundation for Facial Reconstruction supports the Institute of Reconstructive Plastic Surgery at the New York University Medical Center. They maintain a patient-referral service for people suffering facial disfigurements caused by accidents, congenital malformations and diseases. They also provide psychological and financial support services. In 1994, the Foundation published a book titled *Special Faces: Understanding Facial Disfigurement.*

National Foundation for Facial Reconstruction
317 East 34th Street, Suite 901, New York, New York 10016; Phone (212) 263-6656 or toll-free (800) 422-FACE (3223)

The incidence of cleft lip and palate in many developing countries is believed to be three times greater than that in the United States. Operation Smile International is a non-profit, volunteer medical organization which provides reconstructive surgery to needy children and adults who are born with cleft lips and other congenital deformities, disfigurement caused by facial tumors and burns, club feet and sometimes other injury- or disease-caused deformities. Operation Smile also provides education and training to physicians and other healthcare professionals both in and outside of the US.

Medical team members who participate in Operation Smile missions to other countries are selected based on their qualifications and their ability to serve as "Ambassadors" in multi-cultural situations. The majority of the positions on each team are filled by board-certified medical personnel. There are also a few positions for those with no medical background. These positions include coordinators, medical record workers, youth sponsors and youth volunteers.

The medical missions average two weeks in duration and consist of three basic teams. The advance team arrives 3-4 days before the main team in order to prepare the operating rooms for the surgery week and to screen potential Operation Smile patients. With the arrival of the main team, which includes the majority of the medical personnel, the operations begin and last 12-15 hours per day for 5 days. There are also 1-2 days devoted to education for the local medical professionals. The small post-op team remains on site for 3-4 additional days in order to complete the follow-up care necessary to ensure the safe recovery of each and every patient.

To discover the causes of congenital disfigurement, geneticists perform research during the missions and are compiling information on the incidence of cleft lip and palate in developing countries.

Operation Smile's World Care Program identifies patients whose deformities and disfigurements are too severe for treatment in their home countries and brings them to the US for surgery. Operation Smile arranges for surgeons and other medical specialists in the US to volunteer their services and for the free hospitalization and care of the patients.

Operation Smile was founded in 1982 by plastic surgeon William P. Magee and his wife Kathy, an RN and clinical social worker, after they performed surgery on children in the Philippines. Since then, thousands of needy individuals have received surgery at no cost.

While the greatest source of financial support for Operation Smile comes from corporate sponsorship and grants, private individuals provide a substantial amount of financial support needed to support the many mission sites each year.

Operation Smile International
717 Boush Street, Norfolk, Virginia 23510-1501; Phone (804) 625-0375 or 622-7500 or 451-3799

• DOCTORS & SURGEONS — THEIR ACADEMIES, ASSOCIATIONS, BOARDS, FOUNDATIONS AND ORGANIZATIONS

This list contains some of the organizations of surgeons and other physicians. Some of the groups are nothing more than associations, and membership in them does not guarantee education or skills. Some will send out brochures or pamphlets to consumers who request them.

American Academy of Cosmetic Surgery
401 North Michigan Avenue, Chicago, Illinois 60611; Phone (312) 527-6713, toll-free (800) 221-9808

American Academy of Facial Plastic and Reconstructive Surgery
1110 Vermont Avenue, NW, Suite 220, Washington, DC 20005-3522; Phone toll-free (800) 332-3223 outside of Washington, DC or phone toll-free (800) 523-3223 in Canada or phone 842-4500 in Washington, DC

American Academy of Family Physicians
8880 Ward Parkway, Kansas City, Missouri 64114; Phone (816) 333-9700

American Academy of Otolaryngology - Head and Neck Surgery
One Prince Street, Alexandria, Virginia, 22314; Phone (703) 836-4444

American Association for Women Radiologists
1891 Preston White Drive, Reston, Virginia 22091; Phone (703) 648-8939

American Association of Hand Surgery
435 North Michigan Avenue, Suite 1717, Chicago, Illinois 60611; Phone (312) 644-0828

American Association of Neurological Surgeons
22 South Washington Street, Park Ridge, Illinois 60068; Phone (708) 692-9500

American Association of Plastic Surgeons
2317 Seminole Road, Atlantic Beach, Florida 32233-5952; Phone (904) 359-3759

American Association of Plastic Surgery
10666 North Torrey Pines Road, La Jolla, California 92037; Phone (619) 554-9940

American Board of Cosmetic Surgery
18525 Torrance Avenue, Lansing, Illinois 60438; Phone (708) 474-7200

American Board of Family Practice
2228 Young Drive, Lexington, Kentucky 40505; Phone (606) 269-5626

The Advisory Board of Medical Specialties was formed in 1933. In 1970, the name was changed to the American Board of Medical Specialties. The primary function of the ABMS is to maintain and improve the quality of medical care by assisting the member boards in their efforts to develop and use standards for the evaluation and certification of physician specialists.

The ABMS is the official medical certifying group responsible for administrating certification examinations to physician specialists. The intent of the certification process is to improve the quality of patient care. There are 24 specialties that are certified by the ABMS.

One way of checking to see if a doctor has been certified by the ABMS is to check in *The Official American Board of Medical Specialists Directory of Board Certified Medical Specialists*. This book is available in many public libraries and university libraries. It shows whether a doctor has post-graduate education in the specialty they practice in. Because the book is a compilation of information from many sources, some of the information about the doctors listed in the directory may not be accurate.

American Board of Medical Specialties
1007 Church Street, Suite 404, Evanston, Illinois 60201-5913; Phone (708) 491-9091; To find out if a doctor is certified: Phone toll-free (800) 776-2378 (CERT)

American Board of Otolaryngology
5615 Kirby Drive, Suite 936, Houston, Texas 77005; Phone (713) 528-6200

American Board of Plastic Surgery
7 Penn Center 400, 1635 Market Street, Philadelphia, Pennsylvania 19103; Phone (215) 587-9322

Radiologists are doctors who interpret x-rays and help in the diagnostic process. Before letting someone perform an x-ray on you, remember that the person operating the machinery may not be trained, the machinery may not have been inspected recently and may be faulty, you might be exposed to an excessive amount of radiation and any radiation exposure could lead to future health problems to you or your posterity. Many studies have shown that radiologists regularly contradict each other in their interpretation of x-rays. Besides all this, the x-ray might not detect any health problem that could not have been detected by a physical exam or by studying past x-rays or health records, and the only benefit might be to the doctor's pocket book.

American Board of Radiology
300 Park, Suite 440, Birmingham, Michigan 48009; Phone (313) 645-0600 or 643-0300

American Board of Surgery
1617 J. F. K. Boulevard, Suite 860, Philadelphia, Pennsylvania 19103-1847; Phone (215) 568-4000

American College of General Practitioners in Osteopathic Medicine and Surgery
330 East Algonquin, Arlington Heights, Illinois 60005; Phone (708) 228-6090 or toll-free (800) 323-0790

American College of Physicians
Independence Mall West, Sixth at Race, Philadelphia, Pennsylvania 19106-1572; Phone (215) 351-2400

American College of Radiology
1891 Preston White Drive, Reston, Virginia 22091; Phone (703) 648-8902

If your doctor is a Fellow of the American College of Surgeons, he probably has the initials F.A.C.S. displayed somewhere in his office, on his paperwork or on his business card. This is a voluntary organization of surgeons who have agreed to practice under certain professional standards (not that all F.A.C.S. doctors do) and who have completed certain amounts of training and professional preparation. For specific details on how a doctor qualifies to list himself as F.A.C.S., and to find out if your surgeon is a member, contact the

American College of Surgeons
55 East Erie Street, Chicago, Illinois 60611-2797; Phone (312) 664-4050 or 4056

American Federation of Medical Accreditation
522 Rossmore Drive, Las Vegas, Nevada 89110; Phone (702) 385-6886

The American Medical Association has occupied itself with successfully swaying American politicians and laws that govern healthcare since the AMA was founded in 1846. With about 296,000 members composed of county and state medical societies along with representatives from specialty societies, hospitals, and other medical industry professions, the AMA is the nation's largest and most influential organization of physicians.

The AMA publishes a yearly directory of officials and staff. The directory lists various associations, boards and other American healthcare worker groups.

The Physician Data Series, which is operated by the AMA, can provide you with information on a doctor's professional history. When you are provided with any information from the AMA, keep in mind that it is an association of doctors.

American Medical Association
Physician Data Series, 515 North State Street, Chicago, Illinois 60610; Phone (312) 464-5000 or 2000 or toll-free (800) 621-8335

American Osteopathic Board of General Practice
330 East Algonquin Road, Suite 2, Arlington Heights, Illinois 60005; Phone (708) 635-8477

American Osteopathic Board of Ophthalmology and Otorhinolaryngology
405 Grand Avenue, Dayton, Ohio 45405; Phone (513) 222-4213

American Osteopathic Board of Surgery
405 Grand Avenue, Dayton, Ohio 45405; Phone (513) 226-2656

American Osteopathic Hospital Association
1454 Duke Street, Alexandra, Virginia 22314; Phone (703) 684-7700

American Society for Aesthetic Plastic Surgery
3922 Atlantic Avenue, Long Beach, California 90807; Phone (310) 595-4275

American Society for Head and Neck Surgery
P.O. Box 41402, Baltimore, Maryland 21203; Phone (410) 955-3669

American Society for Laser Medicine and Surgery
2404 Stewart Square, Wausua, Wisconsin 54401; Phone (715) 845-9283

American Society for Surgery of the Hand
3025 South Parker Road, Suite 65, Aurora, Colorado 80014-2911; Phone (303) 755-4588

American Society of Contemporary Medicine & Surgery
233 East Erie Street, Chicago, Illinois 60611; Phone (312) 951-1400

The American Academy of Liposuction Surgery offers workshops in liposuction procedures and is associated with the American Academy of Cosmetic Surgery.

American Society of Liposuction Surgery
159 East Live Oak Avenue, #204, Arcadia, California 91006-5249; Phone (818) 447-1579

American Society of Maxillofacial Surgeons
444 East Algonquin Road, Arlington Heights, Illinois 60005; Phone (708) 228-3327

The American Society of Plastic and Reconstructive Surgeons represents approximately 5,000 plastic surgeons or 97 percent of those plastic surgeons certified by the American Board of Plastic Surgery.

American Society of Plastic and Reconstructive Surgeons
444 East Algonquin Road, Arlington Heights, Illinois 60005; Phone (708) 228-9900; Implant Patients' Relations Information: Phone toll-free (800) 635-0635

American Surgical Association
University of North Carolina, Department of Surgery, CB 7245, Chapel Hill, North Carolina 27599-7245; Phone (919) 966-6320

Association of American Physicians and Surgeons
1601 North Tucson Boulevard, Suite 9, Tucson, Arizona 85716; Phone (602) 327-4885

Association of Military Surgeons of the US
9320 Old George Road, Bethesda, Maryland 20814; Phone (301) 897-8800

Canadian Association of General Surgeons
Box 4730, Edmonton, Alberta T6E 5G6; Phone (403) 437-1735

Canadian Association of Radiologists
5101 Buchan Street, #510, Montreal, Quebec H4P 2R9; Phone (514) 738-3111

Canadian Society for Surgery of the Hand
Toronto Western Division, 5 West Wing – 3834, 399 Bathurst Street, Toronto, Ontario M5T 2S8; Phone (416) 369-5448

Canadian Society of Otolaryngology – Head and Neck Surgery
55 MacGregor Avenue, Toronto, Ontario M6S 2A1; Phone (416) 760-8190

Canadian Society of Plastic Surgeons
30 St. Joseph Boulevard East, #520, Montreal, Quebec H2T 1G9; Phone (514) 843-5415

Some lab tests are inaccurate because the people in the labs are overworked or not trained properly or because the equipment they are using is defective.

The College of American Pathologists is the leading authority on lab testing, helps shape state and national regulations governing testing and is responsible for how medical labs are regulated. CAP is financed by medical labs and inspects and accredits labs both in and out of hospitals. CAP does not release its records of mismanaged medical labs to the public (yet another disservice to consumers). Not all labs cooperate with CAP's review and accreditation program and those labs that do participate do it on a voluntary basis.

College of American Pathologists
325 Waukegan Road, Northfield, Illinois 60093-2750; Phone (708) 446-8800

Educational Commission for Foreign Medical Graduates
3624 Market Street, Philadelphia, Pennsylvania 19104; Phone (215) 386-5900

Federation of State Medical Boards of the United States
6000 Western Place, #707, Fort Worth, Texas 76107; Phone (817) 735-8445

Lipoplasty Society of North America
825 East Golf Road, Suit 1141, Arlington Heights, Illinois 60005; Phone (708) 228-9273

National Medical Association
1012 – 10th Street, NW, Washington, DC 20001; Phone (202) 347-1895

Royal College of General Practitioners
Britain; Phone 44-71-224-2236

Royal College of Physicians and Surgeons of Canada
774 Promenade Echo Drive, Ottawa, Canada K1S 5NB; Phone (613) 730-8177 or 6212

Royal College of Physicians and Surgeons of the USA
16126 East Warren, Detroit, Michigan 48224; Phone (313) 882-0641

Royal College of Surgeons
Britain; Phone 44-71-831-5161

Society of University Surgeons
P.O. Box 7069, New Haven, Connecticut 06519; Phone (203) 932-0541

• ELDERLY PERSONS' SUPPORT

Book:
* *Fifty to Forever: The Complete Source Book for Living an Active, Involved, and Fulfilling Second Half of Life,* by Hugh Downs; Thomas Nelson, 1994

Administration on Aging
330 Independence Avenue SW, Room 4284, Washington, DC 20201; Phone (202) 619-2598

American Association of Homes for the Aging
1129 – 20th Street NW, Washington, DC 20036; Phone (202) 783-2242 or 296-5960

American Association of Retired Persons (AARP)
601 E Street, NW, Washington, DC 20049; Phone (301) 427-9611 or (202) 434-2277

American Healthcare Association
1201 L Street NW, Washington, DC 20005; Phone (202) 842-4444

Elderly Support Network
P.O. Box 248, Kendall Park, New Jersey 08824-0248; Phone toll-free (800) 634-7654

Gray Panthers
1424 – 16th Street, NW, Washington, DC 20036; Phone (202) 347-6471

National Association of Area Agencies on Aging
1112 Sixteenth Street, Washington, DC 20036; Phone (202) 296-8130

National Council of Senior Citizens
1331 F Street, NW, Washington, DC 20004-1171; Phone (202) 347-8800

National Institute on Aging
P.O. Box 8057, Gaithersburg, Maryland 20898-8057; Phone (800) 438-4380

Widowed Persons Service (of the AARP)
P.O. Box 199, Long Beach, California 90801; Phone (310) 427-9611

• EYES

American Academy of Ophthalmology
655 Beach Street, San Francisco, California 94109; Phone (415) 561-8500

American Association for Pediatric Ophthalmology
P.O. Box 193832, San Francisco, California 94119; Phone (415) 561-8505

The Van Sickle Surgical Instrument Company sells eye masks that can be frozen and used to help control bruising and swelling.

Van Sickle Surgical Instrument Company
Phone (800) 829-0306

• FATIGUE, COMPULSION AND ANXIETY

Books:
* *Dying of Embarrassment*, by Barbara G. Markway, Cheryl N. Carmin, C. Alec Pollard and Teresa Flynn; New Harbinger 1992
* *Hope and Healing for Chronic Fatigue Syndrome*, by Karyn Freiden; Fireside/Simon & Schuster, 1992
* *The Boy Who Couldn't Stop Washing: The Experience and Treatment of Obsessive-Compulsive Disorder*, by Judith L. Rapoport; Signet, 1991
* *Psychobiology of Obsessive-Compulsive Disorder*, by Joseph Zohar, Thomas R. Insel & Steven Rasmussen; Springer Publishing, 1991
* *Triumph Over Fear*, by Jerilyn Ross; Bantam Books, 1994

Anxiety Disorders Association of America
6000 Executive Boulevard, Suite 513, Rockville, Maryland 20852
P.O. Box 96505, Washington, DC 20077-7140; Phone (301) 231-8368 or for $2 per minute (900) 737-3400

Chronic Fatigue and Immune Disease Center
14441 Memorial Drive, Suite 6, Houston, Texas 77079; Phone (713) 497-7904 or toll-free (800) 972-7904

Chronic Fatigue and Immune Dysfunction Syndrome Association
P.O. Box 220398, Charlotte, North Carolina 28222-0398; Phone (800) 442-3437

National Chronic Fatigue Syndrome Association
3521 Broadway, Suite 222, Kansas City, Missouri 64111; Phone (816) 931-4777

National Headache Foundation
Phone (800) 843-2256

National Institute of Mental Health
Panic Campaign
Room 15C–05, 5600 Fishers Lane, Rockville, Maryland 20857

Obsessive Compulsive Disorder Foundation, Inc.
P.O. Box 9573, New Haven, Connecticut 06535

• HAIR

American Electrology Association (electrolysis = hair removal)
106 Oak Ridge Road, Trumbull, Connecticut 06611; Phone (203) 374-6667

American Hair Loss Council
100 Independence Place, Suite 207, Tyler, Texas 75703; Phone (903) 561-1107

National Committee for Electrologist Certification
96 Westminster Road, West Hempstead, New York 11552; Phone (516) 485-6309

UpJohn is the manufacturer of Rogaine, a prescription medication containing minoxidil (a blood pressure drug). When it is applied to the scalp twice a day it can increase the size of some hair follicles, but is not a permanent solution to hair loss. The UpJohn literature about Rogaine contains some warnings and other clinical information that should be read and analyzed by anyone considering use of the product.

UpJohn Dermatology Division
Phone (800) 635-0655

• HEALTH RESEARCH GROUPS FOR HIRE

THR will do research on any diagnosed medical condition and has often cut the health bills of many clients through finding treatment that is not only more effective, but also less costly.

The Health Resource
564 Locust Street, Conway, Arkansas 72032; Phone (501) 329-5272

Palo Alto Medical Foundation
Palo Alto, California; Phone (800) 999-1999

Planetree Health Research Center operates a consumer health library that concentrates on both conventional and alternative healthcare. They also conduct health research.

Planetree Health Resource Center
2040 Webster Street, San Francisco, California 94115; Phone (415) 923-3680 or 923-3681

• LEGAL ASPECTS OF BEING A PATIENT

Books:
Many books have been written on the subject of legal representation. Look in *Books in Print*, which is available in most libraries, for the books that use the word "malpractice" in their titles.

- *The Consumer Reports Law Book*, Consumer Reports Books (P.O. Box 10637, Des Moines, Iowa 50336 Phone [515] 237-4903)
- *The Consumer's Legal Guide to Today's Healthcare: Your Medical Rights and How to Assert Them*, by Stephen L. Isaacs, JD & Ava C. Swartz, MPH; Houghton Mifflin Co., 1992
- *The Criminal Elite: The Sociology of White Collar Crime*, by James William Coleman; St. Martin's Press, 1985
- *Galileo's Revenge: Junk Science in the Courtroom*, by Peter Huber; Basic Books, 1993
- *Kiplinger's Handbook of Personal Law: Protect Yourself From Everyday Legal Problems that Could Cost You Plenty*, by Jill Rachlin; Kiplinger Books, 1994
- *Representing Yourself: What You Can Do Without a Lawyer*, published by Public Citizen's Health Research Group (Phone [202] 833-3000)
- *Silent Violence, Silent Death: The Hidden Epidemic of Medical Malpractice*, by Harvey Rosenfield; Essential Books, 1994
- *Wrongful Death: A Medical Tragedy*, by Sandra M. Gilbert; W.W. Norton & Company, 1995

The 8-volume *Martindale-Hubbell Law Directory* (630 Central Avenue, New Providence, New Jersey 07974) lists attorneys across the country. Many public libraries carry a copy of it. The American Trial Lawyer's Association also publishes a directory of lawyers.

Courthouse records of medical malpractice cases may point you in the direction of a lawyer who can handle your case. Newspaper articles about medical malpractice are also a good way to find the lawyers in your area who are experienced in medical malpractice.

Check your local courthouse to see what books, pamphlets and other resources they have on hand that may help you in your legal decisions.

The following is a very small portion of the information one would need to consider when malpractice occurs. If you are a victim of medical malpractice, read books on the subject, such as those listed above, and consult with an attorney who specializes in malpractice and who is familiar with the laws in your area.

When a Doctor Was Negligent

Some people approach a doctor's office as if it were a haunted house where life-threatening occurrences take place. To make a visit to a doctor's office seem more inviting the medical community presents advertising with images of happy and caring medical professionals.

In 1976, the Department of Health, Education and Welfare's Malpractice Commission estimated that one-half of one percent of all patients entering hospitals are injured there due to negligence. That estimate would indicate 156,000 such injuries and deaths resulted from doctor negligence in 1988.

> — DHEW Malpractice Commission information from *Journal of Legal Medicine*, February 1976. Calculations by Pamela Gilbert, director of Public Citizen's Congress Watch, in a prepared statement for a Congressional subcommittee hearing, May 20, 1993

As a child we are taught, at least through action, that there are certain authority figures we can trust. One is the teacher, one is the police officer and one is the doctor. Probably the majority of the people who work in these positions are trustworthy and represent their profession to the best their circumstances will allow. Doctors are different than the other authority figures This is because children are told it is okay for a doctor to touch them where no one else is allowed to touch. People depend on that trustworthiness when they turn to doctors in times of need. In the process of being a patient a person lets a doctor see more than what people are used to exposing in everyday life. That is when a person is vulnerable to violation as they place their health in the hands of a medical professional who may sell himself as a caregiver although he may be negligent.

A Los Angeles doctor was sentenced to 13 years in prison for sexually assaulting four female patients. Prosecutors wanted the judge to impose a 37-year sentence. The decertified orthopedic surgeon was convicted of 10 felony and criminal counts of sexual battery and rape, and penetration with a foreign object while the victims were unconscious.

mal•prac•tice (1671) **1**: a dereliction from professional duty or a failure to exercise an accepted degree of professional skill or learning by one (as a physician) rendering professional services which results in injury, loss, or damage **2**: an injurious, negligent, or improper practice : MALFEASANCE

mal•prac•ti•tio•ner (1800): one who engages in or commits malpractice

— By permission. From *Merriam-Webster's Collegiate®
Dictionary* ©1993 by Merriam-Webster Inc., Publisher of the
Merriam-Webster® dictionaries.

**The California medical consumer's rights group Safe
Medicine for Consumers lists the causes of negligent medical
care as the following:**
- Substandard medical care
- Neglect of the patient
- Improper treatment
- Weak doctor regulations by medical boards
- Lack of informed consent by patients
- Poor medical facility maintenance

The tragedy of popular elective surgery procedures is that many people who went in for operations they thought would make their lives better ended up having their quality of life, and sometimes the entire fabric of their existence, disheveled when the surgeries were not successful. Sometimes this is the result of maloccurence (situations out of the doctor's control — in other words: If an operation does not turn out the way you thought it would it does not mean that the doctor was negligent), whereas other times it is caused by the faulty actions (malpractice) of the medical caregivers.

Should one of us go into an emergency room and be asked all the questions that a doctor would ask after an accident, including "Are you allergic to anything?" And you answered "to the best of my knowledge I am not allergic to anything." The doctor proceeded to give you a shot of penicillin. The reaction caused you to go into shock and spend an extra day in the hospital. That, in fact, is malpractice, but it is not negligent. It is just one of those accidents.

On the other hand, had we gone into that same emergency room wearing one of those little medallions that say, "I am allergic to penicillin," and told the person receiving us that we were allergic, they then proceeded not to tell anybody and they still jabbed you with the penicillin. After you had the same reaction, that would be negligent malpractice.

— Congressman Pete Stark, testifying before subcommittee on issues relating to malpractice, May 20, 1993

Actions of a doctor that can be considered negligent:

- Doing things to a patient against the patient's will
- Failing to inform a patient of common risks in a manner meant to deliberately alter the patient's ability to make an educated decision on whether to undergo surgery or other treatment
- Performing an operation without the necessary equipment, medicines, or staff
- Performing an unnecessary operation after misdiagnosing an illness, disease, defect or injury
- Performing a surgery with the knowledge that it is unnecessary
- Causing injury to a patient through faulty practices
  An illness, disease or injury resulting from a doctor's actions is called an "iatrogenic" illness or injury.
  An infection that is acquired during a hospital stay is called a "nosocomial" illness. Nosocomial illnesses are often the result of unclean operating tools, contaminated hospital items, or unsanitary medical workers.
  Birth defects caused by medications are called "teratogenesis" or "teratogenicity" deformities.
- A doctor who is under the influence of drugs or alcohol treating patients
- Approaching a patient sexually
- Fondling or raping a patient while the patient is drugged or unconscious
- Prescribing or administering the wrong medication

- Creating a situation that leads to the death of a patient who did not have a life-or-death condition. This includes complications that result in a suicide.
- Lying to a patient

Many doctors believe it is acceptable to misinform a patient if it is done in a manner that will avoid upsetting or frightening the patient in a way that would interfere with the patient's health and deprive the patient of any hope for a cure.

Some types of doctors regularly have to deal with how to inform a patient about health conditions that might result in the patient's death. It can be a delicate balance of when, what and how to inform the patient in a way that provides for realistic hope. The doctor has to take into consideration what type of person the patient is, how the patient will accept the prognosis and what the patient's capabilities are of calculating the information in a way that is in the patient's best interest. And the doctor has to be prepared for the types of questions the patient might ask while recognizing that statistics do not always dictate how a patient will react to forms of treatment or how long that patient will live.

In September 1993, the California Supreme Court ruled that doctors must give seriously ill patients enough information to make intelligent decisions about treatment but are not obligated to disclose the statistical chances of dying — even if the patient asks to be told the truth about a health condition. The court ruling also held that doctors do not have to inform patients on pertinent details related to patients' non-medical interests, such as survival rates and how much time the patient has to put affairs in order. The ruling states that doctors need to provide statistical mortality rates only if it is a common standard of practice in the medical community.

While misleading a patient or holding information from a patient might be helpful in certain instances where the patient's health would be endangered if they reacted adversely to the truth, it might also alter the patient's ability to focus on the threat to their health. When a potentially life-threatening condition exists, valuable time can be wasted that the patient otherwise could have spent exercising their right to make decisions, doing

research, getting second and third opinions and
considering various available options.

What are the specific damages?

- Pain
- Suffering
- Altered abilities
- Emotional trauma
- Psychological trauma
- Endangerment
- Economic burden
- Altered lifestyle
- Decreased life expectancy
- Damaged or strained personal and professional
  relationships
- Wrongful death of a companion or relative who did not
  have a life-or-death condition

Even after a doctor has been found guilty of gross negligence
that has resulted in the death of one or more of his patients, he
may still be able to continue being a doctor. If a state medical
board investigates a doctor for unprofessional conduct and finds
him guilty, the board might only send the doctor a letter of
reprimand to formally acknowledge the doctor's guilt. This
reprimand probably will not affect the doctor's practice nor will
it be filed in the national database that collects information on
disciplinary actions against doctors. It basically does little if
anything as far as altering the way the doctor treats patients. It
probably will not affect the doctor's standing with insurance
companies or his hospital privileges.

A plastic surgeon who lost his license in one state moved to
Michigan, where he has since been sued dozens of times for
malpractice. He eventually had his medical license
suspended by the Michigan Board of Medicine, which also
fined him $20,000. Some of his former patients say that he
paid a small price for his crimes. In one male breast reduction
operation he left the patient deformed. In one tummy tuck
operation he destroyed the patient's belly button. In another
operation he did a double mastectomy on a woman after
misreading a mammogram. Still, he is legally free to move to
another state and open up shop there.

If you think a doctor who treated you was negligent, one of your options is to consult with a lawyer (before the statute of limitations has run out) who specializes in and is well experienced in malpractice law and who has substantial jury trial experience. You may want to consider taking the doctor to court, not only for personal reasons, but to protect other people from having done to them what was done to you. (People's Medical Society, Public Citizen's Health Research Group, the American Trial Lawyer's Association, the Center for Medial Consumers, the National Center for Patient's Rights, and Safe Medicine for Consumers are groups listed in the Research Resources section of this book that can provide you with information about taking legal action against a medical professional, medical center, or hospital.)

Be careful when choosing a lawyer: like some doctors who sell themselves in a particular specialty when they have not had any special training in that specialty, there are lawyers who market themselves as malpractice lawyers when they have not done any significant amount of research on malpractice law. Ask for the lawyer's resume. Ask the lawyer if they have malpractice insurance and ask to see the certificate of insurance provided by the insurance company.

Upon hiring an attorney, set a requirement that any bill you receive from the lawyer must be itemized with dates, reasons for charges and receipts of any outside charges. Do not let the lawyer charge you for things such as meals, valet parking at restaurants and recreational activities. If the lawyer is hungry he will eat whether or not you let him add food charges to your bill. If he wants to play golf he should play golf but you should not be charged for his golf game on the basis that he was thinking about your case while he played golf. Keep on top of the bills so that you do not end up challenging substantial overbilling charges before the fee dispute service of the county bar association or in a jury trial. (Your chances of winning are greater if you go to a jury trial to dispute overcharges by a lawyer. The fee dispute service of the county bar association is made up of lawyers and some say that the setup there is simply a good old boys' club where the club members always win.)

In choosing a lawyer, experience and fee should be related. One lawyer may charge an hourly rate that, at first, looks cheaper than another lawyer's. However, because of a lack of experience in some area, the less expensive lawyer may charge a larger fee in the long run. Ask for a resume and check references. If you feel overwhelmed, take a trusted friend to the initial meeting to help you keep track as you interview the lawyer about services and fees.

If you retain a law firm, be sure you understand who will work on your case and who will supervise the work. If junior lawyers will handle your work, the fees should be lower. That is fine as long as you know an experienced attorney will be reviewing the case periodically.

Let your lawyer know that you expect to be informed of all developments and consulted before any decisions are made. You may also want to receive copies of all documents, letters, and memos written and received in your case or have a chance to read them in the lawyer's office.

— from US Small Business Administration booklet *Starting and Managing a Business from Your Home,* by Lynne Waymon, in cooperation with the American Association of Community and Junior Colleges

Some of the most popular lawsuits against cosmetic surgeons in the news in the early 1990s included a woman who went in for an eye-lift and ended up having a bad reaction to the anesthesia, became brain damaged, and is now in a wheelchair; a woman who suffered a stroke when she went in for a tummy tuck; a woman surprised to find she received silicone facial implants when she went in for a different procedure; a woman who went in for liposuction and ended up having to get parts of her skin removed after it became so infected it was a threat to her health; and a man who had problems breathing out of his nose and went to a doctor who promised to only repair the breathing and not do any cosmetic changes but ended up doing so, which made his breathing worse, damaged his tear ducts and facial nerves and muscles.

Be cautious about with whom you discuss your feelings about a negligent doctor. The doctor may countersue for trade disparagement (lowering of professional rank), libel and defamation of character. It would be wise to seek legal counsel with an experienced malpractice lawyer before writing any letters or taking any action that involves a negligent doctor or what a negligent doctor did to you.

With the lawyer's guidance (it is not required to have legal advice when filing complaints against a doctor, medical professional, hospital or medical center, but remember that any letter you write can be dug up, taken out of context and thrown in your face in a courtroom), write and send a letter of complaint to the state medical board and any other governing body (administrators of every hospital the doctor is associated with, any school where he teaches, and also to your state legislator who may be working on or familiar with medical regulations) briefly detailing the situation.

Many doctors now work in an employee-type arrangement with HMOs and medical groups. This provides a doctor with a steady income and a more secure work arrangement as the doctor becomes part of a system. HMOs are very cost-conscious, and part of the way they judge a doctor is on a scale of what his way of practicing medicine is going to cost the HMO. If the doctor is a member of an HMO, you may also want to write to an administrator of the HMO. If you are accusing the doctor of performing a surgery that was unnecessary, the HMO may take notice. Any suggestion that the doctor could lose his HMO contract is a serious threat to the doctor's future income.

If the doctor's actions amount to what could be considered criminal activity (drug abuse, rape and other such offenses), you may want to contact the county district attorney's office or the state attorney general.

The state medical board may tell you what steps you should take in filing a complaint against a doctor, and it may require that you fill out specific forms. A letter to the state medical board might trigger disciplinary actions against the doctor and can help pave the way for the doctor's medical license to be taken away. (The process of revoking a doctor's license to practice medicine is rare and usually takes years. State medical boards are composed mostly of doctors. Do not be surprised if your concerns are dismissed by them. In California 12 of the state board's 19 members are doctors.)

> **Reasons another doctor or a hospital might not report or take actions against a bad doctor:**
> - Fear of being sued
> - Financial interest — the bad doctor may be referring a large number of patients to the knowing doctor or may be bringing the hospital a significant amount of business
> - The doctors may get their insurance through the same insurance carrier
> - The doctors may be members of the same medical group or HMO or have other professional/financial links

- Fear of attracting negative attention to the profession, which can result in media reports or stronger regulation by insurance companies or the government

Be prepared to supply the lawyer with your medical history and any information you have to solidify your case. You and your lawyer have to prepare for the time in the courtroom when you exercise your right to present evidence. During this time of preparation remember that everyone deserves a defense and a fair trial and that to protect the innocent from being wrongfully condemned you must prove that the doctor is at fault.

If a doctor is seriously negligent in the treatment of one patient, chances are he has a record of indiscretions and there may be other patients he has mistreated. In California when stories of one bad doctor made their way into the local news, several dozen of his former patients came forward and filed complaints against the doctor. If you know of other people who have had bad experiences with the same doctor, you may want to have a meeting with them and your lawyer.

If the doctor finds out you are taking any type of action that questions his professionalism, he may foresee a possible lawsuit and prepare himself accordingly. Be aware that any letters you send to state medical boards or other governing bodies might be shown to the doctor by the people who receive the letter(s). This can be enough to start a campaign to discredit you as the doctor proceeds to defend his credibility and career.

If you decide to take the doctor to court, be forewarned that a lawsuit can get very involved. The doctor you are suing does not pay legal counsel to make you look like an angel. The other party can dig into your past to find things about your character that may be unflatteringly presented in court to prove your claim is frivolous, that your findings are inaccurate, your reasoning is questionable and possibly that you are mentally incompetent. It is kind of like putting your life under a microscope. Your judgment, morals, memory, honesty, stability, personal history and reputation can be presented in the most unflattering manner, dissected and questioned — all with the goal of portraying your claim as weak. The defense will use any means possible to gather information needed to persuade the jury to rule against you. Private investigators can be hired to spy on you and seek out and question people who know you (or think they know you) to find information that can be damaging to your case. Any information that makes its way into court records is then public record, and other people, including the media, can gain access to it.

Lawsuits against doctors can be very expensive. Before the case goes to court it has to be prepared for the court. This preparation includes filing fees, using the services of other professionals such as court reporters, obtaining and copying records, travel, photocopying, postage, word processing and library and computer research. You will also be required to respond to written questions (interrogatories) from the doctor and his lawyers. Then you will have to go through a deposition where you and your lawyer sit in a meeting room with the doctor's lawyers, a court reporter, and possibly the doctor, and answer questions from the doctor's lawyer under oath. The expenses for all of this are usually your responsibility and can add up into the thousands of dollars. It will be expensive for you and it will be expensive for the doctor's malpractice insurance company as they take actions to defend the doctor. For this reason it would be better for the insurance company if you had died undergoing the surgery because it is likely that it would have been cheaper for them.

Though there is something seriously wrong with a justice system that can be influenced by money, anyone involved with a lawsuit will quickly learn how much influence money can buy in the court system. Chances are that the doctor has more money than you, and one of the privileges of having money is the ability to pay for expensive legal counsel, private investigators and jury consultants. The doctor or his malpractice insurance carrier can probably get a better lawyer than you can — and one who knows how to play all the manipulative legal games. Malpractice insurance is expensive — insurance companies are big money and big money plays tough.

> . . . there has always been a concern about the relatively low rate of official actions against physicians by State boards and a concern that physicians' colleagues were not coming forward or the State boards were not being as aggressive as they ought to be in dealing with negligent providers [doctors]. Perhaps, even that they weren't outreaching to get the information necessary to find out there was a problem [with a doctor].
>
> One interesting development recently is that, as a result of malpractice crises of the mid-1970s, physician-owned insurance companies were developed to provide malpractice insurance.

My understanding is they now provide more than half of the insurance. These companies, owned by doctors, have underwriting committees comprised of doctors and have begun to be somewhat more aggressive in denying coverage or in putting restrictions on the practice of people they insure or in putting surcharges on the physicians they insure. I saw an estimate about that in 1985, of the physicians who sought insurance under these physician insurance companies, 3 percent in that year were under some sort of a restriction. This implies that when you get a group of doctors who have a financial incentive as they own the company, to take a hard look at their peers, they look a little harder than maybe the State boards do.
— Lawrence H. Thompson, Assistant Comptroller General Human Resources Division, US General Accounting Office, during Congressional subcommittee hearing on issues relating to medical malpractice, May 20, 1993

In most States, drivers have to prove they have liability coverage. But in medicine, doctors can practice cosmetic surgery without insurance coverage at all and many do.
— Congressman Ron Wyden during Congressional subcommittee hearings on plastic surgery industry, 1989

Do not expect to win your case on the basis that it resembles a malpractice case where another victim of medical negligence won their case. Each case is judged on its own merits.

If the doctor does not have malpractice insurance (is "going bare"), you may have a difficult time getting a lawyer and you may end up negotiating a settlement with an uninsured doctor. Even if the doctor has malpractice insurance, if he is performing an operation that is outside of his expertise and not covered under his insurance contract, then the insurance company may disclaim responsibility for him and not represent him in the lawsuit. In this scenario he is essentially uninsured, liable for his own actions and will have to pay for his own legal counsel.

If you do get a lawyer to fight your malpractice case, your lawyer (if he is not one of the few lawyers who also has a degree in some area of medicine) will have to consult with a doctor who will explain what it was that was done to you and what was done wrong. You will also need this consulting doctor to testify for you, and this could cost money (expert witness fees).

In its efforts to educate doctors in the legal aspects of medicine, the American Medical Association sells a videotape titled *How to Be an Effective Medical Witness.* The cover of the tape says the tape will teach a doctor to qualify as an expert witness, prepare for testifying, use the available evidence on which to base his opinion, answer questions about his fee, properly state his opinion using "magic" legal words, prepare for and testify at his deposition, deal with trick questions and trial tactics of attorneys, effectively describe complex medical issues, humanize his testimony, deal with conflicting medical reports and opinions and deal with an abusive attorney.

A doctor does not spend years in medical school to have some random patient ruin his career and financial stability with a lawsuit. The doctor, his lawyer, or his insurance company will probably have no difficulty in finding (paying for) another doctor (to be an expert witness) who will testify that the surgery was within acceptable standards and testify to whatever else the doctor wants the jury to hear. Legal magazines are filled with ads placed by experts in every specialty willing to hire out for court cases. There are "jukebox doctors" who make good money by saying whatever they are paid to say when someone deposits the right amount of money in the doctor's pocket. It is your word against theirs and they may be fraudulent, but they have the medical degree and you do not.

On your side of the fence, you may have difficulty finding an expert witness. Many doctors are unwilling to testify against another doctor because they then may be accused of libel or slander or because of some financial interest. If you do find a doctor who recognizes the damage that another doctor has done to you, this doctor might back down from testifying against the negligent doctor based on the fact that both of the doctors get their malpractice insurance from the same insurance company. The insurance company, through its representatives, may suggest that the doctor's insurance can be canceled if he agrees to be your expert witness, or the insurance company may hint about higher insurance premiums. With the issue being cosmetic surgery, you may have difficulty finding a doctor who is willing to defame his profession because you may be thought of as just another cosmetic surgery crybaby who did not get what you wanted. You may also be dealing with a jury who considers any cosmetic surgery to be frivolous and you a fool for letting a doctor do it to you. On the other hand, some people are opposed to cosmetic surgery and the doctors who perform it and this is a bonus for you if you are suing one.

Binding arbitration agreements

Your insurance plan may have limitations on the legal avenues you can take in suing a doctor, including an arbitration clause that limits your right to a jury trial. If you are a member of an HMO, your membership contract probably stipulates that any disputes be resolved through third-party arbitration and not in court. The paperwork you signed when you initially went to the doctor might also contain a binding arbitration agreement. If a patient dies because of negligence, the family is also bound to the arbitration agreement. A pregnant woman who signs this form is binding the rights of her unborn child. A person who changes their mind after signing an arbitration contract has 30 days to cancel the agreement in writing.

If you signed a pre-surgery arbitration agreement at the doctor's office or when you entered the hospital, this may stop your case from being presented before a trial jury. Instead you may be limited to an arbitration panel of three people who are usually lawyers or retired judges who will listen to your case and decide whether any negligence took place and what, if any, award should be given. Each side picks an arbitrator and together they select a third. It is often the third, "neutral," arbitrator who casts the deciding vote. Large awards are rare in the arbitration process and, because arbitration is done in private, there is no public record of the proceedings. Therefore, the malpractice award may not show up on the doctor's state records.

Jury selection can take anywhere from a few hours to a month or more. Men and women summoned for duty are sent in groups to be queried by a judge or the lawyers about whether they can serve for the duration of the trial or if they have any conflicts that could preclude them from being fair. They might be asked to fill out a questionnaire designed to expose their attitudes about issues that will arise at trial. Both sides can remove a certain number of jurors they deem unfit.
— from article titled *Role of Jury Consultants Controversial and Extensive*, by Maura Dolan, Los Angeles Times, September 26, 1994

To win your case, you have to prove to a supposedly fair and impartial jury that the surgery deviated from the accepted standards of practice that exist within the medical community. You may be dealing with a jury who thought you got what you paid for. The jury members do not need to be intelligent or educated; they only need to be 18 years old. Even though people in court are supposed to tell the truth, and nothing but the truth, anyone who has been involved with any kind of serious lawsuit knows that lies exist in courtrooms like wet exists in water. Oftentimes a person can get the feeling that the crooks in the courtroom are not the ones on trial.

The court case can become a display of the expert knowledge held by all of the characters present in the form of legal and medical professionals involved with the case, and the interests of the victim can become lost in this cast of characters who may be using the case to help define their careers. Do not be surprised if the doctor points his finger at you and blames you for the malpractice because of your demands on the doctor. There have been many malpractice cases where the doctor claims he did not want to do the operation but did it only after the patient demanded it against the doctors' better judgment. (Did these doctors also not want the money they made by performing the surgeries?)

> The American Hospital Association, along with other organizations, believes that the medical liability compensation system currently fails to meet its own goals of adequately and fairly compensating injured patients, and at the same time, effectively deterring bad healthcare practices.
>
> Many of our healthcare providers are afraid to practice their trade because of anticipated liability claims and, as a result, resort to defensive medicine, over prescription of tests by providers, et cetera.
>
> Many providers are unwilling to practice in their specialty areas such as obstetrics and emergency room care because of increased malpractice premiums and the threats of unfounded lawsuits. As a result, many communities are left underserved with little or no access to appropriate healthcare services.
>
> People injured by poor quality of care are entitled to fair and prompt compensation for their injuries, but our present system costs far too much and works much too slowly, and

fails to provide fair compensation to most patients injured by medical malpractice, while providing exorbitant lottery-type awards to others.

— from statement of John D. Leech, member, board of trustees, American Hospital Association. Presented at a Congressional subcommittee hearing on issues relating to medical malpractice, May 20, 1993

Duke University Law School's Medical Malpractice Project recently completed a study which attempted to review every malpractice suit filed in North Carolina between July 1, 1984 and June 30, 1987 — 895 cases. The project also collected information on more than 300 other cases filed in a sample of North Carolina counties between July, 1987 and December, 1990. The study found that medical malpractice juries are not consistently pro-plaintiff, nor do they award excessive damages.

According to the study, about 40 percent of the cases reviewed were terminated without any payment to the plaintiff, and about 50 percent were settled. Only about 10 percent of the cases, or 117 cases, were decided by jury.

Out of the 117 cases that went to trial, there were only four large jury awards, ranging in size from $750,000 to $3.5 million (subsequently reduced to 2.9 million). These judgments were awarded in cases involving severe brain damage, permanent paralysis and brain damage, death from suffocation by an intubation tube improperly placed, and a child who suffered brain damage at birth. The study found that the average damage award in cases that plaintiffs won was $367,737. But this number was much inflated by the four large awards discussed above. The median or mid-point award, on the other hand, was only $36,500.

The Duke study also found that injuries are not biased in favor of injured patients. In the cases that went before a jury, the plaintiff prevailed in just one out of five. Furthermore, the juries found in favor of defendants in 18 out of 19 cases that insurers expected to win, and 13 out of 17 cases that insurers rated as questionable. And juries even ruled against plaintiffs in a majority of cases — six out of 11 — that insurers thought they would lose.

— from prepared statement of Pamela Gilbert, director of Public Citizen's Congress Watch, citing Duke University Law School project and with information from "The Unfair Criticism of Medical Malpractice Juries," Neil Vidmar, *Judicature*, October/November, 1992 and "Still Warring Over Medical Malpractice," Kenneth Jost, *ABA Journal*, May 1993.

Presented at a Congressional subcommittee hearing on issues relating to malpractice, May 20, 1993

A US General Accounting Office study of claims closed in 1984 found that the average time to resolve the claim was 25 months. Some took as long as 11 years. In over half the cases, plaintiff legal fees exceeded 30 percent of the payments to the injured party. In addition, the insurers also paid $800 million to investigate and defend the claims closed in 1984 as compared to $2.6 billion that they actually paid in the claims. If you add it all together, it turns out that the lawyers and the overhead account for about almost half of the payments made.

— Lawrence H. Thompson, assistant comptroller general, Human Resources Division, US General Accounting Office. Testifying before Congressional subcommittee hearing on issues related to malpractice, May 20, 1993

Although malpractice victims usually need money immediately, lawsuits can take years to make it through the court system. The medical boards might not take any action against a doctor until there is a ruling against the doctor. During the years it takes to get a ruling, the doctor can harm many other people. The person who was victimized can be awarded a settlement, but this does not mean that collection of the judgment is certain. If the doctor has no insurance company representing him and the patient is suing a doctor directly and the doctor's assets are hidden in financial closets, the patient may not be able to collect a dime.

The patient who sues a doctor can end up owing a lot of money because of lost income and, among other things, legal fees, medical bills and other debts. These costs may amount to more than what was won in the lawsuit. During your trip through the legalities of malpractice hell, you can burn out, which could be what the defense wants so that you drop the lawsuit or take an out-of-court settlement. This could be a good thing, or you may simply be getting taken advantage of again.

The architects of the Clinton health plan considered a proposal that would bar patients from directly suing doctors and instead would allow patients to sue the health insurance providers. The limit, known as "enterprise liability" was designed to mirror other industries where consumers sue the company and not the person or persons who work for the company.

Even if a malpractice victim wins their lawsuit, there is no way to reverse what was done to their body or mind and return it to its original state. It is similar to rape. The victim is the victim because of the negligence, is treated like they are victimizing someone else during the lawsuit, and remains a victim. If there is an out-of-court settlement it can end up protecting the doctor because it will include a secrecy clause that keeps the patient from talking about the settlement. In all, the road to justice (if any is actually built) can make you compromise your goals, can be very time consuming to the point that it interferes with every area of your life and, in the end, can be unsatisfying.

American Bar Association
Phone (312) 988-5000

American College of Trial Lawyers
Phone (714) 727-3194

American Trial Lawyer's Association
1050 – 31st Street NW, Washington, DC 20007-4499; Phone (800) 424-2725 or 2727

International Academy of Trial Lawyers
Phone (408) 275-6767

The International Society of Barristers does not refer people to attorneys. However, the group will confirm if a lawyer is a member of the society.

International Society of Barristers
Phone (313) 763-0165

Since 1969, the National Health Law Program has served as a legal services national support center specializing in health issues for low-income people, minorities, the disabled and the elderly. NHeLP communicates with a variety of Washington-based groups on healthcare access issues. NHeLP has published numerous guides on a variety of health issues including Medicaid, Medicare, state and local indigent healthcare programs, maternal and child health, and civil rights and healthcare.

National Health Law Program
2639 South LaCienega Boulevard, Los Angeles, California 90034; Phone (310) 204-6010

National Women's Law Center
1616 P Street, NW, Washington, DC 20036; Phone (202) 328-5160

National Senior Citizen's Law Project
Phone (202) 887-5280 or (213) 482-3550

Several books put out by the People's Medical Society deal with medical rights.

People's Medical Society
462 Walnut Street, Allentown, Pennsylvania 18102; Phone (215) 770-1670

Public Citizen Books publishes a book titled *Representing Yourself: What You Can Do Without a Lawyer*. The book tells how to solve routine legal problems without a lawyer, how to decide if you do need a lawyer, and how to make sure you are adequately represented. For price information, contact

Public Citizen Books
2000 P Street NW, Suite 605, Washington, DC 20036; Phone (202) 833-3000

• MATERIALS USED IN PLASTIC, RECONSTRUCTIVE, AND COSMETIC SURGERY

Until scientists succeed in their goal of finding a way to grow human tissues such as skin, bone, cartilage and muscle in laboratories, the following materials are being used or are soon to be used to implant into the human body.

Bioplastique: Bioplastique is a man-made material that is not available in the United States because it is not FDA approved. The company that manufactures it, Bioplasty, is headquartered in Minneapolis. Bioplastique has been used in Europe for years to rebuild noses that have been damaged by accident, and to rebuild noses that have been ruined by bad cosmetic surgery. The company describes it as an indictable material that is formed once it has been injected into the skin using a blunt syringe.

Bone from the rib, hips or skull: These can be used to graft onto other bones. Grafts taken from a person's own body are called "autographs." When bone is harvested from the hips, it is taken from the top front of the hip bone area known as the "iliac crest." When it is harvested from the skull, it is usually taken from the back of the head.

Bovine (cow) cartilage: Some doctors have used specially processed cartilage from cows to build up noses and other contour defects of the face and head. Transplanting tissue from one species to another species is called "xenografting."

Cadaver cartilage or cadaver bone: Human skin, bone, cartilage and tendons are used in over 450,000 transplant operations in the United States each year. This is over and above the large number of transplant organs including hearts, lungs, skin, livers, kidneys and eyes that are used in various other operations. Grafts from one person to another are called "allografts."

In 1993, after considering the potential for the spread of infectious diseases through the use of cadaver tissue and finding evidence that some tissue brokers and tissue banks were marketing body parts taken from diseased bodies, and that bodies from questionable foreign countries and other body parts were being sold without proper screening or documentation, the FDA started regulating this area of medicine on an emergency basis granted by Congress. The safeguards included precautions that tissues would be used only after tissue banks had ensured that donors had been adequately tested and screened for infectious diseases.

In some plastic surgery operations, usually those that are done for more than just cosmetic reasons, there is sometimes the need for tissue that the patient is not able to supply — skin transplants for burn victims for example. In this situation one option would be to use donated tissue.

If donated tissue is not available, using transplant tissue may create more risks than are acceptable. Or for other reasons the doctor and patient may elect to use man-made materials.

Calcium phosphate ceramics: A biodegradable polymer material, consisting of hydroxyapetite, a material found in natural bone and biodegradable polymer spheres composed of lactic acid and glycolic acid (poly [lactide-co-glycolide]), which are used in suture material, holds potential as an alternative bone graft material for patients being treated for bone damage or restructuring. The man-made material (researched by orthopedic surgeon Cato Laurencin [now working at the Medical College of Pennsylvania] while at the Massachusetts Institute of Technology) has not yet been used on humans. It is similar in color to bone and has a porous structure that provides temporary scaffolds for bone ingrowth (osteoconduction) of host tissue (the bone) and migration of cells into the interior of the implant. It is produced in sizes of 2cm x 1cm and is carved with a scalpel. When used in a weight-bearing region it needs to be supplemented with a metal plate that fulfills the load-support requirements.

Ear Cartilage: Cartilage harvested from behind or inside the ear has been one of the most common items used in rebuilding or adding to noses. Many people have had ear cartilage grafts placed onto the bridge of their nose and also have had it used to correct problems with the septum. The problem with using ear cartilage is shaping it to the desired form and having it stay that way. Cartilage may also shift out of place and heal improperly. A certain amount of it will fade, and when it is used to build up a nasal bridge it can become lumpy or jagged.

Fascia: Fascia is a thin layer of connective tissue that binds body structures together. While researching this book, I spoke with one doctor who used fascia harvested from the side of the head as a graft to augment the nasal dorsum (the bridge of the nose). Other doctors I spoke with questioned the use of this tissue because they believe it will fade away with time as the body absorbs the grafted fascia.

Gore-tex soft tissue patch: This is a very white leather-type porous material made out of Teflon and is believed to be more inert than silicone rubber. Because the material is porous, there is a lower risk of scar tissue forming around the implant, as may occur with silicone implants. Medical Gore-tex is sold in 1 mm or 2 mm thicknesses and can be layered, glued or sewn together to make an implant. It has been used for decades in various surgeries including open-heart surgery to replace the sack that surrounds the heart. It is also available in mesh form for use in hernia repair and as a gastric wrap for wrapping around stomachs in weight-loss surgery. Many cosmetic surgeons now use it to adhere to the back of cheek and chin implants. The porosity of the material allows for a certain amount of tissue ingrowth, which prevents the implants from moving around. More recently it has been used to augment the bridge of the nose, though many doctors advise against using the material in this manner. It is also available in string or suture form, and doctors have been using it in this form to implant into the lips to make lips more pouty and into facial grooves and deep wrinkles.

Knee Cartilage: A company called Genzyme Tissue Repair (Cambridge, Massachusetts) owns the license to a technique that takes cartilage from the knee and grows cartilage cells in a lab. The cartilage cells are used to repair damaged knees. The new cartilage cells are placed back into the knee and held in place with a piece of periosteum (a tissue that covers bones).

Rib cartilage: When there is a lack of ear and septal cartilage, the ribs can be used a source of cartilage to rebuild a nose or other area. This of course will leave a scar on the torso, but a scar that may fade considerably depending on the person and the type of incision.

A doctor in Beverly Hills, California, Robert Ruder, specializes in constructing ears out of rib cartilage on children who are born with a small nub in place of an ear — a birth defect called microtia.

Sea coral: Coral harvested from the tropical waters of the South Pacific is being used as an alternative when a bone graft is needed. Formerly there were only two choices for a bone graft: bone could either be taken from the patient (usually from the hip) or from another person, usually a cadaver. Coral implants cannot replace entire bones — they can only add to or replace small portions of bone and cannot be relied on for mechanical strength.

The porous microstructure of coral is similar to that of bone and works as a scaffolding for bone to grow into when coral is placed against or inside of bone. Over the following months and years as the new bone grows into the coral implant, degradative cells called osteoblasts eat away at the coral and deposit new bone while blood vessels also establish themselves in the structure.

The two types of coral that have been used are porite, which is used in bones below the neck, and acropora, which is used in neck and head operations. Information put out by the manufacturer, Irvine, California-based Interpore International, states that the coral preparation is a 23-stage "hydrothermal exchange reaction" treatment process that converts the calcium carbonate components of the coral into hydroxyapatite calcium phosphate, the main mineral ingredient of human bone. Research statistics have shown that coral does not activate the body's immune or inflammation responses.

One of the most common uses of coral is for jaw surgery when the jaw is being surgically rearranged and a little extra bone is needed to fill a gap. Other areas where coral has been used are to fill a hole in a bone caused by a bullet injury or to graft onto or into damaged bones.

Some of the significant benefits of using coral bone grafting material are in time savings, because the surgeon does not have to harvest a bone graft from another part of the body, and lowered cost, which is the result of a less time-consuming procedure. The use of coral also lowers the chance of complications that can result from cutting into another part of the patient's body to harvest a bone graft or from using bone from another person who may harbor an infectious disease.

Septal cartilage: This is cartilage taken from the inside center of the nose (the septum) and used to add profile to the bridge of the nose. There is always a chance for nerve damage affecting the senses of taste and smell and the vomeronasal organ, damage to the soft palate, a collapsed nose, and a permanent hole in the septum.

Silicone rubber: This is the solid silicone rubber, not the liquid silicone contained in silicone gel-filled breast implants. It has been used for years as an implant material to augment the nasal bridge (dorsum) and is being used for cheek, chin and other facial implants. It is used in hip replacement and the implantation of other joints. Penile implants used in impotent men are made of silicone, as are the imitation testicles used to fill in for testicles lost to cancer, accident or assault.

Silicone implants for the bridge of the nose have been popular among some Vietnamese women who married American servicemen and other

Asian people who want more of a nasal profile so they will appear more American or Western. These implants on the bridge of the nose and other facial implants may shift position or be driven through the skin if they are bumped hard enough. An infection around the implant can require implant removal.

Skin: A company named Genzyme Tissue Repair (Cambridge, Massachusetts) can grow small pieces of skin for use on patients who have experienced severe burns. The company uses cells from a small piece of the patient's skin. A company named Advance Tissue Sciences (San Diego, California) has developed the technology to grow skin by using cells from the foreskins of circumcised infants.

American Medical Systems is a manufacturer of penile implants.

American Medical Systems
11001 Bren Road East, Minnetonka, Minnesota 55343; Phone (612) 933-4666

Collagen Company
2500 Faber Place, Palo Alto, California 94303; Phone (800) 722-2007

Collagen Biomedical
1850 Embarcadero Road, Palo Alto, California 94303-3308; Phone (800) 227-4004 or (800) 327-1179

Creative Biomolecules is a biotechnology company that has been working on transforming muscle into bone.

Creative Biomolecules
45 South Street, Hopkinton, Massachusetts 01748; Phone (508) 435-9001

Interpore is the American company that processes coral bone implants. They own the patent on the 23-stage procedure of treating coral to convert it into calcium phosphate, which is the main component of human bone. The other company that sells coral for bone implants is called INOTEB and is located in Paris, France.

Interpore Orthopaedics International
181 Technology Drive, Irvine, California 91718; Phone (714) 453-3200 or toll-free (800) 727-4489

LipoMatix is the company that manufactures the Trilucent breast implants that are filled with a natural fat derived from soybean oil and that were introduced in the summer of 1994. The fat is a form of triglyceride which is a natural fat in the body. The implants still use a silicone shell which some experts believe is not good for the body.

LipoMatrix, Inc.
Phone (800) 839-3020

W.L. Gore is the manufacturer of Gore-Tex expanded Polytetraflouroethylene Soft Tissue Patch.

W.L. Gore & Associates, Inc.
P.O. Box 900, Dock A, Flagstaff, Arizona 86002; Phone (602) 779-2771 Sales service center (800) 528-8763; Technical information (800) 437-8181

A manufacturer of permanent makeup pigments:

Spaulding Co.
Route 85, New Scotland Road, Voorheesville, New York 12186; Phone (518) 768-2070

• MENTAL HEALTH, PSYCHOLOGICAL COUNSELING AND THERAPY

Books:
- *Dead Serious: A Book for Teenagers About Teenage Suicide*, by Jane Mersky Leder, Atheneum Books, 1994
- *52 Things You Can Do to Raise Your Self-Esteem*, by Jerry Minchinton, by Arnford House (Vanzant, Missouri 65768, Phone [417] 261-2559), 1995
- *On The Edge Of Darkness: Conversations About Conquering Depression*, by Kathy Cronkite; Doubleday, 1994
- *Self Esteem: The Ultimate Program for Self Help*, by Matthew McKay and Patrick Fanning; MJF Books/Fine Communications, 1987
- *When Good Enough is Never Enough: Escaping the Perfection Trap*, by Steven J. Hendlin; Putnam Books, 1992
- *You Are Not Alone: Words of Experience & Hope for the Journey through Depression*, by Julia Thorn & Larry Rothstein; HarperCollins, 1993

At times of particular stress, even the most steady person will find the assistance of a professional therapist useful. When you reduce your own stress level, you put others at ease too. Visiting with a well-educated therapist with whom you are comfortable and with whom you can also communicate can be beneficial in confronting past or present issues that may be having a negative effect on your life and relationships. There should be a "fit" between your personality and that of the therapist. It pays to seek help from another if you feel dissatisfied or unaided by a particular therapist.

There are many books available in bookstores and libraries that deal with the subject of self-esteem and other personal issues. Many of the books have been written by people who have overcome life problems that may be similar to what you are experiencing. Reading their viewpoint may be helpful to you and sometimes can be of more help than what you can receive from someone who is limited to a textbook knowledge of your problem. By-the-book therapy does not work for everyone, however.

There are also many support groups a person can attend that, along with professional counseling and book reading, can help a person cope with private tragedies with the goal of strengthening the person's coping skills and improving their state of mind.

Because the mind and body are interconnected, a person should not rule out physical health and should seek to improve their diet and level of fitness to create a well-balanced life.

American Association for Marriage and Family Therapy
1100 – 17th Street NW, 10th Floor, Washington, DC 20036; Phone (202) 429-1825 or (202) 452-0109; Phone toll-free (800) 347-2368

American Association of Sex Educators, Counselors & Therapists
435 North Michigan Avenue, Suite 1717, Chicago, Illinois 60611; Phone (312) 644-0828

American Family Therapy Association
2020 Pennsylvania Avenue, Suite 273, Washington, DC 20006; Phone (202) 994-2776

American Mental Health Counselors Association
5999 Stevenson Avenue, Alexandria, Virginia 22304; Phone (703) 823-9800 ext. 383

American Psychiatric Nurses' Association
6900 Grove Road, Thorofare, New Jersey 08086; Phone (609) 848-7990

American Psychosomatic Society
6728 Old McLean Village Drive, McLean, Virginia 22101; Phone (703) 556-9222

American Schizophrenia Association
900 North Federal Highway, Suite 330, Boca Raton, Florida 33432; Phone (305) 393-6167 or toll-free (800) 783-3801

American Schizophrenia Association
900 North Federal Highway, Suite 330, Boca Raton, Florida 33432; Phone (305) 393-6167 or toll-free (800) 783-3801

American Sleep Disorders Association
1610 – 14th Street NW, Suite 300, Rochester, Minnesota 55901; Phone (507) 287-6006

Canadian Psychiatric Association
237 Argyle Avenue, #200, Ottawa, Ontario K2P 1BP; Phone (613) 234-2815

Depression Awareness, Recognition and Treatment Program
The National Institute of Mental Health, Room 15–C–05, 5600 Fishers Lane, Rockville, Maryland 20857

For a free copy of a brochure developed to help people with depression, recognize symptoms and seek treatment options, send a self-addressed, stamped envelope to

Depression Guidelines
P.O. Box 8547, Silver Spring, Maryland 20907

Depressives Anonymous: Recovery From Depression
329 East 62nd Street, New York, New York 10021; Phone (212) 689-2600

Emotional Health Anonymous
Box 63236, Los Angeles, California 90063-0236; Phone (213) 268-7220

Emotions Anonymous
P.O. Box 4245, St. Paul, Minnesota 55104; Phone (612) 647-9712

False Memory Syndrome Foundation
3401 Market Street, Suite 130, Philadelphia, Pennsylvania 19104; Phone (800) 568-8882

Federation of Families for Children's Mental Health
1021 Prince Street, Alexandria, Virginia 22134-2971; Phone (703) 684-7710

International Association of Psychosocial Rehabilitation Services
Sterrett Place, Suite 214, Columbia, Maryland 21044-2626; Phone (410) 730-7190

Manic Depressive Illness Foundation
2723 P Street, Washington, DC 20007

National Alliance for the Mentally Ill
2101 Wilson, Suite 302, Arlington, Virginia 22201; Phone (703) 524-7600 or toll-free (800) 950-NAMI

National Association of Psychiatric Survivors
P.O. Box 618, Sioux Falls, South Dakota 57101; Phone (605) 334-4067

National Depression and Manic Depressives Association
730 North Franklin, Suite 501, Chicago, Illinois 60610; Phone (312) 642-0049 or toll-free (800) 826-2632

National Foundation For Depressive Illness, Inc.
P.O. Box 2257, New York, New York 10116; Phone (212) 268-4260 or toll-free (800) 248-4344

National Institute of Mental Health
Information Resources and Inquiries Branch, 5600 Fishers Lane, Room 15C–05, Rockville, Maryland 20857; Phone (800) 421-4211

National Mental Health Association
1021 Prince Street, Alexandria, Virginia 22314-2971; Phone (703) 684-7722 or toll-free (800) 969-NMHA

National Mental Health Consumers' Association
311 South Juniper Street, Room 902, Philadelphia, Pennsylvania 19107; Phone (215) 735-2465

National Sleep Disorder Foundation
122 South Robertson Boulevard, 3rd Floor, Los Angeles, California 90048; Phone (310) 288-0466

Obsessive-Compulsive Disorder Foundation
P.O. Box 70, Milford, Connecticut 06460; Phone (203) 878-5669 or 874-3834

Support Coalition International
P.O. Box 11284, Eugene, Oregon 11284; Phone (503) 345-9106

• NATURAL COSMETICS AND SKIN CARE

Book:
- *A Consumer's Dictionary of Cosmetic Ingredients: Complete Information about the Harmful and Desirable Ingredients Found in Men's and Women's Cosmetics*, by Ruth Winter; Crown Publishers, 1989

Some cosmetic products contain chemicals such as dyes and scents that may irritate the skin, cause allergic reactions and even cancer. Even common ingredients such as talc may lead to ovarian tumors.

The following companies sell cosmetics that do not contain chemicals or contain a much smaller amount of such chemical additives than cosmetics that are manufactured by the large corporations. Many of their products rely on natural substances such as herbs and oils instead of harsh chemicals such as coal-tar dyes (even if the small print of a hair-dye product lists that the coloring agent is derived from a natural product, it still may contain phenylenediamine-based dyes, and these should be avoided). The products they manufacture are also cruelty free — meaning that they are not tested on animals.

Alba Naturals (skin treatments)
P.O. Box 12085, Santa Rosa, California 95406; Phone (800) 347-5211

Aubrey Organics (send $3.50 for a catalog of 130 hair and skin products)
4419 North Manhattan Avenue, Tampa, Florida 33614; Phone (800) 282-7394

Au Naturel International
P.O. Box 956, Topanga, California; Phone (800) 583-9505

Basically Natural
109 East G Street, Brunswick, Maryland 21716

The Body Shop (call for a catalog)
Phone (800) 541-2535

CamoCare
Phone (800) CAM-OCAR

Earth Science
23705 Via Del Rio, Yorba Linda, California 92678; Phone (800) 222-6720

Jojoba Obispo
P.O. Box 1761, San Luis Obispo, California 93406; Phone (805) 544-3505

Logona USA (non-chemical hair coloring)
554-E Riverside Drive, Ashville, North Carolina 28801; Phone (800) 648-6654

Nature Works
5310 Derry Avenue, Agoura Hills, California 91301; Phone (818) 889-1602

Nature's Gate
9200 Mason Avenue, Chatsworth, California 91311; Phone (800) 327-2012

Nature Safe Products
P.O. Box 14088, South Lake Tahoe, California 96151; Phone (800) 736-8122

Nature's Answer
75 Commerce Drive, Hauppauge, New York 11788; Phone (800) 645-5720 or in New York phone (800) 439-2324

Nutri-Metrics
Pamela Marsen, Inc., P.O. Box 119, Teaneck, New Jersey 07666; Phone (201) 836-7820

Paul Penders
Phone (800) 440-PAUL

Tom's of Maine
Kennebunk, Maine 04043; Phone (207) 985-2944 or (800) 367-8667

For more information on companies that manufacture or distribute products that are not tested on animals and do not contain animal products, contact one of the following

People for the Ethical Treatment of Animals
P.O. Box 42516, Washington, DC 20015; Phone (301) 770-PETA

Research Modernization and Animal Rights
333 Washington Street, Suite 850, Boston, Massachusetts 02108-5100;
Phone (617) 523-6020

Vegetarian Journal ($20 a year)
P.O. Box 1463, Baltimore, Maryland 21203; Phone (410) 366-VEGE

• NURSES

Ask-A-Nurse
Phone (800) 535-1111

American Academy of Nurse Practitioners
Capitol Station, LBJ Building, P.O. Box 12846, Austin, Texas 78711; Phone
(512) 442-4262

American Academy of Physician Assistants
950 North Washington Street, Alexandria, Virginia 22314; Phone (703)
836-2272

American Association of Critical Care Nurses
101 Columbia, Aliso Viejo, California 92656; Phone (800) 899-2226

American Association of Nurse Anesthetists
222 South Prospect, Park Ridge, Illinois 60068-4001; Phone (708) 692-
7050

American Nurses Association
600 Maryland Avenue, SW, Suite 100 West, Washington, DC 20024-
2571; Phone (202) 554-4444 or (800) 274-4ANA

American Nurses Credentialing Center
600 Maryland Avenue, SW, Suite 100 West, Washington, DC 20024-2571;
Phone (800) 284-CERT

American Society of Post Anesthesia Nurses
11512 Allegheny Parkway, Suite C, Richmond, Virginia 23235; Phone
(804) 379-5516

American Society of Plastic and Reconstructive Surgical Nurses
Box 56, North Woodbury Road, Pitman, New Jersey 08071; Phone (609)
589-6247

National Black Nurses Association
1660 L Street, NW, Suite 907, Washington, DC 20036; Phone (202) 673-
4551

National League of Nursing
350 Hudson Street, New York, New York 10014; Phone (212) 989-9393

• PATIENTS' AND CONSUMERS' RIGHTS

Books:
- *The Consumer's Legal Guide to Today's Healthcare: Your Medical
  Rights and How to Assert Them,* by Stephen L. Isaacs, JD, & Ava C.
  Swartz, MPH; Houghton Mifflin Co., 1992
- *Silent Violence, Silent Death: A Consumer Guide to the Medical
  Malpractice Epidemic,* by Harvey Rosenfield; Essential Books, 1994
- *Surgery Electives: What to Know Before the Doctor Operates,* by John
  McCabe; Carmania Books, 1994

- *Wrongful Death: A Medical Tragedy*, by Sandra M. Gilbert; W.W. Norton & Company, 1995

The following are resource organizations that deal with consumer protection, consumer awareness and/or patient's rights. Many of them (unless they are run by the government) are nonprofit and would welcome any donation (check or money order) you can send them. Many (including the government-run organizations) require that when you write them for information you send them a self-addressed, stamped envelope so they do not have to spend their funds on postage.

The Center for Medical Consumers is a health education organization and operates a library in New York City that publishes a monthly newsletter called *Health Facts* that is available for $21 a year.

The Center for Medical Consumers
237 Thompson Street, New York, New York 10012-1090; Phone (212) 674-7105

Citizens for Health works to protect consumers' rights to maintain access to a wide range of healthcare products and services relating to wellness and preventive healthcare. Citizens for Health publishes a newsletter ($25 a year)

Citizens for Health
P.O. Box 1195, Tacoma, Washington 98401; Phone (206) 922-2457 or toll-free (800) 357-2211

The US Government Consumer Information Center distributes a *Consumer's Resource Handbook*. The book tells consumers how to complain to get results. It lists the federal agencies that are responsible for resolving particular consumer problems and tells where help is available in state and local governments and private organizations. Single copies are free and may be obtained by writing to

Consumer Information Center
Handbook, Pueblo, Colorado 81009

Consumer Product Safety Commission
5401 Westbard Avenue, Bethesda, Maryland 20892; Product Safety Line: phone toll-free (800) 638-2772; In Maryland phone toll-free (800) 492-8104

Families USA
1334 G Street, NW, Washington, DC 20005; Phone (202) 737-6340

The Food and Drug Administration has jurisdiction over the content and labeling of foods, drugs and medical devices. The FDA can take law enforcement action to seize and prohibit the sale of products that are falsely labeled. The FDA is a government entity and often bows to the pressure of well-financed lobbyists who represent companies whose interests are in the process of making money — as opposed to protecting the general public.

Food and Drug Administration
Consumer Affairs and Information; 5600 Fishers Lane, HFC–110, Rockville, Maryland 20857; Phone (301) 443-1544; FDA Center for Drugs (301) 594-1012

The Federal Trade Commission has jurisdiction over the advertising and marketing of foods, non-prescription drugs, medical devices and healthcare services. The FTC can seek federal court injunctions to halt fraudulent claims and obtain redress for injured consumers.

The Federal Trade Commission
Correspondence Branch; 6th Street and Pennsylvania Avenue, NW, Washington, DC 20580; Phone (202) 326-2180

Medical Device Reporting Program
Phone (301) 881-0256 or toll-free (800) 638-6725

The National Center for Patients Rights is a non-profit consumer and victim of malpractice advocacy group. They can answer questions about medical misconduct, negligence and malpractice.

National Center for Patients Rights
666 Broadway, Suite 410, New York, New York 10012; Phone (212) 979-6670

National Council on Patient Information and Education
666 — 11th Street, NW, Suite 810, Washington, DC 20001; Phone (202) 347-6711

National Consumers League
815 – 15th Street NW, Washington, DC 20005; Phone (202) 835-3323

National Fraud Information Center Hotline
Phone (800) 876-7060

National Headquarters – Council of Better Business Bureaus, Inc.
4200 Wilson Boulevard, Arlington, Virginia 22203; Phone (703) 276-0100

National Women's Health Network
1325 – G Street, NW, Lower Level, Washington, DC 20005; Phone (202) 347-1140

The People's Medical Society is a nonprofit consumer education organization dedicated to the principles of better, more responsive and less expensive medical care. They work to put previously unavailable medical information into the hands of consumers so consumers can make informed decisions about their own healthcare. The Society keeps records of bad doctors and inadequate health treatment. The Society can provide you with information on how to get copies of your medical records from uncooperative doctors. The Society's books are some of the best ever written about medical rights. Subscription to their newsletter for consumers is included in their yearly $20 membership fee.

Books published by the People's Medical Society:
- *Getting the Most for Your Medical Dollar*
- *Good Operations/Bad Operations*
- *How to Evaluate and Select a Nursing Home*
- *Medicine on Trial*
- *150 Ways to Be a Savvy Medical Consumer*
- *Take This Book to the Gynecologist with You*
- *Take This Book to the Hospital with You*
- *Take This Book to the Obstetrician with You*
- *Your Medical Rights*

If you have any problem locating any of these books at your local library or bookstore, call the People's Medical Society directly.

People's Medical Society
462 Walnut Street, Allentown, Pennsylvania 18102; Phone (215) 770-1670

Public Citizen, an investigative watchdog group, was founded in 1971 by consumer advocate Ralph Nader and has 140,000 members. The group fights for a more open and democratic government, safer consumer products, quality healthcare and a clean environment. The group includes five divisions including a Health Research Group, which is the country's leading consumer awareness group focused on healthcare issues. HRG has long been active in efforts to reform the nation's healthcare system and to improve the quality of medical care. A donation of $35 or more includes a subscription to their monthly *Health Letter*.

Public Citizen Health Research Group has compiled a list called "*10,289 Questionable Doctors.*" It contains some of the names and locations of doctors who have been disciplined by their state medical boards or the federal government. The complete list is available for $200, or a list of doctors in one state is available for $15 plus $2 shipping.

Public Citizen Health Research Group
2000 P Street, Washington, DC 20036; Phone (202) 833-3000

Safe Medicine for Consumers is an advocacy group for patient's rights and for survivors and family members of victims of medical negligence. Although SMC concentrates its efforts in the state of California and on the Medical Board of California, the group will send information to people outside of California to help establish chapters in other states. On request, SMC will supply information on how to successfully file complaints with state medical boards and other agencies.

SMC follows and participates in pending legislation that is in the interest of consumers' medical rights, safety and care. It also works to protect existing public policy issues that promote quality healthcare. SMC helps to educate the public by sending out press releases to the media when there is medical patient legislation that the public should be made aware of. As a way to help expose malpractice, the group regularly connects journalists and news shows with victims of malpractice. The group encourages consumers to get involved with changing the government of the medical industry and to pressure government agencies to react faster and more responsibly to consumer demands for protection from substandard medical care.

Safe Medicine for Consumers
P.O. Box 878, San Andreas, California 95249; Phone (209) 754-4408 or fax (209) 736-2402

The Society of Patient Representatives is associated with the American Hospital Association and advises hospitals on how to set up patient relations programs. Not all hospitals participate.

National Society of Patient Representatives and Consumer
   Affairs of the American Hospital Association
840 North Lake Shore Drive, Chicago, Illinois 60611; Phone (312) 280-6424

• PRESCRIPTION DRUGS

Books:
- *The Complete Drug Reference*; Consumer Reports Books, 1993
- *The Essential Guide to Prescription Drugs*, by James Long; HarperCollins, 1994
- *Worst Pills, Best Pills*; published by Public Citizen's Health Research Group (202) 833-3000

Medications vary in strength. Everyone metabolizes drugs at different rates. Body weight along with age and kidney, liver, heart and lung function, play a part in how a person metabolizes and reacts to a particular drug. The temperature of a room, air conditioning, heating blankets and water beds may cause some drugs to be metabolized differently than intended. Many medications that are believed to be safe for adults can be lethal when given to infants and elderly patients because these groups respond to medications differently and experience more side effects than other patients not in these groups. Part of this is because older people take more drugs than younger people and have more drug residue flowing around in their systems, and when two incompatible drugs match up with each other in the system, there can be an adverse reaction.

Over-the-counter drugs such as Tylenol, Anacin-3, Panadol, and other medications that contain acetaminophen are useful in treating certain ailments, but they can also damage kidneys and lead to kidney failure if taken daily over a long period of time (according to a researchers at Johns Hopkins University). Acetaminophen can cause liver damage and death if taken in too high doses, especially by children.

Taking two over-the-counter medications at the same time that contain the same ingredient can also lead to overdose. When in doubt, ask your pharmacist.

Do not assume that the medication a doctor prescribes has no side effects simply because the doctor did not mention any. Doctors often do not know about all of the side effects, and many lack knowledge about significant risks that exist when patients combine drugs. Much, if not all, of what the doctor knows about a drug is what he learned from the pharmaceutical salesperson or another person who works for the drug manufacturer. The drug company representatives who are in contact with the doctors are known as "detailers" because they explain the details to the doctor about how the drug works and how it is to be prescribed.

Whenever you are given a prescription, unless delaying the intake of the medication would interfere with your health, take time to learn what the drug's side effects are and what the drug is meant to do. Learn how long it works and if it interferes with any other medications that you are taking. Does it have any known long-term risks? Some states have laws that require pharmacists to counsel all patients who ask questions at the time a prescription is filled. Under federal law, pharmacists must offer information on new prescriptions to Medicaid patients.

Some states have laws that require pharmacists to counsel all patients who ask questions at the time a prescription is filled.

Information on drugs can be obtained through the manufacturers; however, do not rely solely on literature put out by them — try finding additional information on the drug at your local library or through the book *Worst Pills, Best Pills* published by Public Citizen's Health Research Group. Also, ask for a copy of the FDA-approval label. This should be available at the pharmacy.

Canadian Society for Clinical Pharmacology
33 Russell Street, Toronto, Ontario M5S 2S1; Phone (416) 595-6119

Consumer Pharmacist Newsletter (subscriptions $48 a year)
ELBA Medical Foundation, P.O. Box 1403, Melairie, Louisiana 70001; Phone (504) 833-3600

To report a doctor, pharmacist or other health professional who is abusing their Drug Enforcement Administration controlled substance (narcotics) license by selling drugs illegally or abusing drugs, contact a diversion investigator at the diversion unit of the nearest field office of the DEA. If you cannot locate the nearest DEA office, contact the national headquarters of the DEA in Washington, DC. The DEA might conduct an investigation into the doctor's handling of controlled substances, or the doctor may be called to present evidence at a DEA administrative hearing. At the hearing the doctor will need to explain his actions and show cause of why his certificate of registration to handle controlled substances should not be revoked.

Drug Enforcement Administration
US Department of Justice, 1405 – I Street, NW, Washington, DC 20005; Phone (202) 401-7834

Food and Drug Administration
Office of Consumer Affairs
Phone (301) 443-3170

The consumer awareness group Public Citizen publishes a book titled *Worst Pills Best Pills*. The book focuses on how to prevent unnecessary illness and risks including untimely death caused by mis-prescribed or over-prescribed medications. It includes easy-to-understand information about many drugs.

Public Citizen has obtained information from the DEA about doctors who have had restrictions placed on or have had their narcotics licenses revoked.

Public Citizen/*Worst Pills Best Pills II*
2000 P Street NW, Washington, DC 20036; Phone (202) 833-3000

The United States Pharmacopeia is an independent regulatory agency that sets standards for the purity and potency of drugs, vitamins and minerals. Compliance with the standards set by the USP is voluntary on the part of manufacturers of these products. Manufacturers whose products correspond to the standards set by the USP can label their product as such. The Food and Drug Administration can take action against the manufacturers of products that carry USP labels but that do not actually correspond to USP standards.

United States Pharmacopeia
Rockville, Maryland; Phone (301) 881-0666

• PROFESSIONAL TITLES

Allergist: Specialist who diagnoses and treats allergic conditions

Allopath: Practices conventional medicine. Allopathic doctors control the American hospital system.

Anesthesiologist: Doctor who administers anesthesia and monitors the patient's vital signs during an operation

A.R.: Assistant Resident

Ayurvedic Doctor: Practices Eastern Indian medical principles encompassing alternative treatments. Considers body type, mood, emotion, lifestyle habits and physical coloring. Includes diet modification; herbal tonics, inhalants and baths; exercise such as yoga; meditation; and changing surroundings to rid your atmosphere of toxic thoughts and substances.

BAc: Bachelor of Acupuncture

CA: Certified Acupuncturist

Cardiologist: Heart specialist

CC: Board Certified Craniopath

CCN: Certified Clinical Nutritionist

CCSP: Certified Chiropractic Sports Physician

Chiropractor: Has a limited license that allows him to do therapies that involve physical manipulation and adjustment of the spine and skeletal system. Treatments may also include massage, traction, hot and cold compresses and ultrasound. Chiropractors do not prescribe drugs and are often opposed to drugs and do not perform surgery. There are 14 accredited chiropractic schools in the US.

CHt: Certified Hypnotherapist

CMT: Certified Massage Therapist

CN: Certified Nutritionist

CNA: Certified Nurses Aid

CNM: Certified Nurse Midwife

CNS: Clinical Nurse Specialist

Cosmetic surgeon: Plastic surgeon who operates on people who want to change their appearance for vanity reasons and are willing to take the risks of surgery to obtain their goals

DAc or DiplAc: Diplomate in Acupuncture. Has passed the national certification exam

DC: Doctor of Chiropractic Medicine

DDS: Doctor of Dental Surgery

Dentist: Doctor who specializes in the care of teeth and gums

Dermatologist: Doctor who specializes in the care of the skin and diseases that affect the skin

DHANP: Diplomate of Homeopathic Academy of Naturopathic Physicians

DHom (Med): Diplomate of the Institute of Homeopathy

DiplAc: Diplomate of Acupuncture

Diplomate: When a doctor is certified by a board he then is a diplomate of that board

DPM: Podiatrist

DO: Doctor of Osteopathy or Osteopathic Physician: A doctor who, in addition to general medical training, has studied manipulative and therapeutic treatments of the musculoskeletal and spinal systems. Their therapies often concentrate on what they call the "neuro-muscular-skeletal system." They are fully licensed physicians who have served internships, passed equivalency exams, are able to prescribe drugs, perform surgery and have the same privileges and responsibilities as a medical doctor (MD). They learn different therapies and have a more holistic approach to treating ailments than allopathic doctors.

Osteopathy was started by Dr. A.T. Still who opened a school of osteopathy in the late 1800s in Kirksville, Missouri. Many people thought of him as a quack. There are currently sixteen osteopathic medical schools in the US. Though there have been massive changes and improvements in osteopathic medicine, many allopathic doctors still do not accept osteopathic therapies. Other allopathic doctors consult with osteopathic doctors on patient care. Most hospitals in America are controlled by allopathic doctors and do not give admitting privileges to osteopathic doctors.

DOM: Doctor of Oriental Medicine: Some state certification boards use this title

DSc: Doctor of Science

EMS: Emergency Medicine Specialist

Endocrinologist: Doctor who specializes in treating disorders and diseases of the endocrine system — the gonads, the adrenal, pituitary and thyroid glands and the pancreas

ENT: Otorhinolaryngologist: Doctor who specializes in treating illnesses and diseases that affect the ears, nose and throat

FACS: Fellow of the American College of Surgeons

FICS: Fellow of the International Craniopath Society

Gastroenterologist: Specialist who treats disorders of the gastrointestinal tract (stomach and intestines)

General Practitioner: Nonspecialist doctor who usually treats general health problems. They often refer their patients to specialists when specific attention is needed. The cost controlling measures implemented by managed care and HMOs that have become dominant in the 1980s and 1990s has placed more influence on giving patients greater access to less expensive general practitioners and less access to more expensive specialist doctors.

GP: see "General Practitioner"

Gynecologist: Specialist doctor who examines and treats disorders of the female reproductive system. They also care for pregnant women.

Hematologist: Doctor who specializes in the blood and the system through which it flows

HMD: Homeopathic Medical Doctor.

Immunologist: Doctor who specializes in treating disorders of the immune system

Intern: Someone who has graduated from medical school and is spending a year of internship in a hospital, clinic, or ambulatory center to gain experience and to learn about taking responsibility for the care of a patient in the role of a physician by interacting and working with doctors in the treatment of patients. The internship year is now called the PGY-1 year. It is organized and sponsored by a single specialty department. Almost all physicians continue their training to complete a residency program to become specialists

Internist: Doctor who specializes in diagnosing and treating diseases

LAc or LicAc: Licensed Acupuncturist. Licensed by the state and has met requirements for national certification

LCSW: Licensed Clinical Social Worker

LD: Licensed Dietitian

LMT: Licensed Massage Therapist

LPN: Licensed Practical Nurse — usually has had less education than an RN (Registered Nurse). Has taken a state license exam.

MAR: Medical admitting resident. A third year resident who is in charge of approving and assigning patients who are admitted into the hospital

MAc: Master of Acupuncture

MD: Allopathic Medical Doctor — has completed a full course of medical training . They often relay on treatments that include chemical drugs and surgery to treat many health conditions. There are 126 allopathic medical schools in the US. Allopathic doctors rule the American hospital system. See "DO" above.

ME: Medical examiner. These are the pros who sign death certificates and conduct autopsies.

Midwife: A nurse-midwife is a specialist nurse who works assisting women during childbirth and may also provide prenatal and postpartum care. Nurse-midwives take state licensing exams and may be a member of a midwife organization. Like all other medical specialists, nurse-midwives can and should remain current in their field by taking continuing education classes.

MPH: Master of Public Health

MT: Massage Therapist

Naturopath: May practice a combination of holistic alternative approaches such as Chinese medicine, Indian and Native American as well as Greek with therapies such as massage, nutrition, herbal medicine, homeopathy, water therapy and even minor surgery to treat the body with an influence on prevention through lifestyle changes and providing the body with what it needs to heal itself. The most popular school for naturopathy is Bastyr University in Seattle, Washington. That school offers a four-year program, bachelor's degrees in the natural health sciences and master's degree programs in nutrition, herbal, homeopathy, botanical medicine and acupuncture. Midwifery, women's healthcare, pediatrics and sports medicine are also taught. Other schools where naturopathic medicine is taught include the Canadian College of Naturopathic in Ontario, the National College of Naturopathic Medicine in Portland and the Southwest College of Naturopathic Medicine in Scottsdale.

ND: Doctor of Naturopathy. See "Naturopath" above.

Nephrologist: Doctor who specializes in kidney problems

Neurologist: Doctor who specializes in diseases of the nervous system

Neurosurgeon: Doctor who specializes in the surgical treatment of brain, nerve, and spinal cord

Nurse's aide: Self-explanatory. Usually has taken a nurse training course at a local or other type of college.

Nurse manager: Head nurse. A head nurse is an RN and is the one who supervises the other nurses who work in a hospital unit.

Nurse Midwife: See "Midwife" above.

Nurse practitioner: Nurse who has received additional medical education and works in the diagnosis and treatment of health problems on a limited level. They also prescribe medications. Some small towns that do not have a local doctor sometimes have a nurse practitioner who they rely on for their care and who is usually supervised by a doctor in a nearby town. There is a strong demand for nurse practitioners because they can perform some of the same tasks as doctors but at a lower cost. Salaries for nurse practitioners range from $45,000 to $65,000 a year.

Nutritionist: Reviews a person's diet, helps them incorporate nutrition into their meals and teaches healthy eating habits.

OB/GYN: Obstetrician Gynecologist

Obstetrician: Specialist who deals with pregnancy and childbirth. On average, obstetricians are sued more than any other kind of doctor.

Ombudsman: Patient representative in the hospital or nursing home area who handles the complaints and other matters related to patient satisfaction

OMD: Oriental Medicine Doctor: Has received an educational degree. Diagnosis from an Oriental Medical Doctor may be the result of conclusions made after examining the eyes, tongue, hair, hearing, voice, body odor and factoring in of diet, age, weight, body shape, posture and capabilities of movement. The harmony of the person is considered and disbalances are treated. Treatments may include acupuncture, massage or other manipulation, exercises, diet changes and various herbal and substance remedies (in other words, traditional Chinese medicine).

Oncologist: A doctor who specializes in the diagnoses and treatment of cancer

Ophthalmologist: Specialist who treats diseases and injuries of the eyes

Optometrist: One who examines the eyes and prescribes corrective lenses such as eye glasses and contact lenses

Orthodontist: Doctor who deals with irregularities of the teeth

Orthomolecular Physician: Usually a medical doctor. Therapies include diet changes, and concentrations on vitamins, minerals, amino acids and other dietary supplements.

Orthopedist: Doctor who specializes in the musculoskeletal system (bone fractures, diseases and malformations)

Osteopathic Physician: see "DO"

Otorhinolaryngologist: Doctor who specializes in treating disorders of the ear, nose and throat (ENT)

PA: Physician's Assistant: Works under a physician's supervision. Has less training than physicians, but some small-town clinics are run by PAs; cannot perform any kind of complicated medical procedure

P-A: Physician-anesthesiologist

Pathologist: Doctor who interprets and diagnoses diseases in tissues

PCT: Patient care technician or nurse extender

Pediatrician: Specialist who cares for babies and young children

Pediatric orthopedist: A children's bone doctor

PhD: Doctor of Philosophy

Physical therapist: A person who helps people rehabilitate from surgery or injury to alleviate pain and restore health to its optimal level. They typically hold at least a bachelor's degree and complete a state licensing exam. They most often work in hospitals, nursing homes, rehabilitation centers, doctors' offices and private clinics. Some physical therapists also visit patients who are recovering at home and others have their own private practice.

Plastic surgeon: Doctor who specializes in treating body parts that have been damaged or that are malformed because of a disease or birth defect; many of today's plastic surgeons sell themselves as "cosmetic surgeons" and occupy themselves with performing unnecessary surgery on people who want to change their appearance for vanity reasons and are willing to take the risks of surgery to obtain their goals

PNC: Psychiatric Nurse Clinician

Podiatrist: Foot doctor, or a doctor of podiatric medicine. Their training is in a two- or three-year course of classes and not an intense training program such as what an MD would be exposed to. Podiatrists treat such ailments as ingrown toenails, bunions and fallen arches. A podiatrist may sometimes perform minor foot or ankle surgery in his office. An MD who treats foot and ankle problems and performs surgery on them is an orthopedic surgeon that specializes in the feet as opposed to an orthopedic surgeon who specializes in the bones and joints on other areas of the body.

Proctologist: Specializes in the diagnosis and treatment of problems with the anus, colon and rectum

Prosthodontist: Specialist in prosthetic dentistry

Psychiatrist: An MD who specializes in the care and prevention of mental illness and emotional and behavior disorders: Has completed post-medical training, has served a residency and is able to prescribe medication; tends to treat more severe mental illness disorders than those treated by psychologists

Psychologist: Doctor who studies the science of mind and behavior: Has a PhD in clinical psychology and tends to work with people who are high functioning and who are usually able to carry on normal life activities but suffer from depression or other less severe disorders than those treated by psychiatrists

Pulmonologist: Lung doctor

RAc: Registered Acupuncturist

Radiologist: Doctor who specializes in the interpretation of x-rays and other diagnostic body images to help diagnose health problems. They also may be involved with radiation treatment of cancer patients and certain testing procedures that use technology that produces diagnostic images such as those created by ultrasound, CAT scans, MRI machines, etc.

RD: Registered Dietitian: A person who has met the educational criteria of the Commission on Dietetic Registration, the credentialing agency for The American Dietetic Association that is located in Chicago, Illinois. Dietitians hold a Bachelor of Science degree in nutrition, have served an internship and are required to complete continuing education courses. Dietitians are employed by hospitals and are also used by schools, nursing homes, food companies, restaurant chains and other companies that are involved in food preparation.

Residency: Next step up from an internship: Period of training in a specific medical specialty; this occurs after graduation from medical school and the length varies from three to seven years, depending on the specialty. Surgical residents have to perform a certain number of specific procedures to become certified in a specialty. To fulfill this requirement they must have patients to operate on; thus they can be too quick to perform operations or simply perform unnecessary operations as they seek to meet the quota requirements of their specialty

Rheumatologist: Specialist who deals with inflammations of the muscles and joints such as arthritis

RN: Registered Nurse: has gone on to receive two or more additional years of education beyond that of a Licensed Practical Nurse to obtain a bachelor's degree in nursing. Registered nurses must pass a state licensing exam

RN,C: Registered Nurse, Certified: Includes certified Registered Nurses who practice in the areas of Medical-Surgical Nurse, Gerontological Nurse, Psychiatric and Mental Health Nurse, Pediatric Nurse, Perinatal Nurse, Community Health Nurse, School Nurse, General Nursing Practice, College Health Nurse, Nursing Continuing Education/Staff Development, Home Health Nurse, and Cardiac Rehabilitation Nurse

RN,CS: Registered Nurse, Certified Specialist: Includes certified Registered Nurses who practice in the areas of Clinical Specialist in Gerontological Nursing, Clinical Specialist in Medical-Surgical Nursing, Clinical Specialist in Community Health Nursing, Clinical

Specialist in Adult Psychiatric and Mental Health Nursing, Clinical
Specialist in Child and Adolescent Psychiatric and Mental Health
Nursing, Gerontological Nurse Practitioner, Pediatric Nurse
Practitioner, Adult Nurse Practitioner, Family Nurse Practitioner,
School Nurse Practitioner

RN,CNA: Registered Nurse, Certified in Nursing Administration

RN,CNAA: Registered Nurse, Certified in Nursing Administration,
Advanced

RPP: Registered Polarity Practitioner

Scrub nurse: Works along with a surgeon as he performs an operation

Social worker: Social workers are on staff at most hospitals. They have
gone through supervised practical training and hold a masters degree
in social work. They help patients and the patient's family with
emotional support and give therapeutic assistance. They can intervene
when a patient is experiencing a problem coping with a medical
condition. They can act as patient advocates and can refer patients to
community or hospital services that may benefit the patient. Much of
their work entails nurturing the independence of the patient. A
patient's nurse or doctor can refer the patient to a social worker.

Societies: Organizations of physicians or medical professionals (nurses,
therapists, etc.) involved in a given field of practice. They represent the
interests of the medical professionals. In most specialty societies, it is
not necessary to be board certified to be eligible for membership

Thoracic surgeon: Operates on those organs within the area between the
neck and the abdomen

Urologist: A specialist whose focus is on the urinary tract including the
bladder and prostate

• PUBLICATIONS

Books of interest to medical consumers:
- *Doctors from Hell*, by Fred Rosen; Windsor Publishing, 1993
- *Ethics on Call: A Medical Ethicist Shows How to Take Charge of Life &
Death Choices in Today's Healthcare System*, by Nancy Dubler &
David Nimmons; Vantage Books, 1993
- *Good Operations, Bad Operations*, by Charles B. Inlander; Viking, 1993
- *The Great American Medicine Show: Being an Illustrated History of
Hucksters, Healers, Health Evangelists, and Heroes from Plymouth Rock
to the Present*, by David Armstrong and Elizabeth Metzger Armstrong;
Prentice Hall/ Simon and Schuster, 1991
- *The Great White Lie; Dishonesty, Waste, & Incompetence in the Medical
Community*, by Walt Bogdanich; Touchstone Books, 1992
- *How to Choose a Good Doctor*, by G.D. Lemaitre; Andover Publishing
Group, 1979
- *Human Rights & Healthcare Law*, by Eugene I. Pavalon; Books on
Demand, 1980
- *Making Medical Decisions*, by Thomas and Celia Scully; Simon &
Schuster, 1987
- *Male Practice: How Doctors Manipulate Women*, by Robert S.
Mendelsohn, MD; Contemporary Books, 1981
- *Medical Malpractice on Trial*, by Paul C. Weiler; Harvard University
Press, 1991
- *Medical Treason*, by Joyce E, Strom-Paikin, RN; Berkeley Publishing
Group, 1992
- *Medicine, Money and Morals: Physicians' Conflicts of Interest*, by
Marc A. Rodwin; Oxford University Press, 1993

- *Men Who Control Women's Health: The Miseducation of Obstetrician-Gynecologists*, by Diane Scully; Teachers College Press, 1994
- *No More Hysterectomies*, by Vickie G. Hufnagel & Susan K. Golant; Plume, 1989
- *Patient or Pretender: The Strange World of Factitious Disorders*, by Marc D. Feldman, Charles V. Ford & Toni Reinhold; John Wiley & Sons, 1993
- *Racketeering in Medicine: The Suppression of Alternatives*, by James P. Carter, M.D.; Hampton Roads Publishing, 1993
- *Smart Patient, Good Medicine: Working With Your Doctor to Get the Best Medical Care*, by Richard L. Sribnick, MD, and Wayne B. Sribnick, MD; Walker Publishing, 1994
- *The Strange Case of Dr. Kappler: The Doctor Who Became a Killer*, by Keith Russell Ablow, The Free Press/Macmillon, 1994
- *Surgery Electives: What to Know Before the Doctor Operates*, by John McCabe; Carmania Books, 1994
- *Talk Back to Your Doctor: How to Demand and Recognize High Quality Healthcare*, by Arthur Levin; Doubleday, 1975
- *The Toadstool Millionaires: A Social History of Patent Medicines in America Before Federal Regulation*, by James Harvey Young; Princeton University Press, 1961
- *When to Say No to Surgery: How to Evaluate the Most Often Performed Operations*, by Robert G. Schneider; Prentice Hall, 1982
- *Wrongful Death: A Medical Tragedy*, by Sandra M. Gilbert; W.W. Norton & Company, 1995
- *You Must Be Dreaming*, by Barbara Noel and Kathryn Watterson; Simon & Schuster, 1992
- *Your Medical Rights: How to Become an Empowered Consumer*, by Charles B. Inlander & Eugene I. Pavalon; People's Medical Society, 1994

The Reader's Guide to Periodical Literature is available in book or computer form in many libraries and lists articles that were written about various subjects and can be very helpful when researching any subject.

The Encyclopedia of Associations is also available in many libraries, lists thousands of organizations and is helpful when trying to find names and addresses of various groups.

Mosey Medical Encyclopedia can be helpful in familiarizing a person with medical terminology.

Boston Women's Health Book Collective
P.O. Box 192, West Somerville, Massachusetts 02144; Phone (617) 625-0271

The Center for the Study of Services is a nonprofit organization that publishes a Hospital Guide that lists the federal mortality rates by hospital and the mortality rates of the most common operations being done. The *Hospital Guide* is available for $12 including postage and handling. Payment can be made by way of check, money order or credit card.

Center for the Study of Services
Hospital Guide, 806 – 15th Street, NW, Suite 925, Washington, DC 20005; Phone (202) 347-7283

Medical Abstracts Newsletter uses easy-to-understand wording to explain various research findings reported in medical journals used by the professionals. All articles in *Medical Abstracts Newsletter* cite the original source of information, including the author's name, journal, volume, page, and issue date so you or your doctor can locate the full report and evaluate its contents. A one-year subscription to the newsletter costs $21. An additional year costs $18. A $4 additional charge should be added per year of subscription for people living outside of the United States.

Medical Abstracts Newsletter
Box 2170, Teaneck, New Jersey 07666; Phone (201) 836-7740

• RARE DISORDERS

Lethbridge Society for Rare Disorders/Canada
515 7th Street South, #100B, Lethbridge, Alberta T15 2G8 Canada; Phone (403) 329-0665

National Organization for Rare Disorders
100 Route 37, P.O. Box 8923, New Fairfield, Connecticut 06812-1783; Phone (203) 746-6518 or toll-free (800) 999-NORD

• RECORDS

Book:
* *The Patients' Guide to Medical Tests*, by Cathey Pinckney; Facts on File Publications, 1986

Most states have laws that provide patients access to their medical records. If any doctor, medical facility or insurance company refuses to give you a copy of your medical records, contact one of the patients' rights groups listed under the Patients' and Consumers' Rights heading of this book and/or contact a malpractice lawyer.

To find out if your state laws address patient access to health information and what those laws are, contact your State Department of Health. For further information send a self-addressed, stamped envelope to

American Health Information Management Association
Professional Practice Division, 919 North Michigan Avenue, Chicago, Illinois 60611-1683; Phone (312) 787-2672, toll-free (800) 621-6828

To find out if the Medical Information Bureau has a medical history file on you that is used by insurance companies and other organizations and to order a copy of this file for your own records, write or call the offices located in Boston. Give them a few variations of your name. For instance, a person named Joseph David Doe may have a file under the name of Joe Doe, Joey D. Doe or Joseph Doe.

Medical Information Bureau (MIB)
P.O. Box 105, Essex Station, Boston, Massachusetts 02112; Phone (617) 426-3660

The People's Medical Society publishes a book titled *Your Medical Rights: How to Become an Empowered Consumer*. The authors are Charles B. Inlander, President of the People's Medical Society, and Eugene I. Pavalon, past President of the Association of Trial Lawyers of America. The book gives detailed information on the rights of a patient and what rights patients have to their medical records, what information doctors and hospitals must disclose before treating a patient, how to avoid unnecessary surgery, and explanations of medical charges and how to have inaccuracies in medical bills corrected.

People's Medical Society
462 Walnut Street, Allentown, Pennsylvania 18102; Phone (215) 770-1670

A book titled *Medical Records: Getting Yours* gives step-by-step instructions on how to get your medical records from private and government medical facilities and doctors, information on why you should obtain your medical records, legal advice on how to demand your medical records, and information on federal and state laws that dictate what medical information you can and cannot gain access to. There is also a glossary of abbreviations that are most commonly used in medical records. As the book states, "Put simply, this book tells you why you should have a copy of your medical records, how to get it, and how to understand what is in it." The book costs $10 plus $2 for shipping from

Public Citizen Publications
2000 P Street NW, Suite 600, Washington, DC 20036; Phone (202) 833-3000

• RELATIONSHIP IMBALANCE

Book:
• *How to Break Your Addiction to a Person: When and Why Love Doesn't Work and What to Do about It*, MFJ Books, 1982

Some people have personality flaws of insecurity that cause them to cling too closely to the people around them. They are often passive and dependent, lack the ability to carry on healthy relationships, depend too much on the people around them or get caught up in taking care of other people and seek to accommodate the needs or wants of others beyond reason and at risk to the quality of their own life.

Co-Dependents Anonymous is a network of support groups set up to help overly dependent people recognize and learn to deal with these traits. To find out about a meeting place near you or to find out how to organize a CODA group, contact

Co-Dependents Anonymous (CODA)
P.O. Box 6292, Phoenix, Arizona 85261; Phone (602) 277-7991
or
P.O. Box 33577, Phoenix, Arizona 85067-3577; Phone (602) 944-0141

• SECOND OPINIONS

Second Surgical Opinion Program
Department of Health and Human Services
330 Independence Avenue, SW, Washington, DC 20201; Phone (202) 690-8056, toll-free (800) 638-6833 or in Maryland call (800) 492-6603

• SEXUAL ISSUES

American Association of Sex Educators, Counselors, and Therapists
435 North Michigan Avenue, Suite 1717, Chicago, Illinois 60611; Phone (312) 644-0828

• SKIN

The skin is the body's largest organ and is made up of two layers — the outer layer called the "epidermis" and the inner layer called the "dermis." Within the skin there is a network of nerves, blood vessels, hair follicles, eccrine sweat glands, apocrine sweat glands and sebaceous glands. All of these work to nourish the skin, protect the skin, let the skin breath and keep the skin moist. The skin and the underlying fat provide insulation and protect the interior tissues.

Damage to the skin from the sun is referred to as "photoaging" or "extrinsic aging." Sun builds up an outer layer of dry skin and can make the skin dull, sallow, and mottled as the connective tissues within the skin are damaged. When the skin tans, the skin cells are actually building up a dark pigment called "melanin," a chemical that is thought to protect the skin from the sun.

The sun gives off ultraviolet (UV) radiation, which comes in two wave lengths — UVA and UVB, and it is this that causes skin damage. UVA speeds up skin aging by causing changes in the skin's elastin and collagen, the proteins in the skin's connective tissue that hold the skin together.

Ultraviolet rays from the sun are also a major contributing factor to skin cancer, which is one of the most common forms of cancer. With more than 700,000 new cases each year, more new cases of skin cancer are diagnosed every year than all other types of cancer combined.

In a study conducted at Boston University and published in the *British Journal Nature*, researchers reported evidence that melanin is produced when the body starts to repair DNA damage caused by overexposure to the sun. It is the damaged DNA that leads to skin cancer.

The most common types of skin cancer are basal cell and squamous cell carcinoma. These two types of skin cancer are believed to be related to cumulative exposure to the sun. A third and the most deadly type of skin cancer, malignant melanoma, can spread rapidly throughout the body. The chances of melanoma forming is believed to be associated with sunburns. People with light skin, a family history of skin cancer, or a number of moles have a greater risk of developing skin cancer. Regardless of skin color, all people are vulnerable to skin cancer, although among very dark-complected people the incidence is very low. For this population, squamous cell carcinoma — which can also be fatal — is the most common.

Today's suntans are tomorrow's wrinkles. To avoid wrinkles and premature aging of the skin, avoid getting sunburn and do not lie out in the sun — especially at midday. Use a sunscreen with an SPF of at least 15 that protects against both UVA and UVB ultraviolet sunlight. Wear a hat that has a rim, and other protective clothing during long periods in the sun. Because UV radiation can also damage the eyes, sunglasses that block UV rays should be worn during extended periods of time spent in the sun. Avoid tanning salons and sunlamps because they also give off UV rays and damage the skin.

> Consult with a dermatologist if you have any unusual blemishes on your skin, such as a mole or other marking that changes in size, depth or color. The sooner skin cancer is found the better the chance that it is caught before it has entered into the dermal layers of the skin where it can spread to lymph nodes in the region and on to the rest of the body.

Alcohol and drug use can contribute to premature aging of the skin. Alcoholic drinks can increase the probability of broken capillaries by causing the blood vessels to expand or dilate, giving the skin an unhealthy redness. People who drink a lot of alcoholic beverages can end up with leathery skin because the alcohol causes the skin to dehydrate. Drugs affect blood circulation, which can make the skin look old and cause acne and fluid retention. Cocaine can destroy the cartilage in the nose. Even the caffeine in sodas, coffee and tea can slow the blood circulation in the skin.

People who have smoked for any length of time have common wrinkles associated with smoking. This pattern of wrinkles that smoking creates is known as "smoker's face." The wrinkles are caused by squinting of the eyes and piercing of the lips. Smoke from cigarettes stains the skin. Nicotine causes the blood vessels in the skin to restrict, which then limits the amount of the oxygen-carrying blood supply that the skin needs to be healthy.

The skin reacts to pleasure and pain. It also reacts to illness and often reflects the health of the entire person. When a person does not eat healthy it can become evident by the condition of the skin. People who find out they are sick often first become aware of it when there is a change in their skin color or texture. When a major health problem exists, such as when a person has a diseased liver, this can also become evident by the appearance of the skin.

The skin is a breathing organ and benefits from exercise, fresh air and cleanliness. To maintain the health of your skin, limit alcohol consumption, do not smoke and stay away from junk food. Avoid skin cleansers and lotions that contain chemicals, synthetic dyes, artificial fragrances and petroleum products. Instead, use skin cleansers and lotions that contain plant extracts, natural oils and vitamins. Wear protective gloves when using detergents and other chemicals.

American Academy of Dermatology
930 North Meacham Road, Schaumburg, Illinois 60168-4014; Phone (708) 330-0230

American Board of Dermatology
Henry Ford Hospital, Detroit, Michigan 48202; Phone (313) 871-8739

American Osteopathic Board of Dermatology
25510 Plymouth Road, Redford, Michigan 48239; Phone (313) 937-1200

American Society for Dermatologic Surgery
930 North Meacham Road, Schaumburg, Illinois 60173; Phone (708) 330-0230 or 9830

National Psoriasis Foundation
6600 SW 92nd Avenue, Suite 300, Portland, Oregon 97223

National Rosacea Society
220 South Cook Street, Suite 201, Barrington, Illinois 60010; Phone (708) 382-8971

National Vitiligo Foundation
P.O. Box 6337, Tyler, Texas 75711; Phone (214) 534-2925

Scleroderma Research Foundation
P.O. Box 200, Columbus, New Jersey 08022; Phone (609) 723-7400 or toll-free (800) 637-4005

• SMELL AND TASTE

Book:
* *The Scent of Eros: Mysteries of Odor in Human Sexuality*, by James Vaughn Kohl and Robert T. Francoeur; Continuum Publishing, 1995

Chemical Senses Clinic at University of California at Irvine
Phone (714) 856-5011

Monell Chemical Sense Center
Philadelphia, Pennsylvania; Phone (215) 898-6666

Smell and Taste Treatment and Research Foundation
845 North Michigan Avenue, Suite 930 West, Chicago, Illinois; Phone (312) 938-1047

• SMOKING CESSATION

Cigarettes stain the teeth; contribute to dental problems; cause bad breath; affect the senses of smell and taste; irritate the eyes;

cause facial wrinkles; impair the immune system; increase the chances of and magnify sicknesses of the sinuses and throat; and change the voice resonance.

Cigarette smoking reduces the blood flow into the small blood vessels that deliver nutrients and oxygen to the bones, and this alters the ongoing process of bone restoration and calcium storage. It also hinders wound healing and this is why it is important to avoid smoking when surgery is planned. The long-term effects of this bone blood supply deficiency can be loss of bone density and eventually osteoporosis, a disease that leads to bone fractures, bone deformities, decreased height and humped back.

American Cancer Society
1599 Clifton Road, NE, Atlanta, Georgia 30329; Phone (800) ACS-2345

American Heart Association
7320 Greenville Avenue, Dallas, Texas 75231; Phone (214) 750-5300

American Lung Association
1740 Broadway, New York, New York 10019-4374; Phone (212) 315-8700

Centers for Disease Control & Prevention
  Office of Smoking and Health
5600 Fishers Lane, Rockville, Maryland 20857; Phone (301) 443-5287

• STATE MEDICAL BOARDS

Association of State and Territorial Health Officials
415 Second Street, NE, Washington, DC 20002; Phone (202) 546-5400

Federation of State Medical Boards of the United States
6000 Western Place, Suite 707, Fort Worth, Texas 76107-4618; Phone (817) 735-8445

Listed below are the state medical boards that license, monitor and discipline doctors in each state. To find out whether a doctor is licensed to practice in your state, contact your state's board. Additionally there are state and county boards that license and supervise dentists, nurses, pharmacies, hospitals and other medical professionals and facilities. Phone numbers of these other boards are available through your state medical board or state capital information operator.

To file a grievance against a medical professional, hospital, or medical center, get in contact with the proper authorities and find out what specific steps to follow. You may need to fill out forms that are supplied by the authority. (To make sure you follow the correct and most effective procedure for filing a complaint, contact the People's Medical Society or the Public Citizen's Health Research Group as they are listed in the Research Resource section of this book under the heading of

Patients' and Consumers' Rights. You may also want to obtain legal advice from an attorney who specializes in malpractice law before you sign your name to any letters or forms that question someone's professional skill, especially if there is the possibility of a malpractice lawsuit.)

If you are seeking to notify authorities of illegal action taken by a medical professional, you may also want to contact your county or state attorney general, who are the chief law enforcement officers in the county and state.

To successfully file a complaint that results in actions taken against a doctor, you will usually need to let the authorities review your medical records.

It may be helpful to contact your elected representatives (senator, congressperson, and state representative) and find out if they are involved with any legislation that will strengthen medical consumers' rights. They might be interested in your story.

It is wise to keep records and a journal of all actions you take in the process of registering a complaint. Keep copies of all forms you sign, records of what office you called, who you spoke with and what the main points of the conversations were along with dates and times.

Alabama State Board of Medical Examiners
848 Washington Avenue, 36104, Montgomery, Alabama 36101-0946; Phone (205) 242-4116; Fax (205) 242-4155

Alaska State Medical Board
3601 C Street, Suite 722, Anchorage, Alaska 99503; Phone (907) 561-2878; Fax (907) 562-5781

Alaska Department of Commerce & Economic Development Division of Occupational Licensing
State Office Building, 9th Floor, 333 Willoughby, Juneau, Alaska 99801; Phone (907) 465-2541; Fax (907) 465-2974

Arizona State Board of Medical Examiners
1651 East Morten Avenue, Suite 210, Phoenix, Arizona 85020; Phone (602) 255-3751; Fax (602) 255-1848

Arizona Board of Osteopathic Examiners in Medicine &Surgery
1830 West Colter, Suite 104, Phoenix, Arizona 85015; Phone (602) 255-1747; Fax (602) 255-1756

Arkansas State Medical Board
2100 Riverfront Drive, Suite 200, Little Rock, Arkansas 72202; Phone (501) 324-9410; Fax (501) 324-9413

California State Medical Board
1426 Howe Avenue, Suite 54, Sacramento, California 95825; Phone (916) 263-2388 or 263-2382; Fax (916) 263-2387

California, Osteopathic Medical Board of
444 North Third Street, Suite A-200, Sacramento, California 95814; Phone (916) 322-4306; Fax (916) 327-6119

Colorado State Board of Medical Examiners
1560 Broadway, Suite 1300, Denver, Colorado 80202-5140; Phone (303) 894-7690; Fax (303) 894-7692

Connecticut Division of Medical Quality Assurance
Connecticut Department of Public Health & Addiction Services, Division of Medical Quality Assurance, 150 Washington Street, Hartford, Connecticut 06106; Phone (203) 566-7398; Fax (203) 566-6606

Delaware Board of Medical Practice
Margaret O'Neil Building, 2nd Floor, Federal & Court Streets, Dover, Delaware 19903; Phone (302) 739-4522; Fax (302) 739-2711

District of Columbia Board of Medicine
605 G Street, NW, Room 202, Lower Level, 20001, Washington, DC 20013-7200; Phone (202) 727-9794; Fax (202) 727-4087

District of Columbia Department of Consumer & Regulatory Affairs
614 H Street, NW, Suite 104, Washington, DC 20001; Phone (202) 727-7823 or (202) 727-7102

Florida Board of Medicine
Northwood Centre, #60, 1940 North Monroe Street, Tallahassee, Florida 32399-0750; Phone (904) 488-0595; Fax (904) 487-9622

Florida Board of Osteopathic Medical Examiners
Northwood Centre, #60, Tallahassee, Florida 32399-0775; Phone (904) 922-6725; Fax (904) 922-3040

Georgia Composite State Board of Medical Examiners
166 Pryor Street, SW, Atlanta, Georgia 30303-3465; Phone (404) 656-3913; Fax (404) 656-9723

Guam Board of Medical Examiners
Department of Public Health & Social Services, Route 10, Mangilao, Agana, Guam 96910; Phone 011 (671) 734-7296; Fax 011 (671) 734-2066

Hawaii Board of Medical Examiners
Department of Commerce & Consumer Affairs, 1010 Richards Street, 96813, Honolulu, Hawaii 96801; Phone (808) 586-2704; Fax (808) 586-2689

Idaho State Board of Medicine
State House Mail
280 North 8th, Suite 202, Boise, Idaho 83720
Phone (208) 334-2822; Fax (208) 334-2801

Illinois Department of Professional Regulation
State of Illinois Center, 100 West Randolph Street, #9-300, Chicago, Illinois 60601; Phone (312) 814-4934; Fax (312) 814-1837
— also —
320 West Washington Street, Springfield, Illinois 62786; Phone (217) 524-2169; Medical Licensing Unit Fax (217) 782-7645

Indiana Consumer Protection
Health Professional Bureau
One American Square, Suite 1020, Indianapolis, Indiana 46282; Phone (317) 232-2386

Indiana Health Professions Service Bureau
402 West Washington Street, Room 041, Indianapolis, Indiana 46204; Phone (317) 232-2960; Fax (317) 233-4236

Iowa State Board of Medical Examiners
State Capitol Complex, Executive Hills West, 1209 East Court Avenue, Des Moines, Iowa 50319-0180; Phone (515) 281-5171; Fax (515) 242-5908

Kansas State Board of Healing Arts
235 SW Topeka Boulevard, Topeka, Kansas 66603; Phone (913) 296-7413; Fax (913) 296-0852

Kentucky Board of Medical Licensure
The Hurstbourne Office Park, 310 Whittington Parkway, Suite 1B, Louisville, Kentucky 40222; Phone (502) 429-8046; Fax (502) 429-9923

Louisiana State Board of Medical Examiners
830 Union Street, #100, New Orleans, Louisiana; Phone (504) 524--6763; Fax (504) 568-8893

Maine Board of Registration in Medicine
State House Station, #317, Two Bangor Street, Augusta, Maine 04333; Phone (207) 287-2480

Maine Board of Osteopathic Examination & Registration
State House Station, #142, Augusta, Maine 04333; Phone (207) 287-2480

Maryland Board of Physician Quality Assurance
4201 Patterson Avenue, 3rd Floor, Baltimore, Maryland 21215; Phone (410) 764-2478 or toll-free (800) 492-6836

Massachusetts Board of Registration in Medicine
Ten West Street, 3rd Floor, Boston, Massachusetts 02111; Phone (617) 727-3086; Fax (617) 451-9568

Michigan Board of Medicine
611 West Ottawa Street, 4th Floor, 48933, Lansing, Michigan 48909; Phone (517) 373-6873; Fax (517) 373-2179

Michigan Board of Osteopathic Medicine and Surgery
611 West Ottawa Street, 4th Floor 48933, Lansing, Michigan 48909; Phone (517) 373-6837; Fax (517) 373-2179

Minnesota Board of Medical Practice
2700 University Avenue West, Suite 106, St. Paul, Minnesota 55114-1080; Phone (612) 642-0538; Fax (612) 642-0393

Mississippi State Board of Medical Licensure
2688-D Insurance Center Drive, Jackson, Mississippi 39216; Phone (601) 354-6654; Fax (601) 987-4159

Missouri State Board of Registration for the Healing Arts
3605 Missouri Boulevard, Jefferson City, Missouri 65109; Phone (314) 751-0098; Fax (314) 751-3166

Montana Board of Medical Examiners
Arcade Building, 111 North Jackson, Helena, Montana 59620-0513; Phone (406) 444-4284/4276; Fax (406) 444-1667

Nebraska State Board of Examiners in Medicine and Surgery
301 Centennial Mall South, 68509, Lincoln, Nebraska 68509-5007; Phone (402) 471-2115; Fax (402) 471-0383

Nevada State Board of Medical Examiners
1105 Terminal Way, Suite 301, 89502, Reno, Nevada 89510; Phone (702) 688-2559; Fax (702) 688-2321

Nevada State Board of Osteopathic Medicine
2950 East Flamingo Road, Suite E-3, Las Vegas, Nevada 89121; Phone (702) 732-2147

New Hampshire Board of Registration in Medicine
Health & Welfare Building, 6 Hazen Drive, Concord, New Hampshire
03301; Phone (603) 271-4501

New Hampshire Licensing Board Office
2 Industrial Park Drive, Suite 8, Concord, New Hampshire 03301-8520;
Phone (603) 2711-1203

New Jersey State Board of Medical Examiners
140 East Front Street, 2nd Floor, Trenton, New Jersey 08608; Phone (609)
826-7100; Fax (609) 984-3930

New Mexico State Board of Medical Examiners
Leamy Building, Second Floor, 491 Old Santa Fe Trail, Santa Fe, New
Mexico 87501; Phone (505) 827-7317; Fax 505 827-7377

New Mexico Board of Osteopathic Medical Examiners
725 St. Michaels Drive, 87501, Santa Fe, New Mexico 87504; Phone (505)
827-7171; Fax (505) 827-7095

New York State Board of Medicine
Cultural Education Center, Room 3023, Empire State Plaza, Albany, New
York 12230; Phone (518) 474-3841; Fax (518) 473-0578

New York Board of Professional Medical Conduct
New York State Department of Health, Room 438, Corning Tower Building
Empire State Plaza, Albany, New York 12237-0614; Phone (518) 474-
8357; Fax (518) 474-4471

North Carolina Board of Medical Examiners
1203 Front Street, 27609, Raleigh, North Carolina 27611-6808; Phone
(919) 828-1212; Fax (919) 828-1295

North Dakota State Board of Medical Examiners
City Center Plaza, 418 East Broadway, Suite 12, Bismark, North Dakota
58501; Phone (701) 223-9485; Fax (701) 223-9756

Ohio State Medical Board
77 South High Street, 17th Floor, Columbus, Ohio 43266-0315; Phone (614)
466-3934

Oklahoma State Board of Medicine Licensure and Supervision
5104 North Francis, Suite C, Oklahoma City, Oklahoma 73154-0256; Phone
(405) 848-2189; Fax (405) 848-8240

Oklahoma Board of Osteopathic Examiners
4848 North Lincoln Boulevard, Oklahoma City, Oklahoma 73105-3321;
Phone (405) 528-8625; Fax (405) 528-6102

Oregon Board of Medical Examiners
620 Crown Plaza, 1500 SW First Avenue, Portland, Oregon 97201-5826;
Phone (503) 229-5770; Fax (503) 229-6543

Pennsylvania State Board of Medicine
Transportation & Safety Building, Room 612, Commonwealth Avenue &
Foster Street, 17120, Harrisburg, Pennsylvania 17105-2649; Phone (717)
787-2381; Fax (717) 787-7769

Pennsylvania State Board of Osteopathic Medicine
Transportation & Safety Building, Room 612, Commonwealth Avenue &
Foster Street, 17120, Harrisburg, Pennsylvania 17105-249; Phone (717)
783-4858; Fax (717) 787-7769

Puerto Rico Board of Medical Examiners
Call Box 13969, San Juan, Puerto Rico 00908; Phone (809) 782-8989; Fax (809) 782-8733

Rhode Island Board of Licensure and Discipline
Department of Health, 3 Capitol Hill , Cannon Building, Room 205, Providence, Rhode Island 02908-5097; Phone (401) 277-3855 or 56; Fax (401) 277-2158

South Carolina, State Board of Medical Examiners of
101 Executive Center Drive, Saluda Building, Suite 120, 29210, Columbia, South Carolina 29221-2269; Phone (803) 731-1650; Fax (803) 731-1660

South Dakota State Board of Medical and Osteo Examiners
1323 South Minnesota Avenue, Sioux Falls, South Dakota 57105; Phone (605) 336-1965

Tennessee State Board of Medical Examiners
287 Plus Park Boulevard, Nashville, Tennessee 37247-1010; Phone (615) 367-6231; Fax (615) 367-6210

Tennessee State Board of Osteopathic Examiners
287 Plus Park Boulevard, Nashville, Tennessee 37247-1010; Phone (615) 367-6281

Texas State Board of Medical Examiners
1812 Centre Creek Drive, 78754, Austin, Texas 78714-9134; Phone (512) 834-7728; Fax (512) 834-4597

Utah Physicians Licensing Board
Division of Occupational & Professional Licensing, Heber M Wells Building, 4th Floor, 160 East 300 South, 84145, Salt Lake City, Utah 84145-0805; Phone (801) 530-6628; Fax (801) 530-6511

Vermont Board of Medical Practice
109 State Street, Montpelier, Vermont 05609-1106; Phone (802) 828-2673; Fax (802) 828-2496

Virginia Board of Medicine
6606 West Broad Street, 4th Floor, Richmond, Virginia 23230-1717; Phone (804) 662-9908; Fax (804) 662-9943

Virgin Islands Board of Medical Examiners
Virgin Islands Department of Health, 48 Sugar Estate, St. Thomas, Virgin Islands 00802; Phone (809) 776-8311; Fax (809) 777-4001

Washington Department of Health
BME/MDB Medical Boards
1300 SE Quince Street, MS: EY-25, Olympia, Washington 98504
Phone (206) 753-2287; Fax (206) 586-4573

Washington Board of Osteopathic Medicine & Surgery
Department of Health, 1300 SE Quince Street, Olympia, Washington 98504-7868; Phone (206) 586-8438

West Virginia State Board of Medicine
101 Dee Drive, Charleston, West Virginia 25311; Phone (304) 558-2921; Fax (304) 558-2084

West Virginia Board of Osteopathy
334 Penco Road, Weirton, West Virginia 26062; Phone (304) 723-4638

Wisconsin Medical Examiners Board
1400 East Washington Avenue, 53703, Madison, Wisconsin 53708; Phone (608) 266-2811; Fax (608) 267-0644

Wyoming Board of Medicine
2301 Central Avenue, 2nd Floor; Barrett Building, Room 208, Cheyenne,
Wyoming 82002; Phone (307) 777-6463; Fax (307) 777-6478

• SUBSTANCE ABUSE

Al-Anon
Family Group Headquarters, Box 862, Midtown Station, New York, New
York 10018; Phone toll-free (800) 344-2666

Alateen
1372 Broadway, New York, New York 10018; Phone (212) 302-7240

Alcoholics Anonymous (AA)
475 Riverside Drive, 11th Floor, New York, New York 10115; Phone (212)
870-3440

Adult Children of Alcoholics (ACA)
World Services Office, 2225 Sepulveda Boulevard, #200, Torrance,
California 90505; Phone (310) 534-1815

American Society of Addiction Medicine
Phone (202) 244-8948

Children of Alcoholics Foundation
P.O. Box 4185, Grand Central Station, New York, New York 10163-4185;
Phone (212) 754-0656

Cocaine Anonymous
3740 Overland Avenue, Suite H, Los Angeles, California 90034-6337;
Phone toll-free (800) 347-8998

Narcotics Anonymous (NA)
World Service Office, 16155 Wyandotte Street, Van Nuys, California
91406; Phone (818) 780-3951

National Association of Children of Alcoholics (NACOA)
11426 Rockville Park, Suite 100, Rockville, Maryland 20852; Phone (301)
468-0985

National Center for Substance Abuse Treatment
Phone toll-free (800) 662-HELP (4357)

National Cocaine Hotline
Phone toll-free (800) COC-AINE

National Institute of Drug Abuse (NIDA)
11426 Rockville Pike, Rockville, Maryland 20852; Phone (310) 443-6245
or toll-free (800) 662-4357

• TEETH, JAW, DENTAL AND ORAL PROBLEMS

Academy of General Dentistry
211 East Chicago Avenue, Suite 1200, Chicago, Illinois 60611-2670; Phone
(312) 440-4300

American Academy of Cosmetic Dentistry
2711 Marshall Court, Madison, Wisconsin 53705; Phone (608) 238-6529
or toll-free (800) 543-9220

American Academy of Implant Dentistry
6900 Grove Road, Thorofare, New Jersey 08086; Phone (609) 848-7027

American Association of Dental Schools
Washington, DC; Phone (202) 667-9433

American Association of Oral and Maxillofacial Surgeons
9700 West Bryn Mawr Avenue, Rosemont, Illinois 60018-5701; Phone (708) 768-6200, toll-free (800) 822-6637 or (800) 467-5268

American Association of Orthodontists
401 North Lindbergh Boulevard, St. Louis, Missouri 63141-7816; Phone (314) 993-1700 or toll-free (800) 222-9969

American Cleft Palate Foundation
1218 Grandview Avenue, Pittsburgh, Pennsylvania 15211; Phone (412) 481-1376

American Dental Hygienists Association
444 North Michigan Avenue, Suite 300, Chicago, Illinois 60611; Phone (312) 440-8900

American Dental Association
211 East Chicago Avenue, Chicago, Illinois 60611; Phone (312) 440-2862

American Society for Dental Aesthetics
635 Madison Avenue, New York, New York 10022; Phone (212) 751-3263

Cleft Palate Foundation
1218 Grandview Avenue, Pittsburgh, Pennsylvania 15211; Phone (412) 481-1376

International Congress of Oral Implantologists
248 Lorraine Avenue, 3rd Floor, Upper Montclair, New Jersey 07043; Phone (201) 783-6300

National Institutes of Health
National Institute of Dental Research
Building 31, 9000 Rockville Pike, Bethesda, Maryland 20892; Phone (301) 496-4261

National Oral Health Information Clearinghouse
9000 Rockville Pike, Bethesda, Maryland 20892; Phone (301) 402-7364

Smile Design Council
Phone (800) 480-4004

TMJ Association (for temporomandibular joint information)
6418 West Washington Boulevard, Wauwatosa, Wisconsin 53213; Phone toll-free (800) 818-8652

TMJ Hotline
Phone toll-free (800) 554-5297

• TISSUE DONATION AND TRANSPLANTS

Every year hundreds of thousands of Americans receive some type of donated tissue transplant. Before these tissues, which range from skin, cartilage, and bone grafts to tendons and heart valves, can be used, they are tested for such diseases as HIV, syphilis and hepatitis. People interested in becoming a tissue donor can get information or a donor card from the

American Association of Tissue Banks
1350 Beverly Road, McLean, Virginia 22101; Phone (703) 827-9582

Red Cross Tissue Donation Services
Phone (800) 272-5287

• WEIGHT AND EATING PROBLEMS

Books:
- *Body Language: The Essential Secrets of Non-Verbal Communication,* by Julius Fast; MJF Books, 1970
- *Body Love,* by Rita Freedman; Harper Collins, 1990
- *Body Traps: Breaking the Binds that Keep You from Feeling Good about Your Body,* by Judith Rodin; William Morrow and Company, 1992
- *Jane Brody's Nutrition Book: A Lifetime Guide to Good Eating for Better Health and Weight Control;* Bantam Books, 1987
- *The Complete Guide to Food Allergy and Intolerance: Prevention, Identification, and Treatment of Common Illnesses and Allergies Caused by Food,* by Dr. Jonathon Brostoff and Linda Gamlin; Crown Publishers, 1989
- *Diary of a Fat Housewife,* by Rosemary Green; Warner Books, 1995
- *Feeding on Dreams: Why America's Diet Industry Doesn't Work & What Will Work For You,* by Diane Epstein and Kathleen Thompson; Macmillan Publishing, 1994
- *The Food Pharmacy Guide to Good Eating,* by Jean Carper; Bantam Books, 1991
- *Get the Fat Out: 501 Simple Ways to Cut the Fat in Any Diet,* by Victoria Moran; Crown Trade Paperback, 1994
- *The Pritikin Permanent Weight Loss Manual,* by Nathan Pritikin; Grosset & Dunlap, 1981
- *The Pritikin Program for Diet and Exercise,* by Nathan Pritikin; Grosset & Dunlap, 1979
- *The Pritikin Promise: 28 Days To A Longer/Healthier Life,* by Nathan Pritikin; Simon & Schuster, 1983
- *Thin for Life: 10 Keys to Success from People Who Have Lost Weight & Kept It Off,* by Anne M. Fletcher; Chapters Publishing (800-892-0220), 1994
- *Today's Healthy Eating: The Guide to Understanding and Using the Healing Powers of Nutrition and Natural Foods,* by Louise Tenney, MH Woodland Publishing (800-777-2665), 1994

Weight problems can be carried from generation to generation because each succeeding generation takes on the same unhealthy diet practices of the generation before. If a person is born to two overweight parents, the person has an estimated 10 times greater chance of becoming overweight than someone born to thin parents. If the person does not keep physically active their chances of becoming overweight increases dramatically. More than anything else, a person's weight is influenced by how active they are and the types of food they eat. (Researchers at Rockefeller University in New York published a study on November 30, 1994 in which they found a gene in mice that the researchers believe is defective in some people and responsible for secreting proteins that signal the brain when the stomach is full. Further studies may show that some people are genetically predisposed to eat too much; however, this will probably be used as an excuse by too many people to continue bad eating habits.)

Fat in the diet is important but nearly all Americans consume too much fat. Having too much or too little fat in the diet can lead to severe health problems. A very healthy range of fat intake for adults is ten to twenty percent of total caloric intake. Babies need a higher percentage of fat than adults for the neurological development that occurs within the first two years of life. Beyond childhood the human body needs a certain amount of fat to survive because fat carries vitamins, provides energy, helps support and protect the organs and nerves, insulates the body, affects water balance and provides other benefits.

Out of the three types of fat, monounsaturated, polyunsaturated and saturated, the monounsaturated fats (found in oils of canola, sesame, olive and avocado) are beneficial to maintaining healthy cholesterol levels. The other two types of fat, polyunsaturated (found in oils of soybean, corn, safflower and cottonseed) and saturated (derived from animal products and tropical oils such as coconut oil) should be restricted because they can clog arteries and cause or contribute to diseases.

Being overweight places additional stress on the heart and can lead to a number of health problems including high blood pressure, stroke, diabetes, various types of cancer, diseases of the cardiovascular and respiratory systems and of the gall bladder and kidneys. Even if a person is not overweight, a high-fat diet or diet that lacks proper nutrition alone can lead to many health problems including cancer.

You cannot lose weight if you do not cut down on the amount of calories you eat or exercise more to burn calories. A healthy body does not come in a can or a powder or a pill. A healthy body is the result of good nutrition and plenty of exercise and this takes constant discipline and work.

Unreliable obesity cures have been sold for centuries, including machines that vibrate fat away and dangerous pills that promise quick weight loss. Many of the fat cures did only one thing — made the manufacturers rich. According to the Institute of Medicine, Americans now spend an estimated $33 billion a year on all types of weight-loss programs and products — many of which are useless — and continue to make manufacturers rich.

Three types of drug treatments being studied for their ability to help people lose or control their weight are Prozac, Orlistat, and a combination of two drugs, phentermine and fenfluramine.

Prozac, the drug used to treat depression, helps maintain a level of serotonin that may be helpful in preventing compulsive eating. Orlistat can reduce some fat absorption, but on a limited scale. Phentermine and fenfluramine have been used in a study conducted by Dr. Michael Weintraub at the University of Rochester. The two drugs were taken by overweight people in combination with a diet and exercise program. All of the drug treatments have not been proven safe or successful for long-term weight loss. Anyone looking into such drug treatments should question what risks to normal nerve formation and chemical reactions within the brain are involved with long-term use of these drugs.

Being thin may be desirable, but an excessive concern over body weight is a sign of emotional illness or disturbance. Most people with eating disorders share certain psychological issues that drive their disorder: low self-esteem, feelings of helplessness, a fear of becoming fat, and often feelings of guilt, disappointment, loss of control and anger.

Two types of severe eating disorders are anorexia nervosa and bulimia. They are often practiced at the same time. A third is uncontrollable "binge" eating that leads to weight gain. All three may give the eater a sense of control and may be a substitute for something missing in the person's life.

Anorexia nervosa is a compulsive desire to lose weight by severely limiting the intake of calories even after suffering hunger pains and becoming dangerously thin. A person with anorexia nervosa is consumed with the fear of gaining weight. People with anorexia tend to be "too good to be true." They often conduct themselves in a manner that they think will please the people around them, keep their feelings to themselves, and tend to be perfectionists, good students and excellent athletes. Some researchers believe that people with anorexia restrict food — particularly carbohydrates — to gain a sense of control in some area of their lives.

Bulimia is the act of achieving weight loss or maintenance goals by vomiting after consuming food. Usually it is done secretly and is accompanied by binge eating, where the person eats large amounts of food. Sometimes the person also uses laxatives and diet pills or other drugs to burn calories. Individuals with bulimia often live in households where there are accusations, blaming, overbearing criticism, and hostility. They are also often impulsive and more likely to engage in risky behavior such as abuse of alcohol and drugs.

Bulimics are more prone to dental problems because they tend to eat junk food, and the constant vomiting associated with bulimia increases tooth decay because the stomach acids destroy tooth enamel. There is also an increased risk of throat cancer. In the long term they have a higher risk of experiencing osteoporosis.

There is a higher than average rate of suicide among anorexics and bulimics. In severe cases of eating disorders the brain can be damaged. Sometimes the person literally starves to death. Scientists believe they have found that acutely ill anorexia and bulimia patients suffer from an imbalance of the chemical messengers, known as neurotransmitters, which control hormone production. People with either anorexia or certain forms of depression also tend to have abnormal levels of cortisol and vasopressin, brain hormones that are believed to be released in response to stress.

Anyone involved with severely uncontrollable or abnormal eating practices should seek professional help. Professionals who are involved in the treatment of people with severe eating disorders are internists, nutritionists, psychotherapists, and psychopharmacologists. Group therapy has also been proven to be beneficial for long-term recovery.

Sensible Weight Maintenance Tips

Losing weight may not be effortless, but it does not have to be complicated. To achieve long-term results, it's best to avoid quick-fix schemes and complex regimens. Focus instead on making modest changes to your life's daily routine. A balanced, healthy diet and sensible, regular exercise are the keys to maintaining your ideal weight.

Although nutrition science is constantly evolving, here are some generally-accepted guidelines for losing weight:

- *Consult with your doctor, a dietitian, or other qualified health professional to determine your ideal healthy body weight.*
- *Eat smaller portions and choose from a variety of foods.*
- *Load up on foods naturally high in fiber: fruits, vegetables, legumes, and whole grains.*
- *Limit portions of foods high in fat: dairy products like cheese, butter, and whole milk; red meat; cakes and pastries.*
- *Exercise at least three times a week.*

— from the pamphlet *The Facts About Weight Loss Products and Programs*, presented as a public service by the FTC, FDA, and the National Association of Attorneys General

The only true diet foods are vegetables, fruits, grains and the like. The only true wonder therapy for controlling weight and having a healthy body is a combination of the right amount of low-fat foods that are rich in nutrients along with exercise and physical activity. Proper diet and exercise take constant discipline and work. You cannot lose weight if you do not cut down on your intake of calories or exercise or otherwise become more active to burn calories. Think of food as fuel. If you put more fuel in than you use, the fuel will be stored in your body in the form of fat. To lose the fat you have to use more fuel than you put in. The higher grade of fuel you put in the engine the better it performs.

Vegetables, fruits and whole grains along with beans and whole rice are the cleanest types of fuel for the body. Oils such as olive oil and canola oil have been shown to be beneficial to health while other oils such as coconut oil and oils derived from animals (butter and lard) have been shown to be harmful to the body and cause or contribute to disease. The body is made up mostly of water, and the body system needs water to clean itself. Gunking up the body system with useless food and not exercising causes the body to become unhealthy. Most foods sold at fast food restaurants (if it can even be considered food), fried foods, foods with a high sugar content, and foods that contain artificial dyes, flavorings and preservatives should be avoided.

Staying physically active through regular exercise burns calories, builds muscles, increases bone strength, raises metabolism, lowers the risks of cancer and heart disease, increases energy and improves overall health. Exercise conditions the body to perform better and is beneficial for people of every age. Regular exercise provides neurochemical changes that reduce fatigue, enhance your state of mind and mood and ultimately your self-image.

You do not have to join an expensive diet club and take part in obsessive/compulsive aerobic dance classes or go to some exotic resort to learn about nutrition and exercise. Your local library probably has plenty of books on the subjects that you can use to teach yourself what foods provide the best nutrition and how to shape up. Joining a gym can be a motivator and some of the equipment found in them can be very effective tools to improve your fitness level — but you do not have to join a gym to get in shape. Going for a brisk walk or a jog every day costs nothing and either one is a good way to begin an exercise program.

Take time to learn how to exercise in a way that will not cause injury. Prevent injuries by warming up before you exercise, and cool down afterward with three to five minutes of casual stretching. Increase your speed and duration of exercise over a period of several weeks before taking up more strenuous forms of exercise and adding some weight training and varieties of physical activity to your routine.

> *Married couples who joined a fitness program together have significantly higher attendance and lower dropout than married adults who join a program without their spouse. These adherence behaviors appear to be influenced by social support more than self motivation. Past literature indicates that spousal support is an important predictor of compliance to medically based exercise programs.*
> — from research study titled: *Twelve Month Adherence of Adults Who Joined a Fitness Program with a Spouse vs. Without a Spouse,* by Janet P. Wallace, John S. Raglin, and Chet Jastremski of Indiana University, Bloomington

One of the most important factors behind a successful fitness program is to eat healthy and exercise regularly — at least three times a week. You should engage in some type of physical activity (Examples: walking, jogging, swimming, bike riding, roller skating, stair climbing, calisthenics, weight lifting, dancing, aerobics, yoga, tai chi, jumping rope, or even playing Frisbee or another casual sport) for a half hour every day to build your endurance and experience the health benefits of exercise. Vary your exercises so you utilize different muscle groups. Include light, controlled stretching exercises throughout every day — but learn the difference between a beneficial *stretch* and a damaging *strain* (see the book *Stretching,* by Bob Anderson. It contains corny but helpful illustrations that show how to stretch). (If you think you are too old for exercise, read the book by Joe Henderson titled *Ten Million Steps* (1994, WRS Publishing [800-299-3366], that tells the true story of Paul Reese, who ran across America at the age of 76.)

American Anorexia and Bulimia Association (AABA)
418 East 76th Street, New York, New York 10021; Phone (212) 734-1114

American College of Sports Medicine
Phone (317) 637-9200

American Council on Exercise
Phone (619) 535-8227

American Dietetic Association
P.O. Box 39101, Chicago, Illinois 60639; Phone toll-free (800) 366-1655

Anorexia Nervosa and Related Eating Disorders Association
P.O. Box 5102, Eugene, Oregon 97405; Phone (503) 344-1144

Anorexics/Bulimics Anonymous (ABA)
P.O. Box 112214, San Diego, California 92111; Phone (619) 685-3344

Bulimia Anorexia Self-Help (BASH)
P.O. Box 39903, St. Louis, Missouri 63139; Phone (314) 991-2274 or toll-free (800) 227-4785 or 762-3334

Center for Child and Adolescent Obesity
UC San Francisco School of Medicine, San Francisco, California; Phone (415) 476-4044

Center for the Study of Anorexia and Bulimia
1 West 91st Street, New York, New York 10024; Phone (212) 595-3449

Cooper Clinic
Dallas, Texas; Phone (800) 444-5764

Duke University Medical Center Diet and Fitness Center
Durham, North Carolina; Phone (800) 362-8446

Foundation for Education about Eating Disorders
P.O. Box 16375, Baltimore, Maryland 21210; Phone (410) 467-0603

Montreux Counseling Center Eating Disorder Program
P.O. Box 5460, Victoria, British Columbia V8R 6S4, Canada; Phone (604) 598-3066

National Anorexic Aid Society &
National Eating Disorders Organization
1925 East Dublin Granville Road, Columbus, Ohio 43229; Phone (614) 436-1112

National Association of Anorexia Nervosa and Associated Disorders
P.O. Box 7, Highland Park, Illinois 60035; Phone (708) 831-3438

National Strength and Conditioning Association
Phone (719) 632-NSCA

Overeaters Anonymous is not a diet club. It does not endorse or provide any food plans. The goal is to help stop people from eating compulsively by providing local support groups that are based on the twelve steps of Alcoholics Anonymous. OA is a nonprofit organization and is self-supporting through member contributions.

Overeaters Anonymous (OA)
P.O. Box 92870, Los Angeles, California 90009; Phone (310) 618-8835 or toll-free (800) 743-8703

Pritikin Longevity Centers (preventative health education hotels)

West coast:	East coast:
1910 Ocean Front Walk	5875 Collins Avenue
Santa Monica, CA 90405	Miami Beach, FL 33140
Phone (310) 450-5433	Phone (305) 866-2237
or toll-free (800) 421-9911	or toll-free (800) 327-4914

Spa Finders is a travel agency that specializes in arranging vacations at health spas. These spas provide classes where guests learn how to eat healthy and exercise effectively and are usually scheduled in combination with swimming or hiking, sauna bathing and massage.

Spa Finders
Phone toll-free (800) 255-7727 in New York call (212) 924-6800

Tufts University *Diet & Nutrition Letter*
203 Harrison Avenue, Boston, Massachusetts 02111; Phone (617) 482-3530 or toll-free (800) 274-7581

Theodore B. VanItallie Center for Nutrition and Weight
    Management at St. Luke's–Roosevelt Hospital Center
New York, New York; Phone (212) 523-8440

Vegetarian Journal (publishes magazine and sells cook books)
Vegetarian Resource Group, P.O. Box 1463, Baltimore, Maryland 21203; Phone (410) 366-8343

• WOMEN'S HEALTH

Books:
- *Body and Soul: The Black Women's Guide to Physical Health and Emotional Well Being*, edited by Linda Villarosa; Harper-Perennial, 1994
- *The Female Heart: The Truth about Women and Heart Disease*, by Marianne J. Legato MD and Carol Colman; Avon, 1993
- *The Hysterectomy Hoax: A Leading Surgeon Explains Why 90 Percent of All Hysterectomies Are Unnecessary, and Describes All the Treatment Options Available to Every Woman, No Matter What Age*, by Stanley West MD with Paula Dranov; Doubleday, 1994
- *Male Practice: How Doctors Manipulate Women*, by Robert S. Mendelsohn, MD; Contemporary Books, 1981
- *The Mother/Daughter Revolution: From Betrayal to Power*, by Elizabeth Debold, Marie Wilson and Idalisse Malave; Addison–Wesley, 1993
- *Outrageous Practices: The Alarming Truth About How Medicine Mistreats Women*, by Leslie Laurence and Beth Weinhouse; Ballantine/Fawcett Columbine, 1994
- *Surgery Electives: What to Know Before the Doctor Operates*, by John McCabe; Carmania Books, 1994
- *Unequal Treatment*, by Nechas and Foley; Simon and Schuster, 1994
- *Women and Doctors: A Physician's Explosive Account of Women's Medical Treatment — and Mistreatment — in America Today and What You Can Do About It*, by John M. Smith, MD; Atlantic Monthly Press, 1992
- *Women's Health Alert: What Most Doctors Won't Tell You About*, by Sidney M. Wolfe and Rhoda Donkin Jones; Addison-Wesley Publishing, 1991
- *Women Under the Knife: A Gynecologist's Report on Hazardous Medicine*, by Herbert H. Keyser, MD; George F. Stickley Company, 1984

Breast Lump & Cervical Cancer Information Hotline
Phone toll-free (800) 4-CANCER; In Alaska phone toll-free (800) 638-6070

A Friend Indeed newsletter focuses on issues relating to women in mid-life and menopause. Ten issues are published each year (monthly except July and August) at a subscription cost of $30.

A Friend Indeed Publications, Inc.
Box 515, Place du Parc Station, Montreal, Quebec, Canada H2W2P1
Or: Box 1710, Champlain, New York 12919-1710; Phone (514) 843-5730

Harvard Women's Health Watch (subscriptions $24 a year)
Harvard Health Publications, 164 Longwood Avenue, Boston,
Massachusetts 02115; Phone (617) 432-1485

National Women's Health Network
224 Seventh Street, SE, Washington, DC 20003; Phone (202) 543-9222 or
(202) 347-1140

National Women's Health Resource Center
2440 M Street, NW, Washington, DC 20037; Phone (202) 293-6045

Older Women's League
666 — 11th Street, NW, Suite 700, Washington, DC 20001; Phone (800)
825-3695

Women's Cancer Resource Center
3020 Shattuck Avenue, Berkeley, California 94705; Phone (510) 548-9272

Women: Midlife and Menopause
7337 Morrison Drive, Greenbelt, Maryland 20770

Final Notes

The body is a very intricate vessel made up mostly of water along with millions of molecules, cells, genes and chemicals that nature has arranged in a precise order. A slight difference in even one of those elements or a slight change in the temperature of the body can throw the whole system off balance to the point where it can die.

Most people believe the body is a type of glove that contains their spirit during what will be a temporary existence on earth. During this earthly existence some people's bodies are not as healthy as others right from the start. Other people will experience various illnesses and physical damage that will alter the way their bodies will function. Still others may reach a point of near physical perfection.

Most of the factors that sketch out physical appearance are determined by the chemical makeup of the body, while a certain amount of what happens to a person during their life, how a person treats their body, and what they put into it will also determine what their body will look like on its path through time. There is nothing that can stop the aging process, but there are ways to alter the way the body ages.

If men and women exercise regularly with their partner, they will both have a better appreciation of just how difficult it is for "real" people to look like airbrushed "babes" or "beefcakes." Real people have real partners, and relationships with real partners are better than magazine centerfolds.
  — from research study titled: *Men's Magazines: the Facts and the Fantasies,* by Dr. Debbie Then, Social Psychologist and Research Scholar, August, 1994

Nothing can replace the benefits of good nutrition, daily exercise and activities that keep the mind active.

•

The author encourages those who want to do something to create a more responsible medical system to support the following groups: **Safe Medicine for Consumers, People's Medical Society, American Silicone Implant Survivors, Coalition of Silicone Survivors, Public Citizen's Health Research Group, National Center for Patient's Rights, Citizens for Health** or **The Center for Medical Consumers**.

The addresses for all of these groups are located in the research section of this book under the heading of Patients' and Consumers' Rights.

•

If you have information you believe should be included in future updates of this book please send it to

Carmania Books
P.O. Box 1272
Santa Monica, California   90406-1272

If sending information on an organization, include the address, phone number, contact person and information on the activities or function of the group.

Additional copies of this book can be ordered by sending a check for $19.95 plus $3 for shipping to the above address. California residents must include sales tax.